Key Concepts in

Medical Sociology

Key Concepts in
Medical
Sociology

THIRD EDITION

LEE F. MONAGHAN & JONATHAN GABE

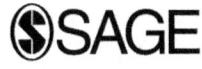

Los Angeles | London | New Delhi
Singapore | Washington DC | Melbourne

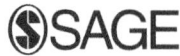

Los Angeles | London | New Delhi
Singapore | Washington DC | Melbourne

SAGE Publications Ltd
1 Oliver's Yard
55 City Road
London EC1Y 1SP

SAGE Publications Inc.
2455 Teller Road
Thousand Oaks, California 91320

SAGE Publications India Pvt Ltd
B 1/I 1 Mohan Cooperative Industrial Area
Mathura Road
New Delhi 110 044

SAGE Publications Asia-Pacific Pte Ltd
3 Church Street
#10-04 Samsung Hub
Singapore 049483

Editor: Alana Clogan
Assistant Editor: Eve Williams
Production Editor: Jessica Masih
Copyeditor: Fern Bryant
Proofreader: Jill Birch
Indexer: Elske Janssen
Marketing Manager: Ruslana Khatagova
Cover Design: Sheila Tong
Typeset by KnowledgeWorks Global Ltd.

Library of Congress Control Number:
2021941241

British Library Cataloguing in Publication
data

A catalogue record for this book is available
from the British Library

978-1-5264-6588-7

CONTENTS

ABOUT THE AUTHORS

EDITORS

Lee F. Monaghan is Associate Professor of Sociology, University of Limerick. He teaches the Sociology of Health and Illness, Classical and Contemporary Sociological Theory, Researching Social Trends and the Sociology of the Body. His writings explore numerous health-related topics, ranging from the war on obesity to COVID-19, and have been published in international journals such as: *Sociology of Health & Illness*; *Social Science & Medicine*; *Social Theory & Health*; *Addiction*; *Health, Risk & Society*; *Critical Public Health* and *Body & Society*. He has also published six edited books and monographs. He is the lead author on a forthcoming book, *Rethinking Obesity: Critical Perspectives in Crisis Times*, to be published by Routledge (with Emma Rich and Andrea Bombak).

Jonathan Gabe is Emeritus Professor of Sociology in the School of Law and Social Sciences at Royal Holloway, University of London. He has had considerable experience of teaching undergraduate and postgraduate students. He has taught modules on Health, Medicine and Society, Sociology of Contemporary Society and Introduction to Sociology to undergraduate students and Sociology of Health and Illness and Health Care Organization to Masters students. His current research interests include pharmaceuticals – especially for sleep and wakefulness, healthcare organization and chronic illness. He has published 17 edited books (including two second editions) and monographs, the latest being *Health and Illness in the Neoliberal Era in Europe* (Emerald, 2020, edited with Mario Cardano and Angela Genova). He has been an editor of the international journal *Sociology of Health & Illness* on two occasions, most recently between 2006 and 2012.

CONTRIBUTORS

Ellen Annandale, Professor of Sociology, Department of Sociology, University of York.

Kirsten Bell, Professor of Social Anthropology, Department of Life Sciences, University of Roehampton.

Gillian Bendelow, Professor Emerita in Sociology of Health and Medicine, School of Applied Social Science, University of Brighton.

Antonia Bifulco, Professor of Lifespan Psychology, Department of Psychology, Middlesex University.

Mary Boulton, Professor Emerita in Health Sociology, Oxford School of Nursing and Midwifery, Oxford Brookes University.

Ivy Lynn Bourgeault, Professor in the School of Sociological and Anthropological Studies at the University of Ottawa and the University Research Chair in Gender, Diversity and the Professions.

Hannah Bradby, Professor of Sociology, Department of Sociology, Uppsala University.

Patrick Brown, Associate Professor of Sociology, Department of Sociology, University of Amsterdam.

Mike Bury, Emeritus Professor of Sociology, Royal Holloway, University of London.

Sarah Cant, Principal Lecturer, School of Law, Policing and Social Sciences, Canterbury Christ Church University.

David Clark, Professor Emeritus of Medical Sociology, University of Glasgow.

Nick Crossley, Professor of Sociology, School of Social Sciences, University of Manchester.

Rebecca Dimond, Lecturer, School of Social Sciences, Cardiff University.

Robert Dingwall, Professor of Sociology, Nottingham Trent University, and Director, Dingwall Enterprises Ltd.

Anne Ellaway, Honorary Professor, Institute of Health and Wellbeing, University of Glasgow.

Eva Elliott, Honorary Research Fellow, School of Social Sciences, Cardiff University.

Mary Ann Elston, Reader Emerita in Sociology, Royal Holloway, University of London.

Bobbie Farsides, Professor of Clinical and Biomedical Ethics, Brighton and Sussex Medical School, University of Sussex.

Alex Faulkner, Professor in Sociology of Biomedicine and Healthcare Policy, Centre for Global Health Policy, School of Global Studies, University of Sussex.

Katherine L. Frohlich, Professor of Public Health, Co-holder of the Myriagone McConnell-UdM Chair on Youth Knowledge Mobilisation, École de Santé Publique, Université de Montréal.

Judith Green, Professor of Sociology, Wellcome Centre for Cultures & Environments of Health, University of Exeter.

Paul Higgs, Professor of the Sociology of Ageing, Division of Psychiatry, University College London.

Sue Hollinrake, Associate Professor of Social Work, School of Social Sciences and Humanities, University of Suffolk.

Jacqueline Hughes, Research Associate, Centre for Trials Research, Cardiff University.

Abbey Hyde, Professor, School of Nursing, Midwifery and Health Systems, University College Dublin.

Anuj Kapilashrami, Professor of Global Health Policy and Equity, School of Health & Social Care, University of Essex.

Gitte H. Koksvik, Researcher in Applied Ethics, Department of Philosophy and Religious Studies, Norwegian University of Science and Technology (NTNU). Affiliate Researcher, End of Life Studies Group, School of Interdisciplinary Studies, University of Glasgow.

Neil Lunt, Professor of Social Policy, Department of Social Policy and Social Work, University of York.

Deborah Lupton, SHARP Professor, Centre for Social Research in Health and the Social Policy Research Centre, University of New South Wales (UNSW) Sydney.

Sara MacBride-Stewart, Reader in Health, Medicine and Society, School of Social Sciences, Cardiff University.

Sally Macintyre, Professor Emerita, Institute of Health and Wellbeing, University of Glasgow.

Per Måseide, Emeritus Professor of Sociology, Faculty of Social Sciences, Nord University.

Nicholas Mays, Professor of Health Policy and Director, Policy Innovation and Evaluation Research Unit, Department of Health Services Research and Policy, London School of Hygiene & Tropical Medicine.

Orla McDonnell, Lecturer in Sociology, Department of Sociology, University of Limerick.

Janice McLaughlin, Professor of Sociology, School of Geography, Politics and Sociology, Newcastle University.

Sarah Nettleton, Professor Emerita of Sociology, Department of Sociology, University of York.

Alison Pilnick, Professor of Language, Medicine and Society, School of Sociology and Social Policy, University of Nottingham.

Jennie Popay, Distinguished Professor of Sociology and Public Health, Faculty of Health and Medicine, Lancaster University.

Gabrielle Samuel, Senior Research Fellow, Faculty of Medicine, University of Southampton.

Jane Sandall, Professor of Social Science and Women's Health, Division of Women's Health, School of Medicine, King's College London, University of London.

Graham Scambler, Emeritus Professor of Sociology, University College London, Visiting Professor of Sociology, University of Surrey.

Sue Scott, Visiting Professor of Sociology, School of Geography, Politics and Sociology, Newcastle University.

Heather Strange, Research Associate, Centre for Trials Research, Cardiff University.

Catherine Theodosius, Senior Lecturer, School of Sport and Health Sciences, University of Brighton.

Julie Vallée, CNRS Researcher in Social and Health Geography, Laboratory Géographie-Cités, Paris-Aubervilliers.

Iain Wilkinson, Professor of Sociology, School of Social Policy, Sociology and Social Research, University of Kent.

Gareth H. Williams (1955–2018) was Professor of Sociology and Director of the Cardiff Institute of Society, Health and Wellbeing, School of Social Sciences, Cardiff University.

Simon J. Williams, Emeritus Professor of Sociology, Department of Sociology, University of Warwick.

INTRODUCTION

Lee F. Monaghan and Jonathan Gabe

First published in 2004 and updated in 2013, the previous editions of *Key Concepts in Medical Sociology* were hugely successful. They proved popular among students of sociology and cognate subjects as well as those undertaking professional training in health-related disciplines. For instance, students of medicine and nursing are often introduced to sociological insights on the relationships between social structures and health inequalities, stigma, the social aspects of bodies or embodiment, death and chronic illness. Hence, as with our own teaching of under- and postgraduate students in the social sciences and future clinicians, we have found it useful to include these texts as key references on our class reading lists.

As might be anticipated amidst broader social transformations, the domains of health and illness are rapidly moving objects for and subjects of sociological analysis. We stated in the second edition that health issues demand ongoing consideration amidst increasing complexity and controversy, or at least people's growing awareness that health, illness and care cannot be taken for granted. That statement also rang true when we were working on this third edition as populations worldwide were living through and seeking to make sense of a 'critical situation' (Giddens, 1979). We are, of course, referring to what transpired following the declaration of the COVID-19 pandemic by the World Health Organization in March 2020, with governments placing restrictions on everyday life (notably recurring 'lockdowns' intended to limit people's mobility and the spread of the virus, SARS-CoV-2, which causes COVID-19). As Dingwall reminds us in this volume and elsewhere (e.g. Dingwall et al., 2013), pandemics and epidemics are just as much social and cultural as they are biomedical phenomena. Outbreaks of infectious disease, inseparable from social definitions and responses, therefore demand sociological attention. One practical consequence of the pandemic for the present volume is that we had to delay the submission of the final manuscript in order to accommodate some of our contributors' altered working situations and lives. However, this delay also enabled authors to engage with issues relating to the pandemic if they deemed these relevant to their entry. Allowing authors and ourselves breathing space in order to 'process the pandemic' (Will and Bendelow, 2020), we believe, renders this volume crucial reading not only in the time of COVID-19 but also in relation to how we might envisage and research medicine, health and society in future.

The decision to revise this text cannot, however, be attributed to the COVID-19 pandemic. We agreed to edit a third edition of *Key Concepts in Medical Sociology* well before the pandemic emerged. Rather, as seen with other popular medical sociology texts, which this book seeks to complement, there is an ongoing need to revise and update the knowledge base under rapidly changing social conditions (e.g. Annandale, 2014; Nettleton, 2020). This book aims to satisfy that mandate, adding to the learning resources available to students via a collection of short, highly focused essays on particular topics. As will be seen, contributors have elaborated, debated and critiqued ideas within what continues to be a lively, thriving and at times controversial area of study. The ongoing theorization of concepts such as 'stigma', 'risk' and 'social class' clearly demonstrates that medical sociology is in good health, so to speak, and as relevant as ever. Essential new concepts and areas of sociological investigation are also included in this third edition, such as 'pandemics and epidemics' and 'pharmaceuticalization' (especially apt as we were finalizing this volume, when governments were aiming to rollout mass vaccination programmes following many months of COVID-related restrictions). As environments, technologies, debates and other social concerns emerge and morph, sociologists' interests also develop whilst remaining indebted to an established canon of key concepts, research and theory.

The aim behind the 'key concepts' approach is to provide readers with systematic, easily accessible information about the building blocks of medical sociology. Our priority has been to present those key concepts (loosely defined here to include substantive issues) that have preoccupied medical sociologists and shaped the field as it exists today. For each one of these concepts, contributors have presented an entry that covers its origin or the background to the issue, an account of its subsequent development and, where relevant, an assessment of its significance to the field. In order to orientate readers, each entry is preceded by a working definition. These were not always easy to write because some of the concepts remain contested within the literature. Each entry then elaborates on the definition, identifying controversies, variations in use and, if relevant, more recent developments in the literature. The entries thus go beyond the inevitable oversimplification of a dictionary, or the passing references that many concepts receive in textbooks. By following cross-references, a picture of the relationship between different concepts can be built up. In addition to a bibliography at the end of each entry, authors provide up to four annotated suggestions for further reading. Our hope is that this book will help guide readers through some of the complexities of the field, encouraging further study and equipping them with the knowledge to understand health and illness, whether as a sociology student, a healthcare professional in training, or an already experienced practitioner.

Before we describe the book's content in more detail, we present a short account of the development of medical sociology, highlighting what is often regarded as its dual orientation towards sociology and healthcare. We hope that this will help the reader to understand the context in which the field and its key concepts have been shaped.

MEDICAL SOCIOLOGY AND ITS DEVELOPMENT

When thinking sociologically it is possible to relate to health and illness in at least two different ways (Bury, 1997). On the one hand, a sociological perspective can be applied to the experience and social distribution of health (disorders) and to the institutions through which care, cures and, increasingly, preventative measures are provided. In this sense, medical sociology can have an applied orientation to understanding and improving health, and can also be seen as one among many disciplines that might appropriately be studied by healthcare providers. On the other hand, the sociological study of health, illness and healthcare can stand alongside analysis of other significant social experiences and institutions, as a means of understanding the society under study. Thus, medical sociology is also a theoretically orientated field, committed to explaining large-scale social transformations and their implications, as well as interactions in everyday settings that bear upon health. These two aspects of medical sociology have, in a well-worn phrase, been characterized as sociology *in* medicine and sociology *of* medicine (Straus, 1957). Most recently, and in viewing Straus' distinction as a heuristic, Mykhalovskiy et al. (2019) propose a third-way that could also be extended to medicine *and* allied health professions – critical social science *with* public health (for an application in the context of COVID-19, see Mykhalovskiy and French, 2020). In so doing, these authors suggest contributors may retain the theoretical distinctiveness of their scholarship whilst also seeking to transform health work so that it is less harmful (similarly, see the entry on 'bioethics' in this volume). Whatever one's position might be in relation to their proposition, the above points to ongoing and lively debate on forms of knowledge and practice that have real-world relevance. Indeed, these are some of the reasons why, in our view, medical sociology is such an exciting, challenging and rewarding field to work in.

The attractions and challenges of medical sociology have a history. In the mid-20th century, medical sociology was a scarcely known subfield of the then controversial but expanding discipline of sociology. Those calling themselves medical sociologists were few and far between. Moreover, they were usually working on applied projects related to public health and social aspects of medicine, often located in medical schools. These sociologists were continuing a long, diverse tradition of research into the relationship between social factors and health in Europe and North America (Bloom, 2000). However, as academic departments of sociology grew in the 1960s, and developed a strongly theoretical orientation, the study of health and illness was sometimes regarded with disdain as being 'an applied activity … lacking in theoretical substance' (Bird et al., 2000: 1). Yet today, medical sociology is one of the largest specialist professional study groups within both British and North American sociology, and thrives in many other parts of the world, notably Australia, New Zealand and the Nordic countries. Sometimes it will be found under alternative designations, such as the 'sociology of health and illness', with the term 'medical' being regarded by some as evoking too strong an association with one particular healthcare profession and with pathology rather than health. But whatever the terminology (and in this volume we have chosen to retain the older title), taught modules which examine sociological aspects of health, disease and healthcare are now almost ubiquitous offerings within undergraduate sociology programmes. This, in turn, has created a demand for myriad textbooks (e.g. Barry and Yuill, 2016; Cockerham, 2021), readers (e.g. Bird et al., 2010; Conrad and Leiter, 2019) and encyclopaedias (Cockerham et al., 2014).

As a result, medical sociology can no longer be regarded as an isolated and applied specialism within its parent discipline. In recent years there has been an increasing rapprochement between long-standing analytical concerns of medical sociology and new issues in sociological theory. Whilst the second edition of *Key Concepts in Medical Sociology* referred to the growing theoretical interest in embodiment, emotions and risk, obvious additions to this list now include digital health (Lupton, 2017) and, as noted above, pandemics and epidemics (Dingwall et al., 2013; Monaghan, 2020). Indeed, we are reminded of Turner's (1992) contention that medical sociology, with its attention to corporeal matters, has the potential to become the 'leading edge of contemporary sociological theory' (p. 163). And it is this concern with sociological theory, or formal conceptual concerns, which serves as a central defining characteristic of medical sociology. Cockerham (2007: 291) writes: 'what makes medical sociology most distinct in relation to other disciplines – like public health and health services research – is its use of sociological theory'. Since 2000, medical sociologists have also been increasingly working across the boundaries with other sociological or interdisciplinary fields, for example, criminology (Timmermans and Gabe, 2003), social studies of science and technology (Faulkner, 2009) and critical weight and fat studies (Monaghan et al., 2022). Consider just one of these examples: criminology. Researchers evidently have much to engage with here given, inter alia, the criminalization of diseases such as HIV (Hoppe, 2018) and what transpired during the COVID-19 pandemic as police enforced mitigation measures and people deemed contagious, including healthcare workers, were reportedly attacked (Sandberg and Fondevila, 2020).

Another growing area of medical sociology research, which travels across disciplinary borderlands, is the study of healthcare organization and health policy. The accessibility and quality of healthcare are significant issues for citizens of any country and, at least in relatively affluent nations, healthcare (public and/or private) is a major component of the domestic economy and one of the largest employers. Moreover, almost all countries in the Global North and increasingly the Global South have experienced major reforms to their healthcare systems since the 1970s. Sociological analysis of these changes and their significance has brought new vigour to the academic study of health policy (Calnan, 2020; Gabe and Calnan, 2009). Calnan (2020), for instance, advances critical sociological insights on health policy through increased attentiveness to powerful structural interests.

Medical sociology has thus now established a secure and prominent place in the social science academe, but not at the expense of its applied institutional roots. In the 1960s and early 1970s, although medical sociologists were mainly to be found in medical schools, their position there was generally a marginal one. Today, the place of social science is far more central in radically revised medical curricula. Sociology textbooks for medical students and other health professionals are now well established and regularly updated (e.g. Denny et al., 2016; Scambler, 2018). And, with the increased incorporation of professional education for nurses and other 'allied health professions' (Nancarrow and Borthwick, 2021) within universities, there has been a burgeoning of medical sociology courses for a wider range of healthcare students. The same holds for qualified professionals, for example through the distance learning programmes of institutions such as the Open University in the UK (similarly, for the USA, see Bloom, 2000).

Today, then, medical sociology is studied by a wide range of students, with some intent on pursuing a career in one of the health professions, and others, at the opposite end of the spectrum, with strong theoretical interests in the constitution of society. One of the impetuses behind this book was our concern that all such students should have the opportunity to learn about the building blocks of their chosen subject. In so doing, a shared community of learners and practitioners should be in a better place to work together to help take the field forward.

EDITORIAL DECISIONS

When editing this text we decided to keep its original structure, as described further below, whilst either seeking updates or deleting previous entries. We also commissioned and authored new material following feedback from the publisher and its reviewers. This edition contains new entries on, for instance, 'intersectionality', 'sexuality', 'the environment', 'neoliberalism', 'medical tourism', 'digital health' and 'professions allied to medicine', in addition to others mentioned above that have particular salience following the outbreak of COVID-19. To inform our editorial decisions we not only drew on our pre-existing knowledge of medical sociology, we also surveyed leading journals (for example, *Sociology of Health & Illness* and *Social Science & Medicine*) and sought the views of colleagues who are established experts in this field. Usually we asked contributors to the previous edition(s) to update their work. Sometimes entries were written afresh by new contributors, or updated by new co-authors. If necessary, we updated entries ourselves, sometimes with the original authors. Throughout, authors were asked where possible to attend to an international context, including the Global South.

When deciding to retain and update entries a key criterion was the continuing discussion about each concept within the broader community of medical sociologists. Often, concepts were retained if there was also scope for their further development and application. For example, whilst 'medicalization' was well defined and explained in previous editions, we have updated it here given, among other things, links to 'pharmaceuticalization'. The latter concept has been viewed as a complex, dynamic, socio-technical process which involves the discovery, development, commercialization, use and governance of pharmaceutical products centred on chemistry-based technologies. As such it can be defined as 'the translation or transformation of human conditions, capabilities and capacities into opportunities for pharmaceutical intervention' (Williams et al., 2011: 711). We have also included material deemed crucial by those working in the field, notably if it has potential to crosscut numerous themes (see, in particular, the new entry on 'sleep' and how it relates to already established areas of study and concepts such as 'gender').

As noted above, we also cut some entries. In part, this was a pragmatic decision given the exigencies of space and our wish to include some new material. Excisions were nonetheless informed by several considerations, including the need to ensure cutting-edge theoretical engagement with globally relevant issues. Some new entries have effectively replaced old ones and have been included in order to capture emerging complexity, contestation and calls for nuanced perspectives (for example, see the new entry on 'neoliberalism'). Furthermore, whilst some concepts have been omitted, relevant discussion is often subsumed under other entries that are of crucial significance in health debates and policy. For example, the previous entry on 'awareness contexts' (articulated in classic sociological studies of processes surrounding end-of-life care) has been replaced with a more inclusive and obvious one on 'death and dying'.

Selecting our key concepts has involved some difficult decisions about what to omit. Other medical sociologists' final list might have looked different but, we believe, only a little. In line with our commitment to offering readers a sense of how medical sociology has developed, we have mainly included classic concepts rather than opt only for those of obvious current (and possibly ephemeral) interest. Talking only in terms of 'concepts' is less than ideal, but in selecting topics we have recognized that, in addition to the key concepts that have been regularly used in medical sociology, there are recurrent substantive issues or particular approaches which should be included.

STRUCTURE AND CONTENTS OF THE BOOK

Entries are organized under five pre-defined themes: (1) the social patterning of health; (2) the experience of health and illness; (3) health, knowledge and practice; (4) health work and the division of labour; and (5) healthcare organization and policy. These themes cover a substantial proportion of medical sociological research and scholarship. There is, of course, some overlap between them. This overlap is reflected in the cross-references made between entries and our strategic positioning of certain concepts, which have generic relevance, earlier in the book. We will outline each of these themes below.

Part 1 focuses on the social patterning of health and includes entries on health inequalities and the social causation of (ill) health. It begins with an entry on 'pandemics and epidemics'. We recognize that entry could have been placed in Part 2, especially given the focus on experiential concerns, but decided that it usefully sets the stage for the remainder of this collection. Other entries in Part 1 explain how social divisions, such as 'social class', are associated with various measures of health status and discuss the ways in which such concepts have been operationalized. The study of inequalities in relation to occupational 'social class' has been particularly prominent in the UK, for instance. However, as the other entries in this section show, the distribution of life chances and health are also patterned by factors such as 'age', 'gender', 'ethnicity' and 'sexuality' – elements of the social structure that increasingly demand a sociological understanding of 'intersectionality' in global context. Furthermore, these entries illustrate how research deploying these concepts has developed through collaborating with other disciplines, such as epidemiology or, as per the new entry on 'environment', natural sciences addressing biophysical and ecological concerns. Of course, understanding how this social patterning of health comes about requires moving beyond statistical correlations. Hence, Part 1 also includes conceptual approaches that have been used to study the causes of health inequalities. Classic sociological debates run through many of these entries; for instance, the relative role in health causation of ideas and values compared to material factors in shaping social change and individuals' actions, and the significance of social integration for health. Such long-standing concerns would likely be recognizable to sociology's founding European triumvirate: Marx, Weber and Durkheim.

Themes in Part 2 include (but are not limited to) those deriving more directly from North American traditions of sociology. These approaches include functionalism and symbolic interactionism, with the conception of illness as a form of deviance linking the two. Sociological studies of the experience and meanings of illness and people's interactions with health professionals have, indubitably, generated concepts that have had a profound impact on both sociology as a discipline and healthcare delivery. 'Medicalization' is a recurrent concept here, denoting possible (partial, contested, revisable) processes that define areas of everyday life as medical problems to be treated. Part 2 also includes the concepts of 'stigma', 'chronic illness' and 'quality of life' which have arguably become so taken-for-granted in discussions of healthcare that their origins in particular concerns and the ways in which their use may have changed can be overlooked. Few sociology students go back, for example, to Parsons' (1951) original formulation of 'the sick role' and, as a result, may not appreciate fully either the context in which Parsons wrote or that this concept was a depiction of normative expectations and not actual behaviours. Other contributions to this section cover concepts such as 'pharmaceuticalization', 'illness narratives', 'embodiment', 'risk' and 'emotions'. In developing and using these concepts, medical sociologists have sought to move beyond one-dimensional accounts of illness as deviance and connect with more general concerns with self-identity and cultural meaning that characterize late or high modern societies. The experience of health and illness can therefore be seen to reflect and contribute to the shaping of contemporary cultures. The emphasis on personal narratives has also expressed this central motif, both for sociology and the wider society.

Part 3 focuses on health, knowledge and practice. Here the entries begin by discussing what has, at times, been regarded as not so much a useful analytical concept but more an object to be attacked: 'the medical model'. Underpinning this model is scientific knowledge about the working of the human body, and the next two entries examine recurrent concerns within medical sociology: the social shaping of this scientific knowledge and its relationship with lay people's knowledge and understanding of health and illness. In healthcare, scientific knowledge and technologies are combined to create forms of practice in which professionals and lay people interact. In recent years, there has been growing sociological interest in how this interaction is shaped, particularly in relation to innovative technologies such as those increasingly involved in the management of 'reproduction' and in genetic medicine or 'geneticization'. New entries on 'medical tourism' and 'digital health' are also included here. Finally, reflecting the influence of the French social thinker Michel Foucault on medical sociology, another highly topical practice is examined, that which is concerned with monitoring and promoting population health. Discussion in this area focuses on the tension between promoting the welfare of patients and the role of healthcare – especially health promotion – in effecting surveillance and disciplinary power over lay people's behaviours/actions/practices. At the same time, modern healthcare is a highly developed set of social processes that are embodied, emplaced and enacted. Healthcare involves many different forms of activity, and is provided by numerous actors, from highly trained professionals to laity engaged in self-care or who offer crucial informal care to others. This complex division of labour is, therefore, the focus of Part 4.

Until relatively recently, medical sociology was preoccupied with doctors, as members of an archetypal, autonomous profession of a particular occupational form and as the dominant group in healthcare provision. The first two entries in Part 4 cover such issues. However, in recent decades sociological research on healthcare providers has developed beyond the study of doctors. This has evolved in three main ways. First, there has been an increase in research on healthcare occupations, especially nursing and midwifery, alongside other 'professions allied to medicine' (for example, pharmacy and rehabilitation professions such as occupational therapy and physiotherapy). Second, particularly since the mid-1980s, sociologists' interest in the rise of medical power and authority has been superseded by a consideration of their putative decline. One possible indication of this is the apparent growth in resorting to non-orthodox medicine, which has revived sociological interest in the concept of 'complementary and alternative medicine'. Third, there has been a shift in emphasis away from specific occupations towards the division of labour itself and the character of healthcare work, wherever it is undertaken. Alongside micro-sociological studies of inter-professional interactions and boundary work, feminism has had an important influence on medical sociology research in this area since the 1970s. On the one hand, it has led to recognition of the value of 'emotional labour' as a relevant concept when studying healthcare as an embodied, relational activity. On the other hand, it has resulted in a wider conception of the location of health and the division of labour, including 'informal care' within the home. We would add, as with the entry on 'health professional migration and integration', that such labour needs to be examined with a close eye on global power relations. Hence, sociological attention should focus not only on relations between health workers and recipients of their care but also on relations between the Global North and the Global South, with care delivered in the former often leaving deficits in the latter.

The final section, Part 5, considers some of the key concepts and issues that have shaped medical sociological research on healthcare organization and policy. As might be inferred from the above discussion, such studies can be focused on different levels: the macro, societal level; the meso level of the formal organizational structure; and the micro interactional level. A concern with these different yet interconnected levels is reflected in our choice of topics, ranging from the hospital and what unfolds therein to the political economy of medicines and the legal systems surrounding healthcare. The key concepts and issues reviewed here fall into three main, albeit overlapping, categories. First are the theoretical concepts used to analyse the major shifts that have been occurring in healthcare across much of the relatively affluent world, such as 'privatization', 'managerialism', 'consumerism', and the reconfiguration of 'citizenship' in relation to healthcare entitlement. Second, there are sociological concepts that have been deployed in the analysis of how some issues become health policy concerns, as exemplified in relation to 'social movements'. Finally, there are concepts relating to institutional processes and organizations that are increasingly prominent in contemporary healthcare, such as 'medicines regulation', 'evaluation' and 'malpractice'. These latter concepts feed back into the discussion of the possible decline of an autonomous and all-powerful medical profession.

REFERENCES

Annandale, E. (2014) *The Sociology of Health and Medicine: A Critical Introduction*, 2nd edn. Cambridge: Polity Press.

Barry, A.M. and Yuill, C. (2016) *Understanding the Sociology of Health*, 4th edn. London: SAGE.

Bird, C.E., Conrad, P. and Fremont, A.M. (2000) 'Medical sociology at the millennium', in C.E. Bird, P. Conrad and A.M. Fremont (eds), *Handbook of Medical Sociology*, 5th edn. Upper Saddle River, NJ: Prentice Hall.

Bird, C.E., Conrad, P., Fremont, A.M. and Timmermans, S. (eds) (2010) *Handbook of Medical Sociology*, 6th edn. Nashville, TN: Vanderbilt University Press.

Bloom, S. (2000) 'The institutionalization of medical sociology in the United States, 1920–1980', in C.E. Bird, P. Conrad and A.M. Fremont (eds), *Handbook of Medical Sociology*, 5th edn. Upper Saddle River, NJ: Prentice Hall.

Bury, M. (1997) *Health and Illness in a Changing Society*. London: Routledge.

Calnan, M. (2020) *Health Policy, Power and Politics*. Bingley: Emerald Publishing Limited.

Cockerham, W.C. (2007) 'A note on the failure of postmodern theory and its failure to meet the basic requirements for success in medical sociology', *Social Theory & Health*, 5 (4): 285–296.

Cockerham, W.C. (2021) *The Social Causes of Health and Disease*, 3rd edn. Cambridge: Polity Press.

Cockerham, W.C., Dingwall, R. and Quah, S. (eds) (2014) *The Wiley Blackwell Encyclopedia of Health, Illness, Behavior, and Society*, 5 volumes. Oxford: Wiley-Blackwell.

Conrad, P. and Leiter, V. (eds) (2019) *The Sociology of Health & Illness: Critical Perspectives*, 10th edn. Newbury Park, CA: SAGE.

Denny, E., Earle, S. and Hewison, A. (eds) (2016) *Sociology for Nurses*, 3rd edn. Cambridge: Polity Press.

Dingwall, R., Hoffman, L.M. and Staniland, K. (eds) (2013) *Pandemics and Emerging Infectious Diseases: The Sociological Agenda*. Chichester: Wiley-Blackwell.

Faulkner, A. (2009) *Medical Technology into Healthcare and Society: A Sociology of Devices, Innovation and Governance*. Basingstoke: Palgrave Macmillan.

Gabe, J. and Calnan, M. (eds) (2009) *The New Sociology of the Health Service*. New York: Routledge.

Giddens, A. (1979) *Central Problems in Social Theory*. London: Macmillan.

Hoppe, T. (2018) *Punishing Disease: HIV and the Criminalization of Sickness*. Oakland: University of California Press.

Lupton, D. (2017) *Digital Health: Critical and Cross-Disciplinary Perspectives*. London: Routledge.

Monaghan, L.F. (2020) 'Coronavirus (COVID-19), pandemic psychology and the fractured society: a sociological case for critique, foresight and action', *Sociology of Health & Illness*, 42 (8): 1982–1995.

Monaghan, L.F., Rich, E. and Bombak, A.E. (2022) *Rethinking Obesity: Critical Perspectives in Crisis Times*. London: Routledge.

Mykhalovskiy, E. and French, M. (2020) 'COVID-19, public health, and the politics of prevention', *Sociology of Health & Illness*, 42 (8): e4–e15.

Mykhalovskiy, E., Frohlich, K.L., Poland, B. et al. (2019) 'Critical social science with public health: agonism, critique and engagement', *Critical Public Health*, 29 (5): 522–533.

Nancarrow, S. and Borthwick, A. (2021) *The Allied Health Professions: A Sociological Perspective*. Bristol: Policy Press.

Nettleton, S. (2020) *The Sociology of Health and Illness*, 4th edn. Cambridge: Polity Press.

Parsons, T. (1951) *The Social System*. New York: Free Press.

Sandberg, S. and Fondevila, G. (2020) 'Corona crimes: how pandemic narratives change criminal landscapes', *Theoretical Criminology*, advance online publication: https://doi.org/10.1177/1362480620981637

Scambler, G. (ed.) (2018) *Sociology as Applied to Medicine*, 7th edn. Basingstoke: Palgrave Macmillan.

Straus, R. (1957) 'The nature and status of medical sociology', *American Sociological Review*, 22 (2): 200–204.

Timmermans, S. and Gabe, J. (eds) (2003) *Partners in Health, Partners in Crime*. Oxford: Blackwell.

Turner, B.S. (1992) *Regulating Bodies: Essays in Medical Sociology*. London: Routledge.

Will, C.M. and Bendelow, G. (2020) 'Processing the pandemic', *Sociology of Health & Illness*, 42 (8): e1–e3.

Williams, S.J., Martin, P. and Gabe, J. (2011) 'The pharmaceuticalisation of society? A framework for analysis', *Sociology of Health & Illness*, 33 (5): 710–725.

PART I

SOCIAL PATTERNING
OF HEALTH

1

Pandemics and Epidemics

Robert Dingwall

> A pandemic is an outbreak of infectious disease on a global scale, as distinct from an epidemic, which is confined to one particular country or regional group of countries.

Pandemics and epidemics received little attention from sociologists until the 1980s, when HIV/AIDS appeared in the USA and other developed countries. The 1918 influenza pandemic, for example, was barely mentioned in contemporary sociology journals, although their publication was much disrupted by the legacy of the First World War and the subsequent economic problems experienced by many countries where the discipline was developing. HIV/AIDS has affected people in most parts of the world, so it qualifies as a pandemic. Ebola in 2013 was confined to a small number of countries in West Africa so it would be described as an epidemic. If we look at the public understanding of these terms, however, the scale of an infection is often confused with its dangerousness: pandemics are thought to be more severe and more likely to present an existential threat to humanity. Both pandemics and epidemics, then, are as much cultural as biomedical phenomena. A popular imaginary is invoked, which may also provide a rich source of metaphors in other spheres (Lavin and Russill, 2010). The World Health Organization (WHO, 1998), for example, has described obesity as a 'global epidemic' as a way to dramatize the health risks that this condition is thought to present and mobilize responses in an effort to prevent it. This frame implies rapidly spreading danger beyond national borders, and obesity scientists are now also using the term 'pandemic' in ways that resonate with the COVID-19 crisis (Monaghan et al., 2022).

An infectious disease may be viral or bacterial. The pandemics and epidemics of bubonic plague that ravaged much of the documented world until the 19th century were caused by a bacterium, *yersinia pestis*. However, the bacterial threat is, at least for the present, contained by the availability of antibiotic treatments. This may change if there is a shift in the evolutionary competition between human efforts to produce antibiotics and the natural selection processes that shape the bacteria. In the modern world, then, pandemics and epidemics are exclusively caused by viruses. There are few specific anti-viral treatments so the main medical intervention is through vaccination to prepare the human body's response to the infection. With long-established viruses, like the major childhood infections, large-scale vaccination has reduced their threat to a very low level in most countries, except where specific population groups have poor access to primary care or community health services or have adopted cultural beliefs that make them reluctant to accept vaccination (Reich, 2016). While such groups are often identified with particular faiths or counter-cultural thinking, they may also be found among wealthy people who consider that they can insulate their children from the everyday risks of mixing with poorer children in schools or elsewhere (Estep and Greenberg, 2020).

HIV/AIDS and influenza illustrate the sources of new viral infections. Although the precise history is still disputed, HIV is generally agreed to be an animal virus that crossed over into human populations in Africa sometime in the early 20th century and which found its way to the USA around 1980. Influenza is an inherently unstable virus, which seems to have a long history in human populations where it is constantly co-evolving with the human immune response. This results in small 'drifts' in its genome, which present more or less annual challenges. Mostly, these just produce another round of mild to moderate seasonal infections. At unpredictable intervals, however, the virus 'shifts' to an extent that the immune system is unprepared to respond. These shifts may come from the inherent instability of the virus or from an exchange of genetic material with the closely related influenza viruses that are carried by other species, particularly pigs and birds. Although there has been growing sociological interest in human/animal interactions, there have been few studies of the implications for disease transmission (Jerolmack, 2013; Procoli, 2004).

It is important to note that, for sociologists, the causative agent is not immediately relevant. Arguably, one of the problems in the management of the COVID-19 pandemic was the way in which it was institutionally captured by specialists in respiratory infections, which limited learning from the experience of HIV/AIDS or other pandemics. The mode of transmission may become important for sociology – a virus that is transmitted by airborne routes may present a different challenge from one transmitted through semen or blood – but this cannot be assumed from the start. Sociologists focus on the societal experience of a pandemic as a context for the impact of the virus rather than on the virus itself. The key elements of such an approach were set out in a paper by Strong (1990). This paper was written as part of a study of the management of HIV/AIDS in the UK, placing it within the context of previous pandemics or epidemics since the Black Death (bubonic plague) swept across Asia, Europe and North Africa between 1346 and 1353. Scholars generally accept that this killed 30–60 per cent of the European population (Benedictow, 2010).

Strong's (1990) analysis started from his observation that pandemics were fundamentally a disruption of social order, which is sociology's core problem as an academic discipline (see also Pickersgill, 2020, and Suggested Further Reading). The assumptions on which everyday life rested were suddenly called into question. One such assumption, extensively documented by ethnomethodologists, is that of trust, namely that interactions with other people are not inherently dangerous. COVID-19 management reversed that assumption. Suddenly, interaction was a risk to be controlled by greater distancing, face covering, etc. If the evidence for the effectiveness of such practices was questioned, some public health specialists argued that they should be continued just to remind people of the riskiness of the social world during a pandemic. The symbolic value of promoting suspicion became as important as the scientific value of effective self-protection. The erosion of trust was a dimension of the first of the three societal pandemics that Strong identified as the accompaniments of any bacterial or viral pandemic: of fear, suspicion and stigmatization; of explanation and moralization; and of action.

The pandemic of fear might be initially justified, in that no-one would know immediately whether a novel infection could wipe out our species or at least have an impact on the scale of the Black Death. Could it disturb our society and economy for generations because of the losses? However, the fear might persist beyond this point and become a basis for suspicion and stigmatization of population groups who were thought to have a particular role in transmitting or sustaining the infection. When COVID-19 was first identified in the UK as a virus originating in China, there were, for example, some boycotts of Chinese restaurants and acts of street violence against people of Chinese appearance.

The pandemic of explanation and moralization describes the competition to explain the appearance of the infection and the reasons why its impact took a particular shape. With COVID-19, for example, its supposed origins in a 'wet market', where live animals and fish were killed and prepared on the spot, could be used by a wide variety of critics of Chinese culture, politics and society. There was an orientalist critique of the 'backward' Chinese who ate a greater range of species than would be common in North America or Europe and did not shut away their slaughter and preparation from public view. This extended into an attack on the Chinese government for permitting such practices to continue, despite the apparent risk of a cross-over of viruses from exotic animals to humans. As sociologists, we might note that the food species considered eatable reflected a society where food availability had often been uncertain and where wet markets were a way to ensure the freshness of food when refrigeration might be scarce. The pandemic of explanation might also encompass some of the 'conspiracy theories' which claimed that the causative agent was not a random infection but emissions from 5G mobile phone networks or germ warfare by the Chinese government.

The pandemic of action refers to the popular expectation or demand that governments will *do something* to protect their populations, regardless of whether this might be expected to be effective. Actions can be driven by their symbolic value in showing official care or concern. Many elements of COV-ID-19 lockdown policies had this characteristic. The risks of outdoor transmission are minimal, for example, so people were usually allowed to walk outside for exercise. If, however, they were carrying golf clubs or tennis rackets, this would often be illegal. In part, this is a cross-over from the pandemic of moralization: these are serious times and no-one should derive pleasure while they are happening by acting in ways that some public health activists might consider frivolous.

There are four particular respects in which the approach outlined by Strong (1990) may benefit from further development in the light of the COVID-19 pandemic, most of which reflect the difference from the early trajectory of the HIV pandemic, which was Strong's principal lens.

First, the pandemic challenge to social order reveals weaknesses in the structures of equality and inequality within societies and the flaws in their healthcare systems. In the COVID-19 pandemic, there was a good deal of patrician policy-making, where people with secure jobs working from big houses with gardens made policies for people in insecure employment living in multi-generational households and overcrowded housing. The UK, in particular, discovered that it had created an 'efficient' health service that normally used its beds and staff more intensively than other developed countries, but then lacked resilience in a crisis of this kind.

Second, fear amplification was short-lived in the HIV pandemic, partly because it quickly became clear that the risk was confined to quite specific groups. In the UK, fear-based messaging was specifically banned by the Chief Medical Officer (Burgess, 2017). With COVID-19, it was adopted early on and sustained throughout. Strong was also sceptical about the use of police powers to enforce controls, because the forces of order would also be vulnerable to infection. COVID-19 saw a great extension of behavioural policing and the penalization of everyday social activities. This was much contested in some countries, particularly the USA and some parts of Europe, but accepted with little protest in others.

Third, fear of COVID-19 became established in the scientific and medical communities to a much greater extent than might have been expected. Again, this was partly because scientists and clinicians working with HIV quickly came to recognize that the infection did not put them at great personal risk provided some fairly routine precautions were taken. It has, indeed, been suggested that they became more preoccupied with the opportunity to win Nobel Prizes than with the patients they were treating or studying (Epstein, 1996). With COVID-19, scientific debates rapidly became caught up with different risk appetites and intensely polarized around issues like face coverings or differential protection of vulnerable groups. Scientists mobilized around petitions and open letters, and publications in political magazines became as important as those in peer-reviewed journals.

Fourth, the COVID-19 pandemic was marked by a particular extension of medical imperialism. Strong (1984) had always been sceptical about this, emphasizing the way in which medicine was surrounded by other sciences that shared its resources and checked its ambitions. In the COVID-19 emergency, however, the polarity was reversed and medicine subordinated other sciences to its own agenda. This started from medicine's moral understanding of disease as a flaw in nature to be corrected, rather than lived with, and then selectively recruited expertise from the existing penumbra of disciplines to promote that agenda. This excluded a range of other sciences. Airborne transmission, for example, became a topic for virologists supported by experts in hospital ventilation. Virology knows about infections within bodies: the space between is a topic for physicists and engineers working in fluid dynamics and social scientists working on proxemics. Patient voices were almost completely excluded, reinforcing a focus on extreme cases. At some points, medical imperialism shaded into claims for iatrocracy, rule by the medically qualified, as if health were the only social good that a society might seek.

In thinking about infectious diseases, it is important to remember that definitions of health and illness always involve moral judgements about desirable and undesirable states of the human body and its relationship with its environment. The management of the COVID-19 pandemic was a good illustration of the dangers of trying to 'follow the science' without asking 'which science' and investigating the values and visions embedded within the prescriptions of scientific advisers. What was the objective: the global eradication of the virus; the elimination of the virus from one country; the acceptance of the virus as an endemic respiratory infection comparable to the 30 or so others that humanity has lived with for millennia? What would be the social, psychological, cultural and economic costs of each goal? Were these proportionate to the benefits? Responses to the pandemic, in short, raise classic questions for the social sciences about who got access to that debate, which voices were included or excluded, what material interests were affected, and how decisions were eventually produced. COVID-19 is a topic for many areas of sociology and calls for medical sociologists to draw fully on the resources of their discipline, and beyond, to prepare a better response to the next infectious virus to emerge.

See also: Emotions; Medicalization; Risk; Stigma; Trust in Medicine.

REFERENCES

Benedictow, O. (2010) *What Disease Was Plague? On the Controversy over the Microbiological Identity of Plague Epidemics of the Past.* Boston: Brill.

Burgess, A. (2017) 'The development of risk politics in the UK: Thatcher's "remarkable" but forgotten "Don't Die of Ignorance" AIDS campaign', *Health, Risk & Society,* 19 (5–6): 227–245.

Epstein, S. (1996) *Impure Science: AIDS, Activism, and the Politics of Knowledge.* Berkeley: University of California Press.

Estep, K. and Greenberg, P. (2020) 'Opting out: individualism and vaccine refusal in pockets of socioeconomic homogeneity', *American Sociological Review*, 85 (6): 957–991.

Jerolmack, C. (2013) 'Who's worried about turkeys? How "organisational silos" impede zoonotic disease surveillance', *Sociology of Health & Illness*, 35 (2): 200–212.

Lavin, C. and Russill, C. (2010) 'The ideology of the epidemic', *New Political Science*, 32 (1): 65–82.

Monaghan, L.F., Rich, E. and Bombak, A.E. (2022) *Rethinking Obesity: Critical Perspectives in Crisis Times.* London: Routledge.

Pickersgill, M. (2020) 'Pandemic sociology', *Engaging Science, Technology, and Society*, 6: 347–350.

Procoli, A. (2004) 'Le temps et la construction du regard sur l'animal de rente. Ethnographie des pratiques et récits des éleveurs bretons', *Cahiers d'Economie et de Sociologie Rurales*, INRA Editions, 72: 91–113.

Reich, J.A. (2016) *Calling the Shots: Why Parents Reject Vaccines.* New York: New York University Press.

Strong, P.M. (1984) 'Viewpoint: the academic encirclement of medicine', *Sociology of Health & Illness*, 6 (3): 339–358.

Strong, P. (1990) 'Epidemic psychology: a model', *Sociology of Health & Illness*, 12 (3): 249–259.

WHO (1998) *Obesity: Preventing and Managing the Global Epidemic.* Geneva: WHO Press.

SUGGESTED FURTHER READING

- Dingwall, R., Hoffman, L.M. and Staniland, K. (eds) (2013) *Pandemics and Emerging Infectious Diseases: The Sociological Agenda.* Oxford: Wiley-Blackwell.

This is also available as a 2013 Special Issue of *Sociology of Health & Illness*, 35 (2). The editors' introduction sets out the case for a sociological approach to pandemics and epidemics, drawing particularly on Strong's (1990) work. The collection illustrates a range of approaches to understanding epidemics and pandemics in the contemporary world.

- Dodsworth, L. (2021) *A State of Fear.* London: Pinter & Martin.

A journalist's well-researched account of the amplification of fear by the UK government and its advisers during the COVID-19 pandemic. Raises important questions about the balance between public health, liberty and bodily autonomy in times of emergency and about the ethics of 'nudging' populations to achieve contested goals.

- Honigsbaum, M. (2019) *The Pandemic Century.* London: Hurst & Company.

This book discusses successive challenges from infectious diseases in the course of the 20th century and is useful as a way to think about their similarities and differences.

- Will, C. and Bendelow, G. (2020) 'Processing the pandemic', *Sociology of Health & Illness*, 42 (8): e1–e3.

Will and Bendelow introduce a Virtual Special Issue (VSI) on the COVID-19 Pandemic: https://onlinelibrary.wiley.com/doi/toc/10.1111/(ISSN)1467-9566.covid-19-content. This VSI includes a review by Monaghan of the relevance of Strong's (1990) work to that pandemic plus subsequent writings on macro-social concerns, drawing from medical sociologists such as Scambler. Other contributions explore issues such as: the symbolic meanings of masks in France, comparing West Nile Virus and COVID-19 and 'the politics of prevention'.

2

Social Class

Graham Scambler

> *Social classes are strata of society defined in terms of (1) the relationship between capital and labour, and extending to (2) aspects of labour market position and work characteristics.*

With the possible exception of the earliest, pre-Neolithic societies characterized by the nomadic lives of hunter-gatherers, human sociability has been marked by enduring hierarchies or strata. Sociologists usually refer to this as 'social stratification'. Even in ancient economies and traditional, 'settled' agricultural societies, systems of stratification were more complex than is commonly thought; but in modern industrial and post-industrial societies stratification is invariably multi-dimensional. Whilst social class is the dimension of stratification that has most often been highlighted and debated, it is far from being the only one. Moreover, as the historian Braudel (1984) has painstakingly shown in his study of Europe from 1400 to 1800, transitions from traditional to modern societies were generally slow and uneven, and, as his focus on the evolution of different forms of market testifies, no modern society is without its pre-modern or feudal residue.

Wright's (2015) classification of different sociological concepts, models and approaches to social class is helpful. He distinguishes between: (1) *the stratification approach*, where class is defined in terms of individual attributes and conditions; (2) *the Weberian approach*, where class is defined in terms of opportunity hoarding; and (3) *the Marxian approach*, where class is defined in terms of domination and exploitation. In the stratification approach, class identifies those economically important attributes of people that shape their opportunities and choices in a market economy, and thus their material conditions of life. Class here is about the *interconnections* between the individual attributes and material conditions of life. The Weberian approach entails a concept of 'social closure'. If a job is to confer special advantages, like a high income, incumbents must have the means to exclude others. This exclusion is often accomplished by forms of educational credentialism (i.e. formal qualifications) alongside other mechanisms (for example, citizenship rights in a global context), leading to unequally (dis)advantaged locations and conflict over resources/rewards/rents. Wright states that private property rights in the means of production constitute the main form of exclusion in a capitalist society, thus pointing to the importance of the Marxian approach to class. This approach is considered the most controversial. 'Domination' in this context refers to the ability to control the activities of others; and 'exploitation' refers to the acquisition of economic benefits from the labouring activity of those who are dominated. All exploitation, then, involves some kind of domination, but not all domination involves exploitation.

Most of the research on class and health can be categorized as the stratification approach, and to a lesser extent the Weberian approach. Socio-economic classifications (SECs), often presented as proxies for more sociological concepts of class, have routinely shown a strong inverse association between occupational standing and health status and longevity. Special mention might be made of a relatively subtle SEC, the broadly neo-Weberian National Statistics Socio-economic Classification (NS-SEC) introduced in England and Wales (see Rose and O'Reilly, 1997). In this scheme, occupations are differentiated in terms of reward mechanisms, promotion prospects, autonomy and job security. It comprises the following: senior professionals/senior managers; associate professionals/ junior managers; other administrative and clerical workers; own-account non-professionals; supervisors, technicians and related workers; intermediate workers; other workers; and never worked/other inactive. The most advantaged NS-SEC 'classes' typically exhibit personalized reward structures, have good opportunities for advancement and relatively high levels of autonomy within the job, and are relatively secure (though with the emergence of 'precarity' in the 21st century hitherto secure jobs are becoming less so). These attributes tend to be reversed for the most disadvantaged or routine 'classes' (Marmot et al., 2020).

In relation to England and Wales, the changes captured through a series of SECs on the one hand and, say, life expectancy on the other, have largely revealed an upward trend for both men and women across the SEC spectrum. However, this has been more rapid among the most advantaged than among those most disadvantaged in the 'socio-economic hierarchy'. Whilst this same pattern has been observed in other developed or high-income countries (Mackenbach, 2005), it should be stressed that this is a dynamic (if not deteriorating) picture and increased life expectancy is never guaranteed, even in 'wealthy' nations. For England, Marmot et al. (2020: 5) express shock that '[f]or part of the decade 2010–2020 life expectancy actually fell in the most deprived communities outside London for women and in some regions for men'.

The above reference to regions is worth underscoring. An earlier study of inequalities in healthy life expectancy (HLE) in England by SEC – this time using the older Registrar General's Classification of Occupations – also distinguished between Local Authorities known to be deprived (called the 'Spearhead group') and others (White and Edgar, 2010). A clear linear relationship was found, with HLEs increasing with SEC group. However, within each SEC group, HLEs for men and women were lower in the Spearhead Local Authorities than in the non-Spearhead Local Authorities. Thus, area of residence matters as well as socio-economic position. Indeed, the salience of 'where you live', nationally, regionally and locally, has been documented in detail by geographer Bambra (2016), albeit with particular reference to high-income nations.

Studies in high-income nations have long pointed to the existence of a 'social gradient' in morbidity and mortality – that is to say, the relationships between SECs and measures of health and longevity are finely graded. Not only are there marked differences between the most and least advantaged in England and Wales, for instance, but the 'higher' one's position is (or level of education, occupational status or housing conditions) the better one's health is likely to be. The following extract from Marmot et al. (2010: 16) is salient here, especially when considering what transpired in the remainder of the decade following Conservative(-led) government austerity policies that reduced/cut welfare:

> These serious health inequalities do not arise by chance, and they cannot be attributed simply to genetic makeup, 'bad', unhealthy behaviour, or difficulties in access to health care, important as these factors may be. Social and economic differences in health status reflect, and are caused by, social and economic inequalities in society.

The entry on social class in the second edition of *Key Concepts in Medical Sociology* explained there is a paucity of material for developing societies, certainly as far as social gradients are concerned. However, drawing from a report from the World Health Organization, it stated there was ample evidence for ubiquitous inter- and intra-national health inequalities, the most dramatic of which appear across the developed/developing, North/South divides. Since then, Marmot et al. (2020: 6) state that the UN has accorded considerable significance to social determinants of health. This is captured in its Sustainable Development Goals, with these authors expressing faith that in a global context 'actions to address inequalities have moved on'.

Such reviews of the evidence and policy are important. However, they emanate from social epidemiology, not sociology and its critical heritage. A sociological perspective on social class, using a Marxian relational approach, introduces, as Wright (2015) contends, issues of exploitation and domination. Whilst there is undoubted sociological utility in the deployment of SECs, some argue that they do not catch enough of the ongoing contradictions between capital and labour that were so pivotal for Marx. Indicators or proxies for class like NS-SEC have raised important issues around the nature of the causal relationship between class and health. Coburn (2009) maintains that SECs themselves reflect class forces in a Marxian sense. The nature of the capitalist class structure, and the outcome of class struggles, for him determine the extent and type of socio-economic inequalities in a given society, and the socio-economic inequalities in their turn shape the pattern of health and healthcare. He urges researchers to 'go far enough up the causal chain to confront the class forces and class struggles that are ultimately determinant' (Coburn, 2009: 44).

For Coburn (2004) it is the growing dominance of neoliberalism from the mid-1970s that is the causal basis of income inequality and its health-compromising sequelae. Global and national political trends have increased the power of the business classes and lowered that of the working classes. However, international pressures towards neoliberal policies have been differentially resisted by nation-states, largely because of their differing historical and institutional structures. Coburn's thesis can be termed a 'class/welfare regime theory'. Countries with less neoliberal – or social democratic – welfare regimes (for example, Finland, Sweden, Norway) have better levels of health than those with more clearly neoliberal regimes (for example, the USA and the UK). Whilst previous analyses have tended to link factors like income inequality and social cohesion with health or well-being, Coburn insists that his version 'deepens' the causal explanation by including economic globalization, neoliberalism and the power of capital, as well as welfare regimes and markets.

Scambler (2018) proffers an account in a similar vein to Coburn's. He argues that the period since the mid-1970s has witnessed a change in what he calls the 'class/command dynamic'. This denotes for him an intensification of (increasing global) class power relative to that of (still largely national, but increasingly privatized and regulatory) state power. Historically, those (men) with money have always been able to buy those (men) with power. Since the mid-1970s they have got more for their money than they did during the post-war era of welfare state capitalism. They have bought the power to shape policy in their own interests. Scambler argues that the expansion in income inequality, new 'flexible' work patterns, job insecurity, welfare cuts, cultural fragmentation and new divisive forms of individualism have their origins in the strategic decision-making of those core financiers, rentiers and Chief Executive Officers (CEOs) of large transnational companies. When, for instance, CEOs clinch excessive remuneration for downsizing workforces, introducing zero hours contracts, substituting part-time for full-time employees, reducing work autonomy in favour of micro-managerial control, outsourcing and terminating final salary pension schemes, they adversely affect the health and longevity of workers and contribute to the growth of health inequalities.

Schrecker and Bambra (2015) have claimed that especially since the 1980s, neoliberalism, or market fundamentalism, has not only dominated economics and politics but has also led to what they call 'neoliberal epidemics'. They have in mind here obesity, insecurity, austerity and inequality, maintaining that each of these constitutes a neoliberal epidemic. Aspects of their thesis have been critiqued (Monaghan et al., 2018). However, such issues have been defined by Schrecker and Bambra (2015) in this way because they are: (1) associated with the rise of neoliberal politics; and (2) are deemed epidemics since they have been 'transmitted' globally at a rate associated with biological contagions. The coronavirus (COVID-19) pandemic that has swept across continents in 2020 might perhaps be regarded as an extreme and more literal instance of contagion facilitated by a globalized, interconnected world committed to market accessibility (see also Arber and Meadows, 2020).

It could be argued that class relations in a Marxian sense play a key role in accounting not just for inter- and intra-national health inequalities but also for the near-ubiquitous failure of governments to tackle them effectively, as well as for some of the flaws to be found in healthcare systems. Revisiting their 2010 strategic review of health inequalities in England, and feeling the need to reiterate their earlier calls for government action in various domains, Marmot et al. (2020: 7) list six key policy objectives:

- give every child the best start in life;
- enable all children, young people and adults to maximize their capabilities and have control over their lives;
- create fair employment and good work for all;
- ensure a healthy standard of living for all;
- create and develop healthy and sustainable places and communities;
- strengthen the role and impact of ill-health prevention.

It is clear from the above that, firstly, having a good healthcare system is only part of the solution to tackling health inequalities and, secondly, social class continues to constitute a major obstacle in achieving greater health equity.

In sum, the concept of 'social class' has utility when exploring the social patterning of health, as evidenced by various measures and proxies. Whether the concept is defined sociologically according to Weberian or Marxian traditions, both have something to offer. The challenge within medical sociology is perhaps to explain the links between social class as a structure or relation, culture and individual behaviour and their implications for health (practices). Graham (1995) showed how seemingly individual decisions to engage in 'risk behaviours' like smoking can be rational by-products of the structured circumstances in which women happen, unwittingly, to find themselves. Arguably, it is the task of sociology to discover more effective ways of: (1) integrating macro-, meso- and micro-sociological theories of health inequalities; (2) facilitating genuinely interdisciplinary approaches to health inequalities; and (3) propagating policies to tackle health inequalities effectively. In view of early sociological commentary on how social class is implicated in COVID-19 (Arber and Meadows, 2020), for instance, and what has subsequently transpired in terms of unequal risks and outcomes, the necessity of this task should be incontrovertible.

See also: Material and Cultural Factors; Neoliberalism; Place.

REFERENCES

Arber, S. and Meadows, R. (2020) 'Class inequalities in health and the coronavirus: a cruel irony?' *The Blog of the Department of Sociology University of Surrey*. Online: https://blogs.surrey.ac.uk/sociology/2020/03/23/class-inequalities-in-health-and-the-coronavirus-a-cruel-irony/

Bambra, C. (2016) *Health Divides: Where You Live Can Kill You*. Bristol: Policy Press.

Braudel, F. (1984) *The Perspective of the World*. London: Collins.

Coburn, D. (2004) 'Beyond the income inequality hypothesis: class, neoliberalism and health inequalities', *Social Science & Medicine*, 58 (1): 41–56.

Coburn, D. (2009) 'Inequality and health', in L. Panitch and C. Leys (eds), *Morbid Symptoms: Health Under Capitalism*. Pontypool: Merlin Press.

Graham, H. (1995) *Unequal Lives: Health and Socioeconomic Inequalities*. Maidenhead: Open University Press.

Mackenbach, J. (2005) *Health Inequalities: Europe in Profile*. Rotterdam: Erasmus MC University Centre.

Marmot, M., Allen, J., Boyce, T. et al. (2020) *Health Equity in England: The Marmot Review Ten Years On*. London: Institute of Health Equity.

Marmot, M., Allen, J., Goldblatt, P. et al. (2010) *Fair Society, Health Lives – The Marmot Review: Strategic Review of Health Inequalities in England post-2010*. London: Institute of Health Equity.

Monaghan, L.F., Bombak, A.E. and Rich, E. (2018) 'Obesity, neoliberalism and epidemic psychology: critical commentary and alternative approaches to public health', *Critical Public Health*, 28 (5): 498–508.

Rose, D. and O'Reilly, K. (eds) (1997) *Constructing Classes: Towards a New Social Classification for the UK*. London: Office for National Statistics.

Scambler, G. (2018) *Sociology, Health and the Fractured Society: A Critical Realist Account*. London: Routledge.

Schrecker, T. and Bambra, C. (2015) *How Politics Makes Us Sick: Neoliberal Epidemics*. Basingstoke: Palgrave Macmillan.

White, C. and Edgar, G. (2010) 'Inequalities in healthy life expectancy by social class and area type: England, 2001–2003', *Health Statistics Quarterly*, 45: 28–56.

Wright, E. (2015) *Understanding Class*. London: Verso.

SUGGESTED FURTHER READING

- Bartley, M. (2017) *Health Inequality: An Introduction to Theories, Concepts and Methods*, 2nd edn. Cambridge: Polity Press.

A useful introductory text, foregrounding social class, income, wealth and culture. It considers various explanations for health inequalities, ranging from behavioural to material factors, whilst also underscoring the lifecourse and social integration.

- Scambler, G. (2018) 'Social class and health inequalities', in G. Scambler (ed.), *Sociology as Applied to Health and Medicine*, 7th edn. London: Palgrave.

Especially salient for students of medicine and allied health programmes, this chapter provides an accessible discussion on social class and health inequalities.

- Smith, K.E. and Schrecker, T. (2015) 'Theorising health inequalities: introduction to a special double issue', *Social Theory & Health*, 13 (3–4): 219–226.

Smith and Schrecker draw out six key themes from 11 articles in this special issue on health inequalities: critical thinking, dynamism/time, intersectionality, imagination, democracy and action. Social class is a key concept that runs through many of these articles and themes.

3

Gender

Ellen Annandale

Gender concerns the social relations within and between groups of men and women, boys and girls. It interacts with biology to shape morbidity and mortality patterns.

Morbidity and mortality are highly sensitive to societal level gender (in)equalities and to normative beliefs about gender-appropriate attitudes and behaviours. When exploring this at the international scale, sociologists draw attention to the associations between the variable and dynamic nature of gender norms and expectations within and across societies and gender differences in health. They emphasize that while biological sex differences need to be taken into account, they interact with social gender-related factors, which typically exert a stronger overall influence on health.

Social relations of gender vary within, between and across countries and regions of the world and over time, which is reflected in different patterns of health and illness. Life expectancy is a robust and commonly used indicator of population-level health. Women have a longer average life expectancy at birth than men across the world, although the extent varies considerably, from just under two years in Zimbabwe to almost 11 years in the Russian Federation, for example (World Health Organization [WHO], 2020a). These figures alone tell us that life expectancy cannot be simply accounted for by differences in male/female biology, since, if this was the case, we would not expect such marked international variations. Transformations in gender differentials in life expectancy over recent decades in different parts of the world illustrate this and point toward the importance of societal gender contexts for health.

First, the UK illustrates shifting gender patterns in the affluent West. Apart from a small downward blip between 2014 and 2015, life expectancy grew throughout the 20th and into the 21st century, to reach an average 79.2 and

82.9 years for men and women respectively in 2016 (Office for National Statistics [ONS], 2018). The number of years that a female might expect to live at birth compared to a male rose from around two additional years for those born in 1841, to reach a historical peak of 6.3 years in 1970. Thereafter, the gender differential has gradually declined to 3.7 years by 2016 (most recent data), a trend broadly mirrored in socio-economically comparable Western countries (Marshall et al., 2019; ONS, 2018). This 'closing gap' has chiefly been due to swifter improvements in life expectancy for males: for example, in the 15 years between 1989 and 2004, men gained 4.0 years and women 2.9 years; by 2005–2010 the equivalent figures had dropped to 1.5 and 1.0 years; and by 2011–2016 they had reached a low of 0.4 and 0.2 years (data derived from ONS, 2018). This male 'catch-up' is primarily due to men's swifter reduction in mortality from cardiovascular disease and (often associated) smoking-related deaths (such as lung cancer) over this period and in the previous decade. Since the 1970s, lung cancer incidence has been declining among men but increasing among women and is associated with historical gender differences in the take-up of smoking, which was much later in women than men and associated with the loosening of social mores in the early decades of the 20th century. However, the time-trend figures signal more than a male catch-up in life expectancy; they also point to a stalling or slowdown in improvements in life expectancy, which began to occur around 2011 (most markedly for the UK, but also in comparator countries). Significantly, the magnitude of this slowdown has been greater for women than for men. Moreover – and highlighting the intersection of gender with other social characteristics – in more socio-economically deprived areas, life expectancy has stalled for men, but has actually declined for women and the mortality rates of older women (over 85) have increased across all areas (Marshall et al., 2019). This gender differential has led researchers to draw associations between the life expectancy slowdown, austerity policies and social vulnerability (of women, the elderly) (Hiam et al., 2018).

A quite different gender–mortality association is observed for our second illustration of the Russian Federation, where, with a life expectancy of just over 66 years for males and just over 77 years for females in 2016, the female advantage of almost 11 years is the largest in the world (WHO, 2020a). The collapse of the Soviet Union in the early 1990s precipitated a mortality crisis of epic proportions, which disproportionately affected men. In the mid-1990s and the highly turbulent years of the transition from a state-managed to a form of market economy, women's average life expectancy was 71.7 years, compared to a lowly 57.4 years for men; that is, a gap of over 14 years (Timonin et al., 2017). The reason why men have particularly suffered is socio-political and connected with the collapse of industrial employment, especially in single-industy towns dominated by male employment, such as the lumber mills of Pitkyaranta. As Parsons (2014) concluded from research in these areas, as countless men became 'unneeded', social collapse translated into negative compensatory health behaviours, such as heavy alcohol consumption (historically associated with normative masculinity) and mortality from cardiovascular disease, alcohol-related causes and suicide.

Yet a further illustration of a very different gender and life expectancy pattern is found in sub-Saharan Africa where, at between two to three years, women's life expectancy advantage over men was small across many countries, such as Cameroon, Chad, Ghana, Sudan and Zimbabwe in 2016 (WHO, 2020a). While this may appear analogous to the situation described for countries of the affluent West, where, as illustrated by the UK, women's life expectancy advantage was just 3.7 years in 2016, the context is very different since average life expectancy is only in the 50s for men and 60s for women in these sub-Saharan countries (WHO, 2020a). Sub-Saharan Africa is geographically and economically diverse, but one of the poorest regions of the world, which undoubtedly accounts for the relatively low life expectancy for men and women alike. Female biological advantages can be countermanded by low social status attributed to girls and women and their limited access to resources that support health and well-being, such as nutritious food and access to healthcare, especially during pregnancy and childbirth, where preventable maternal mortality can be high.

These country and regional illustrations point to complex socio-political factors as the predominant explanation for gender differences in life expectancy, but this does not mean that biological differences have no bearing. Such differences render males and females differentially vulnerable to some causes of death, such as prostate disease in the former and cancer of the cervix and womb and death during childbirth for the latter. The hormone oestrogen can protect females against cardiovascular disease (CVD) in their reproductive years, while testosterone has been associated with weakened immunity and elevated risk of virus effects on the bodies of men. But it is the interaction of these biological factors with gendered social contexts that matters most for health. HIV/AIDS illustrates this. In 2019, approximately 38 million people worldwide were living with HIV, with most residing in low-to-middle-income countries and the majority concentrated in sub-Saharan Africa, where the female/male ratio is 1.7 (WHO, 2020b). HIV is transmitted by contact with fluids, such as blood, semen and vaginal fluid which enter the blood stream by crossing a mucus membrane (for example, of the vagina, tip of the penis, rectum) or by direct injection. Since viral load is higher in sperm than in vaginal secretions and the surface area of the mucus membranes exposed to the virus is higher in females, biology exposes them to higher risk of heterosexual transmission of HIV during intercourse. But it is gendered relations of power, especially where gender-based violence is involved, which renders young women in particular as vulnerable to infection through unsafe sex in the first place – four in five new infections are among adolescent girls and young women aged 15 to 19 in sub-Saharan Africa (UNAIDS, 2019).

The COVID-19 pandemic has also thrown into relief the interaction of social and biological factors in the gender patterning of health and illness. Although at the time of writing in 2020, males and females seem equally likely to be infected by the virus, in most countries more men have died from the disease than women, often by a large margin. Sex differences in biology seem to provide at least part of the explanation, since the angiotensin converting enzyme 2 receptor (ACE2), which has higher levels in men, seems an important risk for severe COVID-19 (Global Health 50/50, 2020). But this is unlikely to provide a complete explanation. Comorbidities are important to the body's response to COVID-19, particularly high blood pressure, CVD, and some lung diseases, all of which tend to have higher age-specific incidence in men internationally.

'Doing health' is a form of 'doing gender' (Saltonstall, 1993). Ironically, the social and political advantages that patriarchy confers on men are often associated with expectations of masculinity that express illness as weakness and vulnerability. What Marcos-Marcos and colleagues (2021: 101) dub the 'negative aftermath of privilege' can impact men's capacity to engage in health-promoting activities, to act on symptoms, and to seek healthcare in a timely manner for all kinds of illness. If timely treatment reduces mortality, this may partially explain higher male COVID-19 death rates. But COVID-19 and other pandemics or epidemics implicate gender beyond differentials in mortality and in ways that disadvantage women. The United Nations Development Programme (UNDP) (Rivera et al., 2020), for example, counsels that the COVID-19 pandemic is hindering progress toward gender equality for women. Food crises (and associated hunger and malnutrition), employment lay-offs, and increased domestic burdens of care for the sick disproportionately affect girls and women globally due to pre-existing structural inequalities. Moreover, gender-based violence against women and girls has increased exponentially during the pandemic as they have been forced into household isolation with their abusers, so much so that this has been widely characterized as a 'shadow epidemic' (Rivera et al., 2020).

Although the patterning of life expectancy provides a vital insight on how health varies by gender, it is only a part of a complex story which also involves the differential experience of illness during men's and women's lifetimes, as illustrated by mental ill-health. While life expectancy is a robust comparative cross-national indicator, self-reports of health are far less valid since health in general, and mental health in particular, can have different cultural meanings. For this reason, in this brief account we will focus on countries of the European Union (EU). According to the latest Eurostat data that were available at the time of writing (the second wave of the European Health Interview Survey, 2013–2015), there was considerable variation in the proportions of men and women suffering from chronic depression across the EU-28 countries in 2014. There were also differences in the extent of the gender difference within a country. However, in each and every instance women were more likely to be chronically depressed than men. The survey also shows that women report more negative feelings such as 'feeling down, depressed, hopeless' and 'feeling bad about self, a failure' than men. Accounting for these patterns, sociologists point to the long historical tendency to equate mental illness with being female and for the expression of mental distress to be more acceptable amongst girls and women than amongst men and boys, although diagnostic bias on the part of health professionals may play a role. But social and material inequalities may also differentially expose women and men to mental ill-health. This may help to explain why, although suicide rates and male/female differentials vary considerably around the world, suicide is more common amongst men in almost all countries (WHO, 2019). The stronger association between risk factors such as loss of a job or home and suicide for men than for women may signal the precipitating role of loss of patriarchal privileges (Rogers and Pilgrim, 2014).

The data drawn upon in this entry assume that gender is a binary phenomenon, underpinned by fixed biological difference. Health surveys in particular have been heavily cisgendered, that is, focused on persons whose gender identity matches their biological sex assigned at birth and who perform a gender identity considered appropriate for this 'sex'. However, this approach is out of step with present-day sociological understandings and with some people's experiences. Sociologists emphasize that a person's gender identity does not necessarily align with a specific biologically sexed body since people may self-identify outside the conventional male/female binary, for example, as transgender or as gender non-binary. Due to normative gender expectations, transgender persons often experience discrimination in everyday life which negatively impacts their health. For example, based on data for 31 US states, Lagos (2018) found cisgender men and women to have the lowest rates of self-rated 'poor health', followed by trans men and women. But the highest rates of poor health by far were amongst trans persons who identify as 'gender non-conforming'.

In conclusion, there are powerful associations between the social patterning of health and gender as it has been studied in terms of male/female differences. While this research is useful, the time has come to reflect more critically on the ways in which gender is conceptualized and measured in order to take account of all forms of gender identity. Importantly, this reminds us that gender is not only constructed in everyday life, but also brought to life in very specific ways by sociologists through the research that they conduct and publish.

See also: Intersectionality; Sexuality; Social Class.

REFERENCES

Global Health 50/50 (2020) *Sex, Gender and COVID-19*. Online: https://globalhealth5050.org/

Hiam, L., Harrison, D., McKee, M. and Dorling, D. (2018) 'Why is life expectancy in England and Wales stalling?' *Journal of Epidemiology and Community Health*, 72: 404–408.

Lagos, D. (2018) 'Looking at population health beyond "male" and "female": implications of transgender identity and gender nonconformity for population health', *Demography*, 55: 2097–2117.

Marcos-Marcos, J., Gash-Gellén, A., Meteos, J.T. and Álvarez-Darde, C. (2021) 'Advancing gender equ(al)ity, lifting men's health: dealing with the spirit of our time', *Journal of Epidemiology and Community Health*, 75: 100–104.

Marshall, L., Finch, D., Cairncross, L. and Bibby J. (2019) *Mortality and Life Expectancy Trends in the UK: Stalling Progress.* London: Health Foundation.

ONS (2018) *Changing Trends in Mortality: A Cross-UK Comparison, 1981–2016.* Online: www.ons.gov.uk/peoplepopulationandcommunity/birthsdeathsandmarriages/lifeexpectancies/articles/changingtrendsinmortality/acrossukcomparison

Parsons, M. (2014) *Dying Unneeded: The Cultural Context of the Russian Mortality Crisis.* Nashville, TN: Vanderbilt University Press.

Rivera, C., Hsu, Y., Pavez Esbury, F. and Dugarova, E. (2020) *Gender Inequality and the COVID-19 Crisis: A Human Development Perspective.* UNDP Human Development Working Paper. Online: http://hdr.undp.org/sites/default/files/covid-19_and_human_development_-_gender_dashboards_final.pdf

Rogers, A. and Pilgrim, D. (2014) *A Sociology of Mental Health and Illness*, 5th edn. Maidenhead: Open University Press.

Saltonstall, R. (1993) 'Healthy bodies, social bodies: men's and women's conceptions and practices', *Social Science & Medicine*, 36 (1): 7–14.

Timonin, S., Danilova, I., Evgeny, A. and Shkolnikov, V.M. (2017) 'Recent mortality trend reversal in Russia: are regions following the same tempo?' *European Journal of Population*, 33: 733–763.

UNAIDS (2019) *Women and HIV – A Spotlight on Adolescent Girls and Young Women.* Online: www.unaids.org/en/resources/documents/2019/women-and-hiv

WHO (2019) *Suicide in the World. Global Health Estimates.* Geneva: WHO. Online: www.who.int/publications/i/item/suicide-in-the-world

WHO (2020a) *World Health Statistics 2020. Monitoring for the SDGs, Sustainable Development Goals.* Geneva: WHO. Online: https://apps.who.int/iris/bitstream/handle/10665/332070/9789240005105-eng.pdf

WHO (2020b) *HIV/AIDS. Key Facts.* Online: www.who.int/news-room/fact-sheets/detail/hiv-aids

SUGGESTED FURTHER READING

- Annandale, E. (2009) *Women's Health and Social Change*. London: Routledge.

A feminist gender theoretical analysis of women's health in different historical time periods. It focuses on women in the Global North, particularly the intersection of gender and capitalism.

- Connell, R.W. (2012) 'Gender, health and theory: conceptualizing the issue, in local and world perspective', *Social Science & Medicine*, 74 (11): 1675–1683.

This article argues for a relational approach, conceptualizing gender as an active social process that generates health consequences. Moving the analysis beyond local arenas, it advances a global perspective by using anorexia and HIV as examples.

- Courtenay, W. (2011) *Dying to Be Men*. London: Routledge.

A wide-ranging discussion of the impact of masculinity on the health of men and boys. The book emphasizes that masculinity is a dynamic concept and experience that is enacted differently within and across societies.

- Singer, T.B. (2015) 'The profusion of things: the "transgender" matrix and demographic imaginaries in US public health', *Transgender Studies Quarterly*, 2 (1): 58–76.

A critical analysis of the use of sex/gender categories in quantitative studies. Singer argues that we need new ways of enumerating gender to highlight the experiences of marginalized people, but also points out that adding more categories inevitably creates additional boxes into which gender identities are confined.

4

Ethnicity

Hannah Bradby

> *Ethnicity refers to a shared social identity that is articulated in terms of common origins and is transmitted from generation to generation with an associated culture.*

Ethnicity is a collective identity justified through common origins and manifested in terms of religion, language, marriage and family patterns, diet and dress. As a social identity, ethnicity can be powerfully felt and acted upon at both the individual and group level, and, furthermore, has been institutionalized in some settings. The concept of ethnicity overlaps with religious, local and national culture and tradition, as was apparent in Zola's (1966) observation of patients' communication, where Italian Americans were said to be expressive and Irish Americans stoic. Despite the criticism of perpetuating ethnic stereotypes, Zola's suggestion that ethnic variation could be explained in terms of cultural (and not socio-economic) difference has been widely cited.

Powerful racialized folk typologies stereotype and essentialize the characteristics of groups that can be described as ethnic, which, in the Global North, means Black and Brown minorities. Meanwhile northern European White ethnic groups are the 'unmarked category' – a norm that does not require explanation, the background terrain against which the epistemological deviancy of Blackness must account for itself. Despite widespread scientific agreement over the lack of evidence for distinct human races, the idea of divisions that have a genetic basis is powerfully persistent. Inequalities by ethnic group in terms of mortality, morbidity and in the experience of healthcare are regularly racialized, whereby a minority ethnic group's shared culture or behaviour is held to be inherent or essential and to be causative. Racialization processes where healthcare structures and organizational routines systematically deprioritize particular minority ethnic groups, for instance Asian and Black groups having lower rates of kidney transplantation, have not been well studied. Thus, how institutional discrimination contributes to minority health deficits is not well understood. Ethnicity has been defined for use in routine and administrative data collection in various settings, including healthcare, and where ethnic patterns can be described they regularly show ethnic minorities to be disadvantaged (Nazroo, 2003). The longstanding essentialist ideas associated with racialized thinking and the routine conflation of race and ethnicity have hampered sociological research into ethnicity and health. This raises the question of how reifying and racializing effects of research into ethnicity should be weighed against the need to document inequity by ethnic group and to explore the inherent sociological interest of how health issues play out with ethnicity.

Medical sociological interest in ethnicity can be divided into three main areas, some of which are more researched and developed than others. First, inequalities in health by ethnic group as indicated by population morbidity and mortality rates and informed by epidemiological approaches. Second, the influence that ethnicity has on health in everyday life. Third, and least studied, the role that ethnicity plays in healthcare settings for both patients and staff as a discriminatory logic that has structured opportunities for and access to healthcare and employment. These three areas are outlined below with critical reference to practices, outcomes and explanations.

Population-based inequality by ethnic group is the first main body of work noted above. The demonstration of ethnic inequalities in health outcomes in statutory, survey or routine data is dependent on the inclusion of an ethnicity variable in such data sets. There are variations in practice in historical, international and national contexts which should first be noted here. For instance, whilst ethnic groups have long been defined in national censuses in Europe, the abuse of these classifications in the 1940s informs France's ongoing rejection of ethnicity as a routine variable on the grounds that it would reproduce earlier anti-Semitic and anti-Roma policies. By contrast, in the UK and Ireland censuses and some other administrative data sets, respondents are routinely instructed to allocate themselves to pre-defined ethnic groups. In the USA both ethnic and racial classifications are used in censuses, while in Australia the current census question asks about 'ancestry', which in earlier versions was ethnic, and earlier still 'racial' origin. Western countries that do not collect ethnicity data use measures of 'migrant background' composed of country of birth and (grand) parents' country of birth as a proxy that can be used in analysis.

While there are both practical and theoretical objections to measuring ethnicity (Bradby, 2003), it is nonetheless demonstrable that where ethnic group is measured against health outcomes, inequalities (which are often also inequities) are found that cannot be explained by socio-economic class. Differences in rates of mortality and morbidity by ethnic/racialized group have been repeatedly demonstrated in the USA (Phelan and Link, 2015) and the UK (see the entry on ethnicity in the second edition of *Key Concepts in Medical Sociology*). Within crudely defined ethnic groups in England, socio-economic gradients in health are evident, whereby better general (self-reported) health is associated with higher household income (Nazroo, 2003). In addition to the familiar socio-economic gradient within ethnic groups, there are gradients between ethnic groups.

Within each class group in data from England, ethnic minority people have lower income than White people, and for the poorest ethnic group – Pakistani and Bangladeshi people – differences were twofold, so equivalent in size to the difference between the richest and poorest class groups in the White population (see Suggested Further Reading below). In settings where ethnicity is not routinely measured, proxies suggest that inequalities exist nonetheless: for instance immigrants of non-European background in Sweden are three to four times more likely than Swedish-born people to suffer from poor, or very poor, health (Hjern, 2012). The economic and social factors that produce health inequalities overwhelmingly disfavouring ethnic minorities are not reducible to class-based disadvantage, refracted as they are through processes of racialization.

The second area of work, noted above, explores *ethnicity's influence on health in everyday life*, and can be considered at the population level through quantitative methods and, using qualitative methods, at the level of interpersonal interactions. The sociological founding father W.E.B. Du Bois researched the subjectivities of African Americans, while also establishing the effects of structural racism on everyday lives. Du Bois' legacy of applying the sociological imagination to health aspects of minorities' everyday life is yet to be developed in medical sociology. Crudely defined ethnic groups used in censuses and surveys are criticized for not capturing the subjective experience of ethnicity (Williams and Husk, 2013). Ethnicity is complex, contingent and dynamic. Political, social and cultural contexts are relevant both in confirming and in disconfirming how it is experienced. The relevance and intensity of different dimensions of ethnicity will vary with time and setting: one's ethnicity might be reinforced when surrounded by a contrasting ethnic group – a Gujerati at a Punjabi wedding, for instance. But equally, depending on social setting, a Gujerati wedding guest might have a sense of commonality with the Punjabi hosts due to a common identity as British Asians living, for instance, in the UK's West Midlands. Outward signs of an ethnic affiliation such as a head scarf, tattoos, jewellery or a beard change the intensity of their meaning and how actively they are interpreted by others.

Despite the contingent and dynamic nature of ethnicity, it is a real collective identity that captures a way of being in the world that can influence health. For instance prohibitions on the use of alcohol and tobacco among Muslims and Sikhs of Punjabi origin have cultural and religious dimensions with complex implications for gendered ethnic identities (Bradby, 2007) and also have real health effects through minimizing consumption levels and delaying the age when consumption first starts. The complex contingency of ethnic identity means that a straightforward link between ethnic identity and health behaviour is unusual, with the contingencies playing out within structural constraints. Insofar as ethnic identities are neither secure nor coherent, they are also open to strategic manipulation (Hall, 1992), indicative of agency. Minority ethnic identity in Western countries is typically associated with migrant labour and refugee status, implying that agency is playing out under the structural constraint of limited socio-economic means and opportunities and, potentially, political opposition and/or repression. Racism is another constraint that is both structural and individualized and that demonstrates agency's limits: 'no amount of strategic manipulation alters the direction of the racist's fist' (Smaje, 1996: 143).

Research into the relationship between health and ethnicity in everyday life is hampered by a tendency to hold features of minority groups' ethnicity accountable for health deficits and to consider individual risk over and above group processes. For instance, minority ethnic people are more likely to be diagnosed as having a severe mental illness than the White majority in the UK: investigations into the causes of these discrepancies have focused on individual risk, overlooking how a person's own experience of socio-economic deprivation, discrimination and exposure to childhood trauma and institutional responses to those experiences, are shaped by structural processes (Nazroo et al., 2020).

The role of the interactions between everyday life experiences, trajectories through health systems and the effects of social structures is what sociology brings to the study of ethnicity and health, which the small-scale approaches of psychology and anthropology do not. The disproportionately high fatality of Black and ethnic minority groups from COVID-19 infection, emergent as the pandemic has played out in northern Europe and the USA, illustrates the need for an approach that includes individuals, systems and the interactions between the two over time. While statistics are still being collated and compiled at the time of writing, Black and ethnic minority people seem to have a disproportionately high risk of being admitted to intensive care and of dying from COVID-19 infection across a range of countries. Public Health England's (2020) rapid review on 'disparities' in the risk and outcomes of COVID-19 found that Black and Asian ethnic groups had higher death rates from COVID-19 compared with White groups, which, crucially, is the opposite of the trend seen in all-cause mortality over previous years. Per capita hospital deaths from COVID-19 for all British minority ethnic groups, except for the Irish, are higher than those of the White British majority, once age, gender and geographic distribution of the population are factored in.

Reasons for the disproportionately high rates of coronavirus infection and of fatality among minority ethnic groups are likely to be multiple but can be summarized as an outcome of racialized socio-economic inequalities, including health inequalities, which amount to structural vulnerability. The population-based inequality by ethnicity described above means that rates of some chronic diseases such as high blood pressure and coronary heart disease are higher for minorities than the general population, and so the outcomes of infection are worse. Structural constraints such as a disproportionately high representation of minorities in overcrowded and poor-quality housing and employment in lower paid and less flexible occupations mean that preventative public health measures such as self-isolation are difficult to achieve and to maintain and so less effective. High levels of employment in essential occupations in the public sector, such as public transport, health and social care provision, may increase the risk of exposure of Black and minority groups to the virus, alongside economic vulnerability as a result of high rates of self-employment, employment in sectors that were shut down and limited financial savings to fall back on (Platt and Warwick, 2020).

The third, albeit under-explored area, addresses *the influence of ethnicity in healthcare settings for both patients and staff.* Racist ideologies intertwine with national ideals around welfare to regulate how medical migrant labour is stratified in statutory health services (Kyriakides and Virdee, 2003). Healthcare systems of wealthy countries have been crucial motors of migration to the extent that a medical training has become a means to enhance personal and family mobility. In the immediate aftermath of the Second World War the UK's National Health Service was staffed by physicians from India and Pakistan and nurses and midwives from the Caribbean. Since then, globalized migration has been an evident trend in the skilled healthcare workforces across the world: between 23 per cent and 34 per cent of practising physicians in New Zealand, the UK, the USA, Australia and Canada have been trained elsewhere (Connell, 2010). The contribution of migrant healthcare workers to maintaining and developing national health systems, despite discriminatory treatment, has begun to be explored (Raghuram et al., 2011). The over-representation of minority ethnic healthcare staff in low status medical specialisms and their high likelihood of working long hours in public-facing roles are ignored in systems that claim to be 'colour-blind'. The ethnic, gendered and occupational inequalities in rates of infection and of mortality are a feature of the COVID-19 pandemic that indicates how interpretations of ethnicity have structured opportunities and access in healthcare settings and beyond (see Suggested Further Reading).

In sum, ethnicity, as a complex and contingent aspect of group and individual identity that is embedded in socio-economic structures and organizational routines, has important effects on the social relations of health and illness. The role of ethnicity has been shown in population data and at the level of lived experience and yet there remains much to be explored. The ways that ethnicity works in combination with other social identities, class structures and racist ideologies, and the circumstances under which it becomes salient for the social relations of health and illness, remain under-researched. The ways that healthcare provision and uptake are patterned by ethnicity are of particular relevance where the occupational structure of healthcare organizations is itself subject to racialized stratification.

See also: Health Professional Migration and Integration; Intersectionality; Material and Cultural Factors; Social Class; Social Divisions in Formal Healthcare.

REFERENCES

Bradby, H. (2003) 'Describing ethnicity in health research', *Ethnicity & Health*, 8 (1): 5–13.

Bradby, H. (2007) 'Watch out for the Aunties! Young British Asians' accounts of identity and substance use', *Sociology of Health & Illness*, 29 (5): 656–672.

Connell, J. (2010) *Migration and the Globalisation of Health Care*. Cheltenham: Edward Elgar.

Hall, S. (1992) 'The question of cultural identity', in S. Hall, D. Held and T. McGrew (eds), *Modernity and its Futures*. Cambridge: Polity Press in association with the Open University.

Hjern, A. (2012) 'Migration and public health in Sweden: the National Public Health Report 2012. Chapter 13', *Scandinavian Journal of Public Health*, 40 (9) suppl.: 255–267.

Kyriakides, C. and Virdee, S. (2003) 'Migrant labour, racism and the British National Health Service', *Ethnicity & Health*, 8 (4): 283–305.

Nazroo, J.Y. (2003) 'The structuring of ethnic inequalities in health: economic position, racial discrimination, and racism', *American Journal of Public Health*, 93 (2): 277–284.

Nazroo, J.Y., Bhui, K.S. and Rhodes, J. (2020) 'Where next for understanding race/ethnic inequalities in severe mental illness? Structural, interpersonal and institutional racism', *Sociology of Health & Illness*, 42 (2): 262–276.

Phelan, J.C. and Link, B.G. (2015) 'Is racism a fundamental cause of inequalities in health?' *Annual Review of Sociology*, 41 (1): 311–330.

Platt, L. and Warwick, R. (2020) *Are Some Ethnic Groups More Vulnerable to COVID-19 than Others?* The IFS Deaton Review VI Inequality. The Institute for Fiscal Studies. Online: www.ifs.org.uk/inequality/chapter/are-some-ethnic-groups-more-vulnerable-to-covid-19-than-others/

Public Health England (2020) *Disparities in the Risk and Outcomes of COVID-19*, August. London: Public Health England.

Raghuram, P., Bornat, J. and Henry, L. (2011) 'The co-marking of aged bodies and migrant bodies: migrant workers' contribution to geriatric medicine in the UK', *Sociology of Health & Illness*, 33 (2): 321–335.

Smaje, C. (1996) 'The ethnic patterning of health: new directions for theory and research', *Sociology of Health & Illness*, 18 (2): 139–171.

Williams, M. and Husk, K. (2013) 'Can we, should we, measure ethnicity?' *International Journal of Social Research Methods*, 16 (4): 285–300.

Zola, I.K. (1966) 'Culture and symptoms – an analysis of patients' presenting complaints', *American Sociological Review*, 31 (5): 615–630.

SUGGESTED FURTHER READING

- Bradby, H. and Nazroo, J.Y. (2021) 'Health, ethnicity and race', in W.C. Cockerham (ed.), *The Wiley Blackwell Companion to Medical Sociology*. Oxford: Blackwell.

The above chapter summarizes USA and UK research findings, in sociological and historical context.

- Smart, A. and Weiner, K. (2018) 'Racialised prescribing: enacting race/ethnicity in clinical practice guidelines and in accounts of clinical practice', *Sociology of Health & Illness*, 40 (5): 843–858.

This article draws on documentary sources and interviews with experts in various health disciplines to examine the racializing role that ethnic group classifications play in clinical guidelines and practice around hypertension in England and Wales.

- Younis, T. and Jadhav, S. (2020) 'Islamophobia in the National Health Service: an ethnography of institutional racism in PREVENT's counter-radicalisation policy', *Sociology of Health & Illness*, 42 (3): 610–626.

Amidst concerns about terrorism in the UK, this article illustrates how the securitization agenda has racialized an ethnic group with profound implications for clinical practice.

- Kapilashrami, A., Otis, M., Omodara, D. et al. (2021) 'Ethnic disparities in health & social care workers' exposure, protection, and clinical managements of the COVID-19 pandemic in the UK', *Critical Public Health,* online first: https://doi.org/ 10.1080/09581596.2021.1959020

This article provides important quantitative evidence on how minority ethnic carers in the UK, compared to White health and social care workers, were much more likely to be exposed to COVID-19 infection. Mindful of systemic racial bias, the authors call for an NHS-wide review in order to evaluate procedural fairness, ensure safe practices and to avert future crises.

5

Sexuality

Sue Scott

Sexuality typically refers to sexual acts and to sexual orientation and/or sexual identity. Sexuality is both private and ubiquitous, important to well-being and potentially risky.

Understanding the social implications of sexuality, including its relationship to health, can be confusing. While medical definitions are usually clear there is often confusion in everyday life about the difference between sex, gender and sexuality. Sex is usually based on medical assessment of a baby's genitals, whereas gender is usually used to denote the social implications of being either female or male (see the entry on 'gender'), and sexuality refers to an individual's sexual preferences/identity. There is added complexity in relation to individuals who consider themselves to be of the opposite gender to that which is usually linked to the sex they were assigned at birth, but this is a matter of gender and not sexuality and therefore will not be dealt with in this entry.

Here, we will focus on sex and sexuality especially in relation to health and illness. Diseases resulting from, or assumed to be related to, sexual behaviour have long been a medical concern, and, since the mid-20th century, the fields of health education and later health promotion have focused on attempting to encourage sexual health. First, however, it is necessary to offer further context and some caveats.

Sexuality includes both the capacity for sexual feelings and an individual's sexual orientation or preferences. However, these two aspects are not preconditions for each other. It is possible to identify as heterosexual, homosexual or bisexual, but have no desire for, or even experience of, sex, *or* as asexual and yet engage in sexual acts *or* to have same-sex sexual relations but not define oneself as homosexual. The definition of 'natural' sexuality is no longer based on religious teachings, although these still circulate, but on biological assumptions that predominate in modern societies. The underlying assumption here is that human sexuality is driven by genes and hormones, and by an innate desire to perpetuate the species – hence the longstanding definition of heterosexuality as normal. However, since the 1970s sociologists have challenged this essentialist view and criticized the assumption that 'natural' sexuality untouched by culture is possible. They argue that people become sexual in specific contexts and that our biographies shape our sexual preferences and practices (Scott and Jackson, 2020). If we look at sexuality historically we find significant differences; for example in medieval Western Europe women were often thought to be full of carnal lust whereas in the Victorian period, in Britain, they were often defined as asexual (Acton, 1865). Likewise, if we take a cross-cultural perspective, we find a wide range of practices which could be, but are not necessarily, viewed as sexual (Herdt, 1981).

Until relatively recently sex was viewed in Western culture as a private matter, only acceptable within marriage, linked to reproduction, and with male heterosexual desire shaping sexual practice. This produced an understanding of sexuality that was both sexist and heterosexist (Scott and Jackson, 2020). Psychoanalysis and related theories, which developed in the early 20th century, argued that attempts to 'repress' these 'natural' sexual urges created problems within the individual psyche, and this thinking influenced the liberation movements of the 1960s.

There are three main strands of explanation in the sociology of sexuality: social interactionism, post-structuralism (primarily shaped by the work of Michael Foucault) and Queer theory – which in turn draws on post-structuralism as well as psychoanalysis and feminism. Feminist work has also been very important. Feminists have drawn on all three kinds of explanation in order to account for the interrelationship between sexuality and gender. In brief, interactionist sociologists argue that there is no innate sexuality; rather, 'being sexual' and 'doing sex' are learnt through the sexual meanings and conventions within social interaction. Feminist interactionist sociologists (Jackson and Scott, 2010) have argued that because children generally develop a sense of their gender before they have access to sexual knowledge they come to understand sexuality through social definitions of gender, which in turn shape our understanding of differences between male and female sexuality. For interactionists sexuality is not fixed, but evolves in relation to biography and cultural context. Foucault (1981 [1978]) argued against the widespread view that sexuality was repressed in the 19th century. Rather, he claimed that sexuality as we now know it was brought into being through the *classification* of various forms of sexual expression, as normal or perverse, and through the *production* of sexuality as an aspect of our inner being. For Foucault, discourses around sexuality encompass aspects of both regulation and liberation, and there is no linear movement from the former to the latter as modernity progresses. Queer theorists stress the importance of individual sexual identity and the range of potential sexual identities. They also argue for the disruption of the binary between heterosexuality and homosexuality (Seidman, 1997). For them 'Queerness' is constituted as marginal, in relation to the heterosexual norm, and therefore all non-normative sexualities come under the umbrella of 'Queer'.

In order to fully understand sexuality sociologically, we need to explore how it is affected by various social factors. These factors include the interrelationship of social structures, other social divisions and positions, everyday social and sexual practices, as well as the meanings attached to sexuality within cultural discourses and individual subjectivities. Sociological and *some* everyday accounts of sexuality do focus on its social construction, but essentialist explanations have not disappeared. Indeed, they have seen a revival. As sexuality has become ever more closely linked to individual identities it has also been increasingly understood as a fundamental aspect of the self. Also, developments in genetics and neuroscience have led to attempts to find a 'gay' gene and a 'gay' brain. Some lesbians and gay men do indeed understand their sexuality as a fundamental aspect of their biology, whereas others draw more on biographical and cultural explanations and/or see it as a matter of collective identity. The sociological questions, in this context, are: why are some explanations more dominant/acceptable at any given time? What are their implications? Why is heterosexuality still relatively unproblematized? Sociologists are also interested in understanding what we might call the 'specialness' of sex – the way it is seen as a central aspect of everyday life *and* raised above the quotidian. Recent sociological research into asexuality has argued that sex is not at all important for some people (Scott et al., 2014). The case has also been made that a great deal of sexual activity is neither risky nor exotic, but rather mundane, every day and possibly marginal (Jackson and Scott, 2010).

As noted above, sex has been related to health as well as to sickness. Modern medicine, while defining 'normal' sex as a natural biological function, classified homosexuality and many other sexual practices as perversions. It is worthy of note that homosexuality was only finally removed from the World Health Organization's International Classification of Diseases in 1990. Treatment regimens were devised for 'sexual deviants' aimed at curing them through a variety of means – castration, aversion therapy, Electroconvulsive therapy (ECT), drugs and psychotherapy – at different points in time from the late 19th century onwards. It is significant that psychological and psychotherapeutic interventions have, in more recent years, shifted from 'treating' homosexuality towards supporting lesbians and gay men who are suffering from mental health problems, primarily as a result of continuing discrimination and abuse. Such research as there is, on the general health of lesbian and gay individuals, suggests poorer overall health, particularly in relation to mental health, than the heterosexual population (Meads et al., 2012).

The so-called 'liberation' of sex and sexuality in the 1960s, epitomized by legal changes regarding homosexuality and abortion, was, from the start, countered by crises and panics about, for example, gay sexual behaviour and teenage pregnancy. These concerns became entangled with changing ideas about risk and danger. Previous perceptions of a world fraught with hazards, which humans could do little about, had shifted towards an increased expectation that we would/should be able to obviate risks. Expectations grew that this would be done through scientific and social developments, coupled with management of individual behaviour (Gabe, 1995).

This focus on risk was clearly played out in relation to HIV/AIDS in the 1980s and 1990s. HIV was seen as a problem of (not just for) gay men because the initial spread in the Global North was through the gay community. There was a backlash against homosexuals for allegedly causing the pandemic through 'casual' sex. Sociological and anthropological research countered some of these assumptions and ensured that epidemiologists and public health professionals were better informed about the social contexts of HIV transmission (Bloor, 1995). It was widely assumed that the gay community should be targeted with information. However, this completely missed the many men who identified as heterosexual but sometimes had sex with men and who would be much less likely to go to the places where information and support were available (Deverel and Prout, 1999). It was also generally assumed that gay men who had high numbers of sexual partners were most at risk of becoming infected. However, as Hunt et al. (1991) showed, gay men tended to be more willing to use condoms with casual partners than within an established relationship, even if one, or both, partners was/were non-monogamous.

Sex can be viewed and/or experienced as problematic throughout the life-course. There are currently public health concerns about the sexual behaviour of midlife and older heterosexuals. The incidence of sexually transmitted infections (STIs) has increased in this age group as a result of the breakdown of long-term relationships and the opening up of opportunities through internet dating (Dalrymple et al., 2016). Children and young people have also been a major focus of anxiety in relation to sexual risk. In this context there has been much debate about sex education (Buston et al., 2001), with more liberal opinions in tension with the view that children should be protected from too much sexual knowledge. Sociologists have argued that keeping children in ignorance, or only teaching them the 'facts', fails to prepare them to deal with sex and relationships (Jackson and Scott, 2015). Such 'protection' potentially puts young people at risk of abuse and STIs and, in the case of girls, of sexual coercion and pregnancy.

As contraception made it possible to separate heterosex from reproduction, and as gay and queer sexualities became more visible, a shift occurred in our understanding of what sex is for. Sexual activity is increasingly seen as being for leisure and pleasure, reinforcing the view that good sex is healthy and can improve one's life and well-being. However, not having 'good' sex is increasingly seen as a personal failing and something to be rectified. Also, while in the past sexual competence was seen to be primarily an issue for men, the increases in women's autonomy and the options available to them have encouraged a greater focus on female pleasure but also raised expectations of their performance. In this context the options for improving the situation are both personal (for example, partner change and self-help manuals) *and* professional (for example, therapy, counselling and pharmaceuticals). Drugs, such as Viagra, are used to sustain male sexual performance, while the search for a safe equivalent for women continues. The way in which Viagra works means that, once again women are expected to be available to respond at the appropriate moment, thus rendering equality in the practice of sexuality problematic – another example of the non-linear process of social change in relation to sexuality (Potts et al., 2003).

The liberalization of sexuality carries a contradictory kernel of anxiety. There is a struggle between the desire for sex to be liberated from normative constraints while at the same time redefining what is seen as normal, to widen the range of socially acceptable sexual expression. A good example of this latter move is the legalization of gay marriage which, besides increasing equality, has the effect of rendering gay relationships more respectable without actually unsettling heterosexuality (Richardson, 2004).

Tensions between sex as healthy and sex as risky continue to play out in the media, within health promotion and in personal relationships. For sociologists, however, sex is neither intrinsically good nor bad, healthy nor unhealthy. What *is* of sociological interest are the particular ways in which sex acts, sexual relations and sexual identities are socially ordered and the continuities and changes in these over time. Specifically, in relation to the relationship between sexuality and health, more sociological research is needed on: sex and sexuality in later life; the relationship between sexual identity and sexual experiences; the mental health and general health status of the wider population of LGBTQ+ individuals plus continued critical analysis of the field of sexual health promotion.

See also: Ageing and the Lifecourse; Gender; Risk.

REFERENCES

Acton, W. (1865) *The Functions and Disorders of the Re-productive Organs in Youth, in Adult Age, and in Advanced Life, Considered in their Physiological, Social, and Moral Relations*. Held by the British Library, London.

Bloor, M. (1995) *The Sociology of HIV Transmission*. London: SAGE.

Buston, K., Wight, D. and Scott, S. (2001) 'Difficulty and diversity: the context and practice of sex education', *British Journal of the Sociology of Education*, 22 (3): 352–368.

Dalrymple, J., Booth, J., Flowers, P. et al. (2016) 'Socio-cultural influences upon knowledge of sexually transmitted infections: a qualitative study with heterosexual middle-aged adults in Scotland', *Reproductive Health Matters*, 24 (48): 34–42.

Deverel, K. and Prout, A. (1999) 'Sexuality, diversity and community: the experience of MESMAC', in R. Parker and P. Aggleton (eds), *Culture, Society and Sexuality: A Reader*. London: UCL Press.

Foucault, M. (1981 [1978]) *The History of Sexuality, Volume One*. London: Pelican.

Gabe, J. (ed.) (1995) *Medicine, Health and Risk: Sociological Approaches*. Oxford: Blackwell.

Gagnon, J. and Simon, W. (2004) *Sexual Conduct*, 2nd edn. New Brunswick, NJ: Aldine Transaction.

Herdt, G. (1981) *Guardians of the Flutes.* New York: McGraw Hill.

Hunt, A.J., Davies, P.M., Weatherburn, P. et al. (1991) 'Changes in sexual behaviour in a large cohort of homosexually active men in England and Wales 1988–1989', *British Medical Journal*, 302: 505–506.

Jackson, S. and Scott, S. (2010) 'Rehabilitating interactionism for a feminist sociology of sexuality', *Sociology*, 44 (5): 811–826.

Jackson, S. and Scott, S. (2015) 'A history of researching childhood and sexuality: continuities and discontinuities', in E. Renold, J. Ringrose and R.D. Egan (eds), *Children, Sexuality and Sexualisation*. London: Palgrave.

Meads, C., Camona, C. and Kelly, M.P. (2012) 'Lesbian, gay and bisexual people's health in the UK: a theoretical critique and systematic review', *Diversity and Equality in Health and Care*, 9: 19–32.

Potts, A., Gavey, N., Grace, V.M. and Vares, T. (2003) 'The downside of Viagra: women's experiences and concerns', *Sociology of Health & Illness*, 25 (7): 697–719.

Richardson, D. (2004) 'Locating sexualities: from here to normality', *Sexualities*, 7 (4): 391–411.

Scott, S. and Jackson, S. (2020) 'Sexuality', in G. Payne and E. Harrison (eds), *Social Divisions: Inequality and Diversity in Britain*. Bristol: Policy Press.

Scott, S., McDonnell, L. and Dawson, M. (2014) 'Asexual lives: social relationships and intimate encounters', *Discover Society*, Issue 9, 3 June. Online: https://discoversociety.org/2014/06/03/asexual-lives-social-relationships-and-intimate-encounters/

Seidman, S. (1997) *Difference Troubles: Queering Social Theory and Sexual Politics*. Cambridge: Cambridge University Press.

SUGGESTED FURTHER READING

- Parker, R.G., Aggleton, P. and Thomas, F. (eds) (2015) *Culture, Health and Sexuality: An Introduction*. London: Routledge.

This collection explores a range of topics relating to social and cultural aspects of sexuality and sexual health: sex and gender, sexual diversity, sex work, migration and sexual violence. It includes conceptual and empirical material and is global in its scope.

- Jackson, S. and Scott, S. (2010) *Theorizing Sexuality*. Maidenhead: Open University Press.

This book provides an overview of the field of sexuality and develops a feminist sociological position in evaluating debates and theories in relation to the wider development of modernity. It considers the biographical, interactional and institutional contexts of our sexual lives as well as examining the cultural meanings and everyday practices of sexuality.

- Kneale, D., Becares, L. and Weeks, H. (2020) 'How are LGBTQ+ people faring during the COVID-19 pandemic?' *Discover Society*: Covid-19 Chronicles, 7 May. Online: https://discoversociety.org/2020/05/07/how-are-lgbtq-people-faring-during-the-covid-19-pandemic/

This short article argues that the restrictions relating to the COVID-19 pandemic are likely to exacerbate existing health inequalities for LGBTQ+ people. While there is a paucity of research, what does exist suggests that LGBTQ+ individuals may have higher levels of chronic illness, which could lead to poorer outcomes for those infected with the virus.

- Mercer, C.H., Tanton, C., Prah, P. et al. (2013) 'Changes in sexual attitudes and lifestyles in Britain through the life course and over time: findings from the National Surveys of Sexual Attitudes and Lifestyles (Natsal)', *The Lancet*, 382 (9907): 1781–1794.

This article discusses the findings from the best available large-scale longitudinal overview relating to sexuality in Britain, providing useful background and context for reading more in-depth and specific studies. The survey does cover sexual health in relation to sexual orientation but there is still a lack of information about the wider health status of LGBQ individuals.

6

Intersectionality

Anuj Kapilashrami

Intersectionality is a lens and political tool to conceptualize and act on social inequalities. The concept and associated theorizing challenge the belief that we lead single-issue lives and have universal experiences of oppression and disadvantage.

Intersectionality has evolved as a set of theoretical positions that reject the idea that our social relations are experienced as separate phenomena and that people, their lives and struggles, can be reduced to one singular identity. Such a rejection makes visible important differences within population groups otherwise considered homogeneous, and the 'multiple positioning that constitutes everyday life and the power relations that are central to it' (Phoenix and Pattynama, 2006: 187). In short, intersectionality promotes an understanding that humans are shaped by the interaction of different identities or categories of difference (for example, 'race'/ethnicity, religion, gender, class, sexuality, disability among others) and the material and affective conditions associated with these.

The use of the term 'intersectionality' is traced back to the Black feminist critique of how feminist and anti-racist discourses served to marginalize and over-stabilize the lived realities of intersectional identities such as 'women of colour'. Although first coined by Crenshaw (1991), a critical race scholar and civil rights advocate, when articulating the need to examine the 'intersecting oppressions' of race and patriarchy, the concept has a longer and richer genealogy. Intersectional thinking and examining the relationship between social factors and modes of oppression have been a longstanding feature of various social justice struggles against heteronormative patriarchy, colonialism and slavery, dating back to 19th-century writings and activism in both the Global South and North (John, 2015). Contemporary thinking on intersectionality has since been informed by feminist attempts to locate 'difference' in marginalized women's struggles (for example, the *Dalit* women's movement in India in the 1970s), challenging orthodox understandings of gender and the essentialism in mainstream political movements. The aim is to reveal and confront sites and dynamics of power at the intersections of multiple structural positions, alongside hegemonic masculine power.

The distinctive contribution of intersectionality as a concept lies in two closely related core tenets. First, it makes clear that different social divisions interact in ways that are complex, mutually constituting and not merely additive. Thus, when examining the intersection of gender with race and class, an intersectional perspective sensitizes researchers to how gender performativity and relations are racialized (i.e. constituted differently along racial lines), and linked to the (trans)formations of social class in a globalized economy. In other words, the interaction of gender, race and class is greater than the sum of its parts. The second tenet is that these interactions occur in, and are mediated by, multiple sites and levels of power constituted by wider socio-political-economic processes (for example, of neoliberal globalization, imperialism, colonialism) and institutions such as laws/policies, state, market and religion. Intersectionality therefore demands analysis of inequalities to be embedded in the multiple levels of the social ecology – from individual factors to wider institutional and structural processes – that determine privilege and oppression.

Such analyses can produce a more nuanced understanding of the pathways and processes that influence the health and well-being of differently situated persons within and outside a social group. Yet, despite the rapidly expanding body of work on intersectionality, its application has not reached its full potential in health research and policy. This may be attributed to several factors, most notably the continued preoccupation within public health on studying 'disease' causation by examining individual-level risk factors narrowly defined in biological, genetic and behavioural terms, with limited attention paid to wider social determinants of health. Consequently, population-level health interventions informed by such evidence tend to rely on deficit and paternalistic models that blame vulnerable populations, and in the process increase inequalities. Second, health inequalities research and policy overwhelmingly focus on the social gradient in health, explained primarily by socio-economic differences. Such a focus obscures the influence of other categories of difference (for example, gender, ethnic/Indigenous/caste/minority status, disability, sexual orientation, immigrant status, rural residence) despite the mounting evidence of their association with morbidity and mortality (Baru et al., 2010; Sen and Östlin, 2008). Such neglect became evident in the early responses to the COVID-19 pandemic that continued to ignore the higher infection rates and mortality among minority ethnic groups in the USA and UK, or the excess burden on migrants and refugees. Research on other categories of difference has often advanced in silos, overlooking the interactional dynamics between these social divisions. A further dissonance arises from the positivist methodologies more commonly utilized in population health research, which are less aligned with an intersectional focus on generating situated and embodied knowledge. This problem is compounded by the absence of the sophistication necessary in quantitative research to go beyond measuring the unequal average distribution of health (or illness) between groups to analyse relational processes and structural dynamics of power (Wemrell et al., 2017). However, more recent efforts in *social* and *eco* epidemiology are promising in exploring ways to capture diversity in measures of health outcomes and social characteristics (Wemrell et al., 2017). These attempts complement the range of qualitative methodologies utilized to study the complexity of social location, power and their influence on health. Together, these developments increase intersectionality's appeal and, to some degree, its integration in population health studies to achieve more specificity in mapping health inequalities.

Intersectionality has travelled widely across diverse theories and praxis – feminist, Indigenous, *Dalit* feminist, Queer and postcolonial theories – offering a fertile ground for the concept to grow. In migrating across diverse geographical, institutional and epistemic sites, intersectionality has increased in scope and strength, and witnessed wider uptake to inform equity-related policy and practice. However, such extensions also generated critical dilemmas, broadly grouped under two main concerns related to its application and analytic scope. First, dangers are associated with its wide endorsement by agencies, such as the United Nations, and inconsistent usage. Arguably, attempts to mainstream intersectionality have not been accompanied by the necessary reforms of institutions that are inherently patriarchal, racist, predominantly White (or majoritarian), neo-colonial and oppressive. Scholars caution against a mere listing of differences that are often reduced to 'protected characteristics' or identities as it risks oversimplification and threatens the very political project intersectionality is intended to serve. Southern feminists add to this critique by drawing attention to the 'imperialism of categories', implicit in the intersectional analysis originating in the North, which disregards non-Western politics of identity and worldviews (Menon, 2015). Second, early writings questioned whether intersectionality is a 'theory of marginalized subjectivity' that reveals the production of difference and disadvantage among oppressed groups or a 'generalized theory of identity' (Nash, 2008: 10) relevant to all subject positions, including the relatively privileged (for example, White middle-class heterosexual woman). A focus on different social categories led to questions around which social divisions matter and whether all matter equally, often leading to competing claims about the relative importance of one group over the other and reifying individual differences.

The above critiques and questions have prompted a breadth of theoretical developments and attempts to define the analytical scope of intersectionality. Yuval-Davis (2006: 195) helpfully reminds us that rather than focusing on 'how many' or on the nature of interaction (additive, interlocking or mutually constitutive), the debate must concern 'conflation or separation of the different analytic levels in which intersectionality is located'. It is these levels that I now turn to before outlining various applications of intersectional analysis with reference to population health research, public health policy and programmes. My discussion refers to a time before and after the outbreak of the COVID-19 pandemic, with the latter energizing concerns about the unequal patterning of illness and, by extension, the necessity of intersectional analyses.

Several scholars have attempted to answer the question 'what intersections are under examination and at what levels do they operate?' Dhamoon and Hankivsky (2011) identify four kinds of interactions: identities of an individual or a social group, notably the oppressed (for example, transgender person); the social 'categories' of difference (race, gender, sexuality); the processes of production of differences (racialization, gendering); and the wider systems of domination (colonialism, racism, patriarchy). While much research has examined one or more of these, treating them as distinct, it is important to be reminded that inequalities are often produced and situated in the complex interactions between these multiple dimensions of social life comprising determinate structures and subjects.

McCall's (2005) work offers useful insights on this complexity and workings of 'categories' of analysis. She describes three delineations of intersectional analysis based on how they utilize analytical categories. The first approach, termed *anti-categorical*, rejects any form of categorization, emphasizing inherent fluidity of social categories and identity; the second, *intra-categorical*, focuses on differences within a social group; while the third, *inter-categorical*, examines linkages *between* the categories to document relationships of inequality (and their changing configurations) across social groups. All these iterations converge on three points: the need to move beyond categories to focus on social dynamics; recognition that social divisions not only constitute (inter)subjective experiences of in/exclusion, subordination and emancipation but are also (simultaneously) expressed at institutional and systemic levels; and the importance of analysing spatial–temporal contexts.

With regard to population health, an intersectional lens offers a wide range of applications – for collecting data, as a methodology and epistemological approach in research, and to inform public health policy and programmes. The research applications can be broadly grouped under three areas. First, there are studies that examine the distribution, access and uptake of healthcare services and the differences in material and affective conditions that result in inequalities in their provision and use. For example, in studying women's reproductive choices and contraceptive uptake in rural Tanzania, Carroll and Kapilashrami (2020) reveal the dynamic interactions between individual factors (age, marital status, rural residence) and the gender–power relations and social controls experienced within households and institutions that shape reproductive disadvantage among women. Besides similarities resulting from the shared experiences of poverty and geography, the authors also report differences among women. For example, they identify a greater risk of exclusion from public health services and reproductive entitlements among *Sukuma* and *Maasai* women, tracing these to their historic marginalization and displacement. A second set of studies examines the influence of social location on wider determinants (work, nutrition) and health risks (gender-based violence). The third group comprises explorations of self-reported or observed health outcomes. These studies include qualitative and quantitative (*inter-categorical*) assessments of conditions such as hypertension risks and ischemic heart diseases, among others (Wemrell et al., 2017).

Most intersectionality-informed research foregrounds experiences of minority groups, as in the focus on migrant women in Hanley et al.'s (2019) study of intersecting risks of health and homelessness in Canada. Another is Doyal's (2009) research on HIV-positive, Black African women and men who migrated to London – a study that examines subjectivities arising at the intersections of multiple marginal positions. Doyal reveals the distinctive experiences of stigma and discrimination associated with HIV amongst women (linked to the moral and social dimensions of motherhood), heterosexual men (linked to access to work, money and power), and gay and/or bisexual men (linked to sexual deviance). Sen and Iyer (2012) also alert us to the importance of studying the 'middle groups' in the gender and economic class spectrum (for example, non-poor women and poor men), exploring how they leverage class or gender in securing entitlements – in this case, treatment for chronic conditions in India.

While class, gender and race/ethnicity in the case of the USA and Europe have been the 'traditional triumvirate' of intersectional analysis, more recent studies have examined these along with sexual orientation, disability, immigrant status as well as other structural dynamics relating to homelessness and unemployment. An example of the latter is a Participatory Action Research study undertaken with multiple disadvantaged groups (identity based as well as those with shared experience of homelessness, migration and/or unemployment) in Scotland (Kapilashrami and Marsden, 2018). The study involved participants in identifying health-enabling resources and access barriers. While the authors found general consensus in the notion of 'healthful living' among differently situated population groups, variance emerged in the value placed on these resources and the material and affective conditions that shaped their ability to translate these into improved health.

The ongoing COVID-19 pandemic at the time of writing, and the social inequalities that it exposes and amplifies, creates a moral imperative for researchers, policy-makers and advocates to address the health needs and rights of those most affected. Urgent appeals from scholars to move 'beyond silos' in examining the risks and burden of the pandemic and the need for a radical new conception of our praxis on the road to recovery bring renewed attention to intersectionality (Hankivsky and Kapilashrami, 2020). Realizing the bold vision of 'build(ing) back fairer' (Marmot et al., 2020) will require adopting this lens to collect diverse data, undertake analyses to identify those most at risk, and design policies targeting intersectional disadvantages. An area particularly lacking is the empirical and discursive analysis of the formulation and implementation of health and social policies (including pandemic preparedness and recovery plans) utilizing an intersectional lens.

In summary, intersectionality has come to occupy an increasingly visible position in sociological analysis of difference and stratification. The multi-level analysis it promotes allows linking the micro-level experiential and intersubjective understandings of individuals and groups with social processes and systems that pattern health. In so doing, intersectional studies may produce useful understandings to inform structural level interventions, directing attention away from reductionist behavioural solutions that fail to address the fundamental causes of health inequalities. Such thinking enables us to move beyond mere descriptions of differences in distribution of resources to unpack the shared mechanisms of causality comprising the unequal power relations that underpin health. Intersectionality, as a key concept in medical sociology, offers scope for novel enquiry in and responses to health inequalities that are vital in these challenging times.

See also: Ethnicity; Gender; Health Professional Migration and Integration; Place; Sexuality; Social Class.

REFERENCES

Baru, R., Acharya, A., Acharya, S. et al. (2010) 'Inequities in access to health services in India: caste, class and region', *Economic and Political Weekly*, 45 (38): 49–58.

Carroll, A. and Kapilashrami, A. (2020) 'Barriers to uptake of reproductive information and contraceptives in rural Tanzania: an intersectionality informed qualitative enquiry', *BMJ Open*, 10 (10): e036600.

Crenshaw, K. (1991) 'Mapping the margins: intersectionality, identity politics, and violence against women of color', *Stanford Law Review*, 43 (6): 1241–1299.

Dhamoon, R.K. and Hankivsky, O. (2011) 'Why the theory and practice of intersectionality matter to health research and policy', in O. Hankivsky, S. de Leeuw, J. Lee et al. (eds), *Health Inequities in Canada: Intersectional Frameworks and Practices*. Vancouver and Toronto: UCB Press.

Doyal, L. (2009) 'Challenges in researching life with HIV/AIDS: an intersectional analysis of black African migrants in London', *Culture, Health & Sexuality*, 11 (2): 173–188.

Hankivsky, O. and Kapilashrami, A. (2020) 'Intersectionality offers a radical rethinking of Covid-19', *thebmjopinion*, 15 May. Online: https://blogs.bmj.com/bmj/2020/05/15/intersectionality-offers-a-radical-rethinking-of-covid-19/

Hanley, J., Ives, N., Lenet, J. et al. (2019) 'Migrant women's health and housing insecurity: an intersectional analysis', *International Journal of Migration, Health and Social Care*, 15 (1): 90–106.

John, M.E. (2015) 'Intersectionality: rejection or critical dialogue?' *Economic & Political Weekly*, 50 (33): 72–76.

Kapilashrami, A. and Marsden, S. (2018) 'Examining intersectional inequalities in access to health (enabling) resources in disadvantaged communities in Scotland: advancing the participatory paradigm', *International Journal for Equity in Health*, 17 (1): 1–14.

Marmot, M., Allen, J., Goldblatt, P. et al. (2020) *Build Back Fairer: The COVID-19 Marmot Review. The Pandemic, Socioeconomic and Health Inequalities in England*. London: Institute of Health Equity.

McCall, L. (2005) 'The complexity of intersectionality', *Signs: Journal of Women in Culture and Society*, 30 (3): 1771–1800.

Menon, N. (2015) 'Is feminism about "women"? A critical view on intersectionality from India', *Economic & Political Weekly*, 50 (17): 37–44.

Nash, J.C. (2008) 'Re-thinking intersectionality', *Feminist Review*, 89 (1): 1–15.

Phoenix, A. and Pattynama, P. (2006) 'Intersectionality', *European Journal of Women's Studies*, 13 (3): 187–192.

Sen, G. and Iyer, A. (2012) 'Who gains, who loses and how: leveraging gender and class intersections to secure health entitlements', *Social Science & Medicine*, 74 (11): 1802–1811.

Sen, G. and Östlin, P. (2008) 'Gender inequity in health: why it exists and how we can change it', *Global Public Health*, 3(S1): 1–12.

Wemrell, M., Mulinari, S. and Merlo, J. (2017) 'Intersectionality and risk for ischemic heart disease in Sweden: categorical and anti-categorical approaches', *Social Science & Medicine*, 177: 213–222.

Yuval-Davis, N. (2006) 'Intersectionality and feminist politics', *European Journal of Women's Studies*, 13 (3): 193–209.

SUGGESTED FURTHER READING

- Hankivsky, O. and Jordan-Zachery, J.S. (eds) (2019) *The Palgrave Handbook of Intersectionality in Public Policy*. Basingstoke: Palgrave Macmillan.

This edited volume addresses a gap in intersectionality research by highlighting key challenges, possibilities and critiques of intersectionality-informed approaches in improving public policy. It offers a global perspective across a range of geographical contexts and public policy issues, including: suicide prevention, education, mental healthcare, gender-based violence and equality policy. The volume demonstrates both the added value and 'how-to' of intersectionality-informed policy approaches that aim to advance equity and social justice.

- Kapilashrami, A., Hill, S. and Meer, N. (2015) 'What can health inequalities researchers learn from an intersectionality perspective? Understanding social dynamics with an inter-categorical approach', *Social Theory & Health*, 13 (3–4): 288–307.

Critiquing the overwhelming attention to socio-economic position (and other single axes of difference) in health inequalities research, the authors draw on scholarship and activism on race/ethnicity, gender and caste-based differences in health to make a case for the adoption of intersectionality theory. They argue for an inter-categorical conceptualization of social location that recognizes differentiation without reifying social groupings – thus encouraging researchers to focus on social dynamics rather than social categories.

- Heard, E., Fitzgerald, L., Wigginton, B. and Mutch, A. (2020) 'Applying intersectionality theory in health promotion research and practice', *Health Promotion International*, 35 (4): 866–876.

This article provides an overview of the diverse applications of intersectionality theory in public health. The authors discuss specific examples of intersectionality as a methodological and epistemological approach and as a tool for action and intervention, calling for wider uptake of this theory among health promotion researchers and practitioners.

- Gkiouleka, A., Huijts, T., Beckfield, J. and Bambra, C. (2018) 'Understanding the micro and macro politics of health: inequalities, intersectionality & institutions – a research agenda', *Social Science & Medicine*, 200: 92–98.

The paper posits an analytical framework that integrates intersectionality with institutional approaches to studying health inequalities. It also discusses methodological implications of considering the interplay between individuals and institutions, arguing that quantitative designs can incorporate an intersectional institutional approach.

7

Place

Katherine L. Frohlich, Julie Vallée,
Sally Macintyre and Anne Ellaway

Place refers to a socially significant or socially constructed location in geographical space.

While place has arguably received most attention within disciplines such as geography, both geographers and sociologists have explored the relevance of place in our understanding of health variation and inequality. Place constitutes, as well as contains, social relations and physical resources (Cummins et al., 2007). While there is no single definition within medical geography, geographers have tended to define place as being a socio-cultural location, with space being a natural and physical construct relating to geometric location. According to Gesler, 'place is studied with an eye to its meanings for people; space is analyzed in terms of its quantifiable attributes and patterns' or, in other words, place is 'a space filled with people acting out their lives' (quoted in Kearns and Joseph, 1993: 712). In the recent past, there has been a tendency to focus nearly exclusively on place of residence in much of place and health research. We will expand this focus to include more contemporary and relational notions of place, shifting the emphasis to nodes in networks, rather than discrete and autonomous bounded spatial units. Relational theories posit that places are produced and maintained by the activities of 'actors', proximate or distal to a particular place, who operate individually or in concert across a wide range of geographical scales (Conradson, 2005; Cummins et al., 2007). After elucidating the historical background of the idea of place and health, and pointing out the concerns of disciplines such as epidemiology and geography, we highlight the current relevance of the concept of 'place' in medical sociology with reference to some recent research.

An early text on the influence of place on health was *Airs, Waters, Places* in the Hippocratic Corpus from the fifth century BC. The three elements in the title refer to features of climate and topography, believed to influence the prevalence and types of disease found in different places. In Britain, social regularities in death rates were first studied systematically in the 17th century by John Graunt, whose 'Natural and political observations upon the Bills of Mortality' was published in 1662. Graunt was interested not only in the direct effects of the environment on physical health, but also in its effects on mental health and human behaviour. During the early 19th century, contagionist and anti-contagionist explanations of disease causes opposed one another, while variations of miasma theory still predominated. According to that theory, geographic health disparities were due to topographical factors such as differences in altitude and climate. A pioneer in the sociology and geography of health, the French doctor Louis-René Villermé (1782–1863) adhered to anti-contagionist explanations of disease causation and demonstrated the association between poverty and mortality by studying the variations of mortality rates across the city of Paris. Villermé famously demonstrated that death rates in 12 arrondissements varied by population density and income. The impact of industrialization in the 19th century generated a considerable amount of interest in the social and geographical patterning of disease in the UK, Germany and the USA. In Britain, for example, William Farr examined the social patterns of mortality by comparing the death rates of different localities. He drew up life tables for 'healthy districts' which could be compared and served as a basis for inferring that much premature mortality was due to environmental conditions and therefore preventable. Friedrich Engels' work on the conditions of the working class in England was undertaken in the spirit of scientific discovery, social justice and reform, as was Rudolf Virchow's work on typhus in Upper Silesia during this same period.

Since this time, the respective influence of people and place on health is often called into question. An increased emphasis on the role of individualism in studying the relationship between people and health emerged after the second half of the 20th century. This followed on the heels of the epidemiological transition (the replacement of infectious diseases by chronic diseases due to improved hygiene, healthcare and disease prevention), and the consecutive focus on chronic diseases and individual lifestyle choices (particularly the 'big four' of smoking, drinking alcohol, diet and exercise). Emphasis on people also expanded in the political realm: priority groups, such as the poor, migrants, and others, defined as 'high risk' subpopulations, also became the target of national health policies around this time. This increased focus on people, however, detracted attention away from a more structural and collective understanding of the conditions that shape health outcomes. Concomitantly, place, particularly in the form of local areas, neighbourhoods and Healthy Cities, gained importance, for example in the Ottawa Charter for Health Promotion (WHO, 1986). In this context, the creation of 'supportive environments' (referring to settings where people live, learn, work and play) was identified as one of the five key action areas of health promotion.

This focus on local areas resulted from two rationales: places merit exploration because they either concentrate people affected by health problems (e.g.

spatial segregation) or because they are themselves involved in the production of health problems (e.g. neighbourhood effects). These two rationales echo two former competing hypotheses about the relative importance of 'breeder' and 'drift' communities. The 'drift' hypothesis suggests that ill individuals gravitate towards specific areas while the 'breeder' hypothesis suggests that such areas generate illness in their residents. These two rationales also echo the introduction of multi-level (i.e. mixed effect regression) models into health and place research in the 1990s. This methodological formalism led to a significant amount of empirical research seeking to separate out the effects of neighbourhood contexts from the background characteristics of residents – otherwise known as context vs. composition.

A compositional explanation for area differences in health involves analysing the role of individual characteristics of residents in a particular area (e.g. the collective age, sex or socio-economic status of people living in a neighbourhood). A contextual explanation of area differences in health, on the other hand, involves analysing the role of the characteristics of an area (such as access to amenities and facilities to support a healthy life), over and above those of the individual residents (Bernard et al., 2007; Diez-Roux, 2001; Macintyre and Ellaway, 2003; Riva et al., 2007). Place effects, however, often continued to be treated as a black box of people–place interactions. The frequent use of ecological indices to measure material advantage or disadvantage in residential areas (famously through deprivation indices based on postal or census geography) is a case in point. In research using these ecological indices, it remains unclear if they are used as proxies for neighbourhood social structures shaping health status and behaviours, or as proxies for individual social profiles. The latter case involves the ecological fallacy – the inference of individual-level relationships from associations observed at the aggregate level. A number of influential sociological papers in the 1950s (e.g. Robinson, 1950) warned that the ecological fallacy could lead to entirely incorrect inferences being made because ecological and individual correlations between the same variables can differ markedly, even in different directions.

Competing interests between individual and place explanations of health lead to a false dualism about the respective importance of context and composition (and of breeder and drift hypotheses), thus failing to recognize that they may mutually reinforce each other. In his book *The Truly Disadvantaged*, Wilson (1987) brought attention to the fact that individual poverty matters more strongly in neighbourhoods where the population is overwhelmingly socially disadvantaged. Introducing the notion of 'concentration effects', he suggested that disadvantaged people often deal with a double burden: they must grapple with the multiple problems arising from their own lack of income as well as the social effects of living in a disenfranchised neighbourhood. The idea of concentration effects has developed in more recent health and place research by considering the reciprocal relationship between people and place.

Recent advances in relational theory help us understand this reciprocal relationship by viewing places as dynamic ecosystems. The relational approach to place views places and the resources they provide as shaped by political powers, social networks, regulation by various actors, and local interactions with people (Cummins et al., 2007). A relational conception of place allows us to concentrate on the processes and interactions occurring between people, places and their health over time. Fostering a relational perspective requires a reassessment of existing articulations of location and scale typically used in the study of health and place in the past. Relational geography rejects the structure–agency dichotomy, for instance. Additionally, these theories posit that populations engage in important place-to-place mobility on a daily basis, as well as over the lifecourse. This implies that individuals often influence, and are influenced by, conditions in multiple spatial locations over multiple time scales: over the years – the 'life course of place' (Pearce, 2015) – as well as over 24-hour periods – the 'daycourse of place' (Vallée, 2017). Places are contemplated from a non-Euclidean perspective where place boundaries are fluid and distances are relative. Relational theories have thus moved beyond their former focus on neighbourhood effects on health.

Recent empirical examples of relational place considerations involve the exploration of people's experience of place. The concept of 'activity spaces' – understood as the multiple settings where people study, work, or otherwise spend time in the course of their daily activities – has been introduced to gain insight into the role of daily mobility in place exposure and in the production of (social) health inequalities (Shareck et al., 2014). An alternative relational consideration of place involves the exploration of neighbourhood experiences. Empirically, this can involve asking people to draw and discuss their own self-defined neighbourhood, for instance. By allowing people to self-define their neighbourhoods, information can be gathered about past and future spatial behaviours in relation to health; they capture an individual's effective past access as well as potential future access to neighbourhood resources (Vallée et al., 2020).

The COVID-19 pandemic has brought to the fore the inequitable effects of activity spaces and neighbourhood conditions on exposure to the virus. For more privileged people, easy access to parks, other green spaces, summer homes and areas where one could safely visit and do exercise with minimum exposure to other people has led to lesser exposure to the virus. For those less privileged, the experience of crowded housing and neighbourhoods, the need to use public transport to go to work, and the type of work required during the pandemic has put them at a higher risk of contracting COVID-19, leading to important inequities in both who contracted and died from the disease.

Whereas sociologists conducted many of the early health-related community studies, sociology and sociological theory have been less apparent in the recent literature on the role of place and health, dominated largely by epidemiologists and medical geographers. Yet relational theory, and other relevant theories of pertinence to sociology, such as phenomenology, post-humanism, and others, could be of great utility in helping us better understand how place shapes the distribution and experience of health and illness. Future work in medical sociology, we would argue, should therefore pay heed to its classic heritage and not leave the concept of 'place' solely to other disciplines.

See also: Environment; Material and Cultural Factors; Psychosocial Factors; Social Class.

REFERENCES

Bernard, P., Charafeddine, R., Frohlich, K.L. et al. (2007) 'Health inequalities and place: a theoretical conception of neighbourhood', *Social Science & Medicine*, 65 (9): 1839–1852.

Conradson, D. (2005) 'Landscape, care and the relational self: therapeutic encounters in rural England', *Health & Place*, 11 (4): 337–348.

Cummins, S., Curtis, S., Diez-Roux, A.V. and Macintyre, S. (2007) 'Understanding and representing "place" in health research: a relational approach', *Social Science & Medicine*, 65 (9): 1825–1838.

Diez-Roux, A. (2001) 'Investigating neighborhood and area effects on health', *American Journal of Public Health*, 91 (11): 1783–1789.

Kearns, R.A. and Joseph, A.E. (1993) 'Space in its place: developing the link in medical geography', *Social Science & Medicine*, 37 (6): 711–717.

Macintyre, S. and Ellaway, A. (2003) 'Neighborhoods and health: an overview', in I. Kawachi and L.F. Berkman (eds), *Neighborhoods and Health*. Oxford: Oxford University Press.

Pearce, J. (2015) 'Invited commentary: history of place, life course, and health inequalities-historical geographic information systems and epidemiologic research', *American Journal of Epidemiology*, 181 (1): 26–29.

Riva, M., Gauvin, L. and Barnett, T.A. (2007) 'Toward the next generation of research into small area effects on health: a synthesis of multilevel investigations published since July 1998', *Journal of Epidemiology & Community Health*, 61 (10): 853–861.

Robinson, W.S. (1950) 'Ecological correlations and the behavior of individuals', *American Sociological Review*, 15 (3): 351–357.

Shareck, M., Frohlich, K. and Kestens, Y. (2014) 'Considering daily mobility for a more comprehensive understanding of contextual effects on social inequalities in health: a conceptual proposal', *Health & Place*, 29: 154–60.

Vallée, J. (2017) 'The daycourse of place', *Social Science & Medicine*, 194: 177–181.

Vallée, J., Shareck, M., Le Roux, G. et al. (2020) 'Is accessibility in the eye of the beholder? Social inequalities in spatial accessibility to health-related resources in Montréal, Canada', *Social Science & Medicine*, 245: 112702.

WHO (1986) *The Ottawa Charter for Health Promotion*. Online: www.euro.who.int/__data/assets/pdf_file/0004/129532/Ottawa_Charter.pdf

Wilson, W.J. (1987) *The Truly Disadvantaged: The Inner City, the Underclass, and Public Policy*. Chicago: University of Chicago Press.

SUGGESTED FURTHER READING

- Kawachi, I. and Berkman, L.F. (eds) (2003) *Neighborhoods and Health.* Oxford: Oxford University Press.

This book brings together a wide range of theoretical, methodological and empirical research not only from the fields of public health and epidemiology, but also from sociology, psychology and social policy. It illustrates the prominence of the ongoing 'context' versus 'composition' debate and is a reference textbook for many scholars involved in neighbourhood-level research.

- Moon, G. and Pearce J. (2020) 'Twenty-five years of *Health & Place*: citation classics, internationalism and interdisciplinarity', *Health & Place*, 61: 102202.

This article discusses some of the key articles and themes from *Health & Place* over the last 25 years of its existence. This interdisciplinary journal offers comparative perspectives on the difference that place makes to the incidence of ill-health, the structuring of health-related behaviour, the provision and use of health services, and the development of health policy.

8

Environment

Sara MacBride-Stewart

In health terms, the environment is two things: it is where people live, work and recreate; and it is nature, the 'wild' or the biophysical. Human health is a consequence of these societal–biophysical interactions; the result of the influence of the natural environment on how we live, and the influence that humans have on the natural environment.

The concept of the environment is used in different ways by different disciplines. Natural scientists define it in biophysical terms, as the context that sustains life. Social scientists treat it as the social context for human action (Fox and Alldred, 2018). Health scientists regard the environment as a source of human harm, describing it either as the socio-cultural, economic and institutional context responsible for human disease and illness, or the physical, chemical (abiotic) or living, biological (biotic) and biophysical environment that exists as a resource for human life, a habitat for survival and the repository for waste. A biophysical understanding suggests human health rests in the physical, natural, nonhuman world, which is mediated through human senses, emotions and bodies. It is the socio-cultural environment that is of key concern for medical sociologists, as a passive background for health, and the context for social action that shapes the social causes of disease and illness, and their inequalities.

When conceived as a passive background, the natural and social environment can be a source of harm to human health (Gislason, 2013). Social scientists ensure that the external context (what is outside humans and human action) is recognized as much as a contributor to illness and health as human physiology (or the internal context). In the literature on the hazards and benefits to human health, attention is given to short-term externalities (for example, flooding or an hour spent in nature) as well as longer-term changes to the natural environment, such as climate change, deforestation and urbanization (Gislason, 2013).

As the context for social action, attention is given to the social, cultural and economic environment, described as the places in which people live, work and socialize. The environment here is a social system or process that can shape human action and identities, and that can be harmful or beneficial to human health (as shared values and collective consciousness). The attention given to social structures and institutions can be used to understand the divisions that are created between people or groups, or more fundamental divisions between the social and the natural world (Gislason, 2013). The capacity of humans to affect and shape the biophysical and social environment, on which they depend for health, is explained through the social and constructed nature of human health. While natural processes can also affect the social context, additional effort is needed to recognize the role of the natural environment in shaping health (rather than being determined by these institutions).

When the natural environment is taken into account, there is evidence that improvements in life expectancy (mortality) and years lived in poor health (morbidity) are worsening as a direct result of climate change (increased global temperatures due to fossil fuel consumption) and land use change (Franchini and Mannucci, 2015). Research into the causes of severely infectious diseases like COVID-19, SARS and Ebola suggest that human activity has impacted on the natural world (deforestation, transportation), thereby escalating the likelihood of their emergence and spread (United Nations Framework Convention on Climate Change [UNFCCC], 2017). To understand how to sustain levels of health, researchers are encouraged to build an awareness of humans' impact on the environment. This awareness includes understanding: (1) threats to human health, (2) improvements that enhance human health, (3) threats to natural resources used to improve health or deliver healthcare, and (4) health inequalities caused by uneven environmental impacts of human activity.

Before moving forwards, it is worth noting how medical sociologists understand the role of the social determinants model of health. A substantial body of evidence shows how the distribution of money, power and resources is largely responsible for health inequalities at local, national and global levels (Bradby, 2012). By drawing on perspectives and ideas from epidemiology, medical sociology almost exclusively regards social and economic factors as key to the conditions under which environmental decline is experienced and contributes to disease. This model remains focused on (and may be becoming outdated in this respect) the social context and all its norms, institutions and inequalities that shape the relationship to the natural environment (Bradby, 2012). For medical sociologists, the social environment is a wide set of structures and processes that largely sit outside medicine, like access to transport, housing or education, on which health depends. While more critical approaches distance themselves from the broader and historical traditions of (medical) sociology, particularly those associated with (Parsonian) functionalism and symbolic interactionism, it is this social environment, the successful functioning of society and its norms, that dominates discussions about what contributes to human health.

Ecological models (also called 'eco-social' and 'socio-ecological') have prompted a conceptual shift in the social determinants literature. They address the gap in understanding how disturbances in the natural world, i.e. pollution, declines in biodiversity or flooding, affect human and planetary health. Using both linear (eco-social) and dynamic and multi-layered (socio-ecological) approaches for understanding the 'causes' of disease, these models propose that the natural environment (its biodiversity, degradation and management systems), along with inequalities in access, use and provision of it, is a contributor to illness (McLaren and Hawe, 2005). Alternately, health or an 'adaptive capacity' to respond to environmental change is also possible (see Rayner and Lang, 2012, for a discussion). The socio-ecological health approach has been widely taken up in health policy; for example, the World Health Organization (WHO) includes urbanization and effects on living conditions as one of nine overarching social determinants integral to health and well-being (Hordyk et al., 2015). Socio-ecological health models also consider how globalization and consumption processes at the global level are consequential for and are shaped by local behaviours and actions, and vice versa (McLaren and Hawe, 2005).

Notably, questions about the wider ecological processes that govern humans (for example, seasons, pollination of food crops), and the capacity of nonhuman animals, plants or processes (i.e. earthquakes) to have independent actions that can affect human health, have largely been left to earth scientists and biologists. Environmental sociology draws attention to a conceptual 'turn to nature', recognizing that social factors alone cannot explain the intricate relationships between the natural environment and human health. While the devastating impacts of human activity warrant further study, so too do efforts showing how mutually beneficial ecological–social relationships can improve health (see suggested read: Kimmerer, 2013). Core ideas converge here, to regard health as embedded in socio-ecological processes that reflect interrelationships between the natural environment and its ecological, social and economic dimensions (McLaren and Hawe, 2005).

The problem with social determinants and ecological approaches becomes apparent when considering environmental injustice (Pellow and Brehm, 2013). Critical development studies assume that environmental conditions are a matter of poor (economic but also social) development, but that development that includes the use of natural resources will improve health outcomes. This claim is supported by research findings that link global development to improvements in population health. Yet missing from the analysis is how improvements in access, use and autonomy over the natural environment can also have negative health outcomes, particularly evident when considering the deleterious effects of consumption (of natural resources) by the Global North on the South. This gap in the social determinants model struggles to explain how chronic, infectious diseases and mortality rates, along with health issues resulting from severe events (for example, flooding, storms), are increasing for some people and places but not others. While medical sociology may have been slow to grasp how human activities (deforestation, land use change, burning of fossil fuels) have shaped this new 'epidemiological transition', it is possible that the global COVID-19 pandemic might lead to new perspectives on health and environmental inequalities from a social sciences lens.

The 'turn to nature' signals a new set of interdisciplinary relationships that are needed to understand the scope of the environment–health relationship. Geographical, evolutionary and psychological approaches can help address shared concerns about for whom in society, how and under what conditions the natural environment benefits human health. This contemporary concern about the environment–health relationship includes asking what new understandings of existing sociological concepts and approaches are needed, such as expanding social determinants to include environmental capital as well as social capital, or including environmental policies in the analysis of health policy. It may also involve socio-ecological analysis of existing psychological and environmental concepts and theories, *so that they are viewed critically through a sociological lens* (see also Maller et al., 2008). Attention could be directed here at concepts such as 'resilience' and 'restoration' (relating to the capacity of individuals and nature to manage environmental change), 'biophilia' (the innate, evolutionary affiliation to natural environments) as well as 'stress reduction theory' (the physiological impact of nature contact).

Within medical sociology, references to nature and the environment, present in the work of its early contributors, are only now being rediscovered. As already explained, attention to the natural environment has encouraged thinking more broadly about the influences (social and natural) that contribute to health. For Foucauldian medical sociologists (with their interest in how knowledge is produced and shapes our understandings), the re-emergence of the natural environment may be an expression of the politics that currently shape our health and healthcare services (Bradby, 2012). The value of the natural environment for health, for example, has re-emerged in popular discourse and academic research (Maller et al., 2008) at a crucial moment for society where health systems worldwide are subject to chronic under-resourcing (or profiteering). The natural environment has come to represent a potential alternative for preventing ill-health as the discourse of environmental benefit and threat has become visible with the declaration of a 'climate emergency'. Understanding the discourses of health, and the role of medicine, in the context of this combined health and environmental crisis may be needed now, more than ever.

In medical sociology thinkers in the new materialism camp have cautioned against only focusing on health discourses (Fox and Alldred, 2018). They argue that in a new era of environmental politics, social constructionist accounts struggle to address our material experience of the world outside of these health discourses. For new materialists, the concept of the environment must be revised to include the importance that material and other nonhuman (or ecological) processes have on human health. By integrating human and nonhuman aspects, they argue that medical sociologists would be better placed to consider how existing human relationships to nature impact on society and the natural environment. They propose that a radical ontology is needed, one that addresses the tendency to separate human (cultural) processes from natural ones, and that avoids discussing the natural environment (or indeed any physical entity) as an object. Health, human bodies and health systems are instead conceived of as processes that gain meaning around specific events and people (MacBride-Stewart, 2019). Drawing together human and nonhuman processes, new materialism aims to breakdown distinctions, seeing health and medicine relationally via a focus on patterns of connections between them. In this approach health is never an outcome; rather, it is a process, intimately tied up in associations and relationships that regard environments not as states but as capacities for action. Ecological health therefore is one which starts from the idea that environments and bodies are entangled. In their contribution to the debate over the privileging of human action over nature's agency, new materialist sociologies have argued that human and nonhuman health has the potential to be expressed in different, possibly as-yet-unknown, ways.

To conclude, the concept of the environment in medical sociology has long been considered as the background or context in which health and disease emerge. However, an interdisciplinary and relational understanding of the environment has contributed new perspectives to explain how intersecting societal–biophysical processes contribute to both human and planetary (including nonhumans') health. Medical sociology is adapting its conceptual tools and understanding to grasp these new ideas. Certainly COVID-19 provides an important route for medical sociologists to contribute their insights and learning about the existing societal–biophysical conditions that precipitated and accelerated a global pandemic. Questions remain about the role for medical sociology in reducing human impacts on the environment for human and planetary health, but new materialist thinking seems to offer a promising way forward for bringing the natural world into closer focus.

See also: Material and Cultural Factors; Place.

REFERENCES

Bradby, H. (2012) *Medicine, Health and Society.* London: SAGE.
Fox, N.J. and Alldred, P. (2018) *Sociology and the New Materialism: Theory, Research, Action.* London: SAGE.
Franchini, M. and Mannucci, P.M. (2015) 'Impact on human health of climate changes', *European Journal of Internal Medicine*, 26 (1): 1–5.
Gislason, M.K. (2013) *Ecological Health: Society, Ecology and Health.* Bingley: Emerald Group Publishing.
Hordyk, S.R., Hanley, J. and Richard, É. (2015) '"Nature is there; it's free": urban greenspace and the social determinants of health of immigrant families', *Health & Place*, 34: 74–82.

Maller, C., Townsend, M., Leger, L. et al. (2008) *Healthy Parks, Healthy People: The Health Benefits of Contact with Nature in a Park Context – A Review of Relevant Literature*, 2nd edn. Deakin University and Parks Victoria, Melbourne, Australia. Online: www.deakin.edu.au/__data/assets/pdf_file/0016/310750/HPHP-2nd-Edition.pdf

MacBride-Stewart, S. (2019) 'Atmospheres, landscapes and nature: off-road runners' experiences of well-being', *Health*, 23 (2): 139–157.

McLaren, L. and Hawe, P. (2005) 'Ecological perspectives in health research', *Journal of Epidemiology & Community Health*, 59 (1): 6–14.

Pellow, D.N. and Brehm, H.N. (2013) 'An environmental sociology for the twenty-first century', *Annual Review of Sociology*, 39: 229–250.

Rayner, G. and Lang, T. (2012) *Ecological Public Health: Reshaping the Conditions for Good Health*. Oxon: Routledge.

UNFCCC (2017) Climate change impacts human health. *United Nations Framework Convention on Climate Change*. Online: https://unfccc.int/news/climate-change-impacts-human-health

SUGGESTED FURTHER READING

- Barry, J. (2007) *Environment and Social Theory*, 2nd edn. London: Routledge.

Part of the 'Routledge Introductions to Environment Series', this book provides an in-depth account of how social theory has understood 'nature' and 'the environment'. Earlier chapters address the historical management of these ideas while later chapters address concepts of risk and risk society. This book is essential reading for students seeking to understand the contested concept of the environment and nature in social theory.

- Kimmerer, R.W. (2013) *Braiding Sweetgrass: Indigenous Wisdom, Scientific Knowledge and the Teaching of Plants*. London: Penguin Random House.

This book combines attentiveness to nature, cultural knowledges and ways of doing things, with botany and natural history. Sociological concepts like 'gift', 'community', 'family and kin' are used to bring both scientific knowledge and the natural world to life. Kimmerer interweaves the social and natural sciences, showing the possibilities of an integrated approach.

- Marsden, T. (ed.) (2019) *The SAGE Handbook of Nature*. London: SAGE.

This four-volume anthology includes important background reading for students. Specific sections and chapters on the environment include: Part Two: Natural and socio-natural vulnerabilities: interweaving the natural and social sciences (see Larner) and Part Eleven: Biosensitivity – an integrative approach to the health of people and planetary systems (see Capon).

- Nading, A.M. (2014) *Mosquito Trails: Ecology, Health and the Politics of Entanglement*. Berkeley: University of California Press.

This is an excellent critical ethnological study of a disease – Dengue Fever – which is one of the world's most prevalent mosquito-borne illnesses. Nading blends medical anthropology, political ecology and science and technology studies in an innovative analysis of local environments, global disease, people and mosquitos. It is a must-read for any student wanting to know what the field of socio-ecology and environmental health looks like, or should look like.

9

Material and Cultural Factors

Graham Scambler

> *Material factors refer to those natural or social structures that can have a causal bearing on population and individual health and longevity, while cultural factors denote the 'frames' in terms of which groups and individuals make sense of their lives and take decisions that can similarly impact on their own and the population's health.*

It is important to recognize this distinction between material and cultural factors when considering the social patterning of health. This is because despite the strong interrelations between them they can and do influence each other, making it crucial that they are distinguishable in theory and in empirical research. It has been rightly noted that once clearly distinguishable material factors, invoked by structural concepts of social class for example, have become progressively blurred in the face of a growing salience of cultural factors. This is reflected in the studies of class conducted by Savage (2015) and manifest in the Great British Class Survey that was their popular progeny. But while it is true that people's identities, their sense of self and of what is and ought to be the case, no longer straightforwardly reflect their class position, class as a structural factor cannot be reduced to culture and identity. To reiterate, material factors, rooted in structure, must be distinguished from cultural factors if their interrelations and contributions to the patterning of health are to be properly assessed.

The publication of the Black Report (DHSS, 1980) marked a turning point in the understanding of health inequalities in the UK and beyond. Black and his colleagues ranked material factors as of primary importance for explaining health inequalities, with cultural factors (giving rise to individual 'risk behaviour') in second place. In short, the Black Report allotted a higher priority to the 'hard' material underpinnings to people's lives – for example, their incomes, housing and quality of neighbourhood spaces – than to 'soft' culturally-informed healthy versus unhealthy lifestyles. This hard/soft division has political overtones. Through the 1980s and beyond, the UK, the USA and most other 'developed' societies have been characterized by party political divisions between a social democratic or left-of-centre focus on hard material factors and, increasingly, a neoliberal or right-of-centre focus on soft cultural factors. The underlying logics are unambiguous. Political parties presenting as social democratic/left-of-centre express a commitment to 'collectivist' government interventions targeting material redistribution, while those espousing a neoliberal/right-of-centre programme advocate a philosophy of 'individualism' predisposed to allow individuals to assume personal responsibility for their health-related behaviours. The French philosopher/sociologist Michel Foucault has deployed the terms 'technologies of the self' and 'governmentality' to suggest that people have come to internalize the idea that they are personally responsible for their health status, with the consequence that they now police their own health-related behaviours. This, he concludes, represents a new form of governance (Foucault, 1988).

The material/cultural distinction might retain an analytic value, as well as exposing differences in political ideology, but it has an increasing number of critics. Health inequalities research since the Black Report has shown that if people's everyday circumstances, lives and health behaviours are examined in detail, no hard and fast line can be drawn between the causal influence of material versus cultural factors. Individual decisions to smoke, purchase cheap 'fast foods', adopt sedentary lifestyles, consume alcohol and drugs and so on, have a lot to do with people's differential access to material resources, both in the present and in the futures they can anticipate for themselves and their families. Smoking can seem a relatively cheap and reasonable way of handling stress and *getting by* if you are a single mum with three children under the age of five trying to live on Universal Credit in the post-welfare state era (Marmot et al., 2020).

It does not follow from this that cultural factors reduce to material factors. Culture is pervasive and its values and norms inevitably frame and underpin day-to-day preventive health behaviour, illness behaviour and sick role behaviour among individuals as well as at the societal level of healthcare systems. Quah (2010) makes three important points about the study of culture in health and illness. First, she emphasizes the need to recognize culture as an independent phenomenon, if not an entirely autonomous one (for example, while it is affected by material factors it cannot be reduced to them). Second, she rightly insists that there is significant intra- as well as inter-cultural variation, and that this extends to healthcare systems. Many systems lack internal consistency, with the different subgroups – for example, doctors, nurses and managers – having different perspectives and interpretations of its values and principles and how they might be optimally implemented (i.e. possessing their own distinctive subcultures). This point has special relevance to the changes made to the National Health Service (NHS) following the Health and Social Care Act of 2012, which encourages the growth of provision from private providers in England. Quah refers, third, to what she calls 'pragmatic acculturation', by which she means borrowing from other cultures and subcultures to solve specific practical problems. This is found across all aspects of behaviour around health and illness. It has particular resonance in the context of the COVID-19 pandemic, where expertise in China, where the outbreak emerged, is informing action across many other countries.

Culture is generally taken to refer to a reasonably coherent set of beliefs, values, attitudes and habits or behavioural dispositions. Any given society might have a distinctive cultural 'profile', but each also has a set of overlapping subcultures: an Afro-American or Afro-Caribbean teenager from a household with no family members having been in employment for several years might have remarkably little in common with the son or daughter of a white lawyer or doctor. To recognize this is not to lend credence to cultural 'stereotypes'. Stereotypes – for instance, associating (material and) cultural disadvantage or impoverishment with risk behaviours for health – invariably embody errors of omission or commission; and they also of course gloss over exceptions. Teenagers from disadvantaged or impoverished households do become lawyers and doctors, even if this is statistically exceptional. It is one thing to uncover statistical trends and quite another, and more complex, matter to provide sociological explanations for what is going on, and why.

Sociologists have often had a primary focus on material factors, while anthropologists, by contrast, have written mostly about culture. In recent years, however, much of the socio-epidemiological and sociological literature on health inequalities has asserted the existence and significance of culture-based 'psychosocial pathways'. The notion of 'social capital' popularized by Putnam (2000), which refers to the positive, health-bestowing effects of people's supportive networks of family, kin, friends, neighbours and acquaintances, has often been cited in this context. Wilkinson (1996) triggered a series of studies by contending that material and cultural factors combine to promote health inequalities and, in so doing, he extended Durkheim's classic argument about the social genesis of suicide to disease and death more generally, focusing on what makes *societies* rather than *individuals* healthier. His contention was that high-income inequality leads to social fragmentation and dislocation and a breakdown of reciprocity and trust in people's dealings with each other, and thenceforth to differential rates of morbidity and mortality (as well as to many other social pathologies; see Wilkinson and Pickett, 2009).

Such matters cannot be divorced from biology and psychology. Some commentators claim that prolonged stress due to psychosocial factors results in an increase in allostatic load: if too many negative changes occur too rapidly, bodily adjustment is compromised, resulting in overload and exhaustion (McEwen, 1998; Saxbe et al., 2020). An inconsiderate manager would be harder to accommodate in an office or workplace that was too hot, cold or noisy, or when a worker had been on an inadequate diet. There is in this literature prima facie evidence for an association between material factors and allostatic load. In such complex ways are material, cultural and psychosocial factors intertwined.

Scambler (2018) has sought to avoid choosing between material and cultural factors by proposing a notion of 'asset flows'. He suggests that adopting this approach allows (1) for both material and cultural factors to influence a person's life chances and prospects for health and longevity; and (2) for their relative contributions to vary over time. He lists six asset flows, as follows:

- biological (positive/negative 'body capital');
- psychological (resilient/vulnerable);
- social (networked/isolated);
- cultural ('high' insider/'low' outsider positioning);
- spatial (depressed/affluent neighbourhoods);
- material (high-income/low-income household).

This conceptualization acknowledges not only variation over time (for example, an unexpected redundancy due to COVID-19 can drastically reduce household income), but also for compensation between flows: a weak flow of spatial assets might be compensated for by a strong flow of psychological or social assets.

It is clear then that material and cultural factors both influence health and longevity. It is not a question of 'either/or'. Wilkinson and Marmot (2003) put this well when they insist that the effects of both material and cultural factors extend to most diseases and causes of death. Disadvantage, they state, has many forms and can be absolute or relative. It can take the form of possessing a paucity of family assets, poor schooling during adolescence, insecure employment, being stuck in a dead-end job, bringing up a family in inauspicious circumstances or surviving on an inadequate pension. They add that these disadvantages tend to concentrate among the same people and that their effects accumulate over the lifecourse. The longer people live in stressful material and psychosocial environments, the more pronounced the physiological wear and tear and the less likely they are to experience a healthy old age.

The work of social theorists like Bourdieu (1977) is relevant at this point. It is apparent that material and cultural factors pertinent for health involve ideas of structure and agency. Bourdieu's notion of *habitus* was initially formulated and applied in relation to social class. He argued that a structural, class-based habitus can be discerned empirically from people's everyday orientations and decision-making. Their day-to-day lives bear witness to sets of behavioural dispositions to see things and to act in certain ways. Whether they are aware of it or not, their agency, or ability to 'decide for themselves', is socially structured (though not structurally determined). In this way, it can be maintained, people's health behaviours can only be comprehensively explained if full account is taken of their social positioning (for Bourdieu, principally their class location).

If agency is structured in this way, it can only be exercised in the cultural contexts in which people find themselves. Cultures and subcultures provide recipes and scripts for action. The 'choices' that people make, as well as the 'symbolic' resources available to make them – comprising those pre-established cultural beliefs, values and attitudes they absorb as if by osmosis during socialization – are themselves more socially structured or 'shaped' than they are likely to appreciate. Culture too, in other words, is structured, though like agency not structurally determined (Scambler, 2018). Cockerham (2010) deploys a framework that owes much to Bourdieu and his idea of habitus when he discusses the social bases of what appear to be lifestyle decisions that have a critical bearing on health. Individuals who internalize similar life chances, he argues, share the same habitus because they are more likely to have similar shared experiences. Consequently, there is a high degree of affinity in health lifestyle choices. Stressing Bourdieu's emphasis on class habitus, Cockerham suggests that while health lifestyle choices may depart from class standards, personal styles are never more than a deviation from a style of class that relates back to the common style by its difference.

In conclusion, it can be argued that material and cultural factors alike exercise a crucial influence on health, illness and healthcare; that there is invariably a two-way or dialectical relation between them; and that both are linked in their genesis to the deep social structures of any given society. Going forward, and as the world emerges from the COVID-19 pandemic that is radically exposing the fissures of 'the fractured society', medical sociologists could contribute critical insights on how material and cultural factors are implicated in the social patterning of health. In so doing, attention should also be given to government responses, which, even in relatively wealthy nations, have proven far from adequate (see, for example, Scambler, 2020).

See also: Psychosocial Factors; Social Capital; Social Class; Surveillance and Health Promotion.

REFERENCES

Bourdieu, P. (1977) *Outline of a Theory of Practice*. Cambridge: Cambridge University Press.

Cockerham, W. (2010) 'Health lifestyles: bringing structure back', in W. Cockerham (ed.), *The New Blackwell Companion to Medical Sociology*. Oxford: Wiley-Blackwell.

DHSS (1980) *Inequalities in Health: Report of a Working Group (The Black Report)*. London: HMSO.

Foucault, M. (1988) *Technologies of the Self: A Seminar with Michel Foucault*. L.H. Martin, H. Gutman and P.H. Hutton (eds). Amherst: University of Massachusetts Press.

Marmot, M., Allen, J., Boyce, T. et al. (2020) *Health Equity in England: The Marmot Review Ten Years On*. London: Institute of Health Equity.

McEwen, B.S. (1998) 'Stress, adaptation, and disease: allostasis and allostatic load', *Annals of the New York Academy of Sciences*, 840 (1): 33–44.

Putnam, R. (2000) *Bowling Alone: The Collapse and Revival of American Community*. New York: Simon & Schuster.

Quah, S. (2010) 'Health and culture', in W. Cockerham (ed.), *The New Blackwell Companion to Medical Sociology*. Oxford: Wiley-Blackwell.

Savage, M. (2015) *Social Class in the 21st Century*. London: Penguin.

Saxbe, D.E., Beckes, L., Stoycos, S.A. and Coan, J.A. (2020) 'Social allostasis and social allostatic load: a new model for research in social dynamics, stress, and health', *Perspectives on Psychological Science*, 15 (2): 469–482.

Scambler, G. (2018) *Sociology, Health and the Fractured Society: A Critical Realist Account*. London: Routledge.

Scambler, G. (2020) 'COVID-19 as a "breaching experiment": exposing the fractured society', *Health Sociology Review*, 29 (2): 140–148.

Wilkinson, R. (1996) *Unhealthy Societies: The Afflictions of Inequality*. London: Routledge.

Wilkinson, R. and Marmot, M. (2003) *Social Determinants of Health: The Solid Facts*, 2nd edn. Copenhagen: WHO.

Wilkinson, R. and Pickett, K. (2009) *The Spirit Level*. London: Allen Lane.

SUGGESTED FURTHER READING

- Bartley, M. (2017) *Health Inequality: An Introduction to Theories, Concepts and Methods*, 2nd edn. Cambridge: Polity Press.

Bartley usefully explores material and behavioural-cultural factors and their relation to health inequalities alongside other factors (for example, psychosocial and lifecourse effects). This second edition also connects with more recent thinking and evidence on 'individual characteristics for health inequality'.

- Hinote, B. (2015) 'William C. Cockerham: the contemporary sociology of health lifestyles', in F. Collyer (ed.), *The Palgrave Handbook of Social Theory in Health, Illness and Medicine*. London: Palgrave Macmillan.

Emphasis is often given to the effects of lifestyles on health, though the focus tends to be individualistic at the expense of social factors. Hinote offers a detailed account of what medical sociology has to offer in these debates, with reference to Cockerham's pioneering 'health lifestyle theory'. According to such theorizing and associated research, individuals and social structures are inextricably connected and health outcomes must be critically analysed in view of these dynamic relations.

10

Psychosocial Factors

Antonia Bifulco

'Psychosocial factors' is a summary label used to characterize socio-environmental and personal conditions or attributes that increase or decrease risk of illness over the lifecourse.

Psychosocial factors have been a focus of research on the causation of disease in both medical sociology and health/clinical psychology. Traditionally there has been polarization with medical sociology emphasizing the role of socio-environmental factors such as rapid social change, social anomie or low socio-economic status and material deprivation. Health or clinical psychology has stressed the importance of personality (for example, Type A, which is aggressive and competitive), and cognitive-emotional factors such as coping (for example, locus of control) or self-esteem. The challenge within health models has been to see how these sets of factors intertwine and to investigate their interaction. Health effects can be direct, for example where poor living conditions increase risk for respiratory infections, or less direct, for example migrant populations who are at increased health risk through social separation and changes in dietary habits.

Both sociological and psychological lines of enquiry have a common interest in the investigation of adverse childhood experience as a precursor to poor adult health status. Socio-environmental factors such as loss of parent, exposure to childhood neglect and abuse, and broken or deprived family settings have been associated with a range of poor health outcomes, both physical and psychological. Lifespan psychosocial models show adverse childhood experience is also associated with a range of adult risk factors such as perpetuated lower socio-economic status, being a single parent, becoming a victim of domestic violence, worse educational attainment and poorer employment record. Such experiences are, in turn, related to psychological factors such as lower self-esteem, reduced ability to relate to others and poorer coping with stress. Two models are evident in the literature: one emphasizing dose-effects (the amount of exposure to childhood adversity) in affecting health (see below, the ACE studies), a second emphasizing psychosocial risk pathways comprising different trajectories. Both involve identifying key mediating or moderating factors. Psychosocial models of illness now also examine resilience, identifying, for example, the mediators of childhood adversity such as emotional dysregulation, and how these can be nullified by resilience factors to avert clinical disorder.

In considering physical health, risk factors in these models include smoking (risk for cardio-vascular and lung disease), alcohol consumption (risk for diseases of liver, stomach and central nervous system), obesity (risk for diabetes mellitus, cardiovascular disease) and physical inactivity (risk for cardiovascular disease). Causes of these have been sought in both socio-environmental and psychological domains. The former include, for example, social class, marital status, dietary habits and social support whilst the latter include, for example, risk-taking, Type A behaviour and attachment avoidance. Whilst there is accruing evidence of the importance of factors in both domains, sociologists question the attribution of individual responsibility in lifestyle and health, indicating the substantial role played by socio-economic status and culture, particularly in early years. Such reasoning is also evidenced in social epidemiology and public health (Marmot, 2020). Psychologists point to the greater specificity of their models in terms of identifying which individuals will succumb through cognitive-emotional or behavioural features, but also through the impacts of clinical disorders such as depression and anxiety (Khayyam-Nekouei et al., 2013).

Determining a *causal* role for psychosocial factors and illness involves the following:

Timing and duration: Psychosocial risk factors can act as antecedent, perpetuating or residual factors of ill-health. For example, in the work domain, initial loss of job can trigger mental or physical health problems, and the ensuing lack of employment can aggravate existing disorders. Conversely, chronic unemployment is often a residue of the associated long-term ill-health. Similar distinctions can be made about the impacts of marital/partner status, where health differences between marital groups can result from both an effect of health on marital status (through selection of healthy functioning in partners) and an effect of marital status on ill-health (stress induced by unhappy relationships, which leads to health problems).

Varying risk factors: A causal factor is one which, when manipulated, can be shown to change risk of outcome. In the study of psychosocial factors, adequate distinction is rarely made between fixed and varying risks. A fixed marker is unchangeable, and encompasses aspects such as race, gender and year of birth. Although these aspects might be distally associated with health outcomes, they are unlikely to account for the timing of a disorder, nor can they be manipulated to change a health outcome. Varying risk factors, on the other hand, can either change spontaneously within a subject (such as age or pubertal status), or be changed by intervention (for example, self-esteem or social skills) or by intention (for example, marital status). The change potential for psychosocial risks is important not only in understanding causal agency for disorders but also for devising interventions. Many health studies, due to single-time point measurement, underestimate the degree to which psychosocial risks are varying.

Dose-effects: Causality of risks can be determined by dose-effects – the more the exposure to or 'dose' of risk, the higher the likelihood of the illness outcome. This model has been applied very effectively in the investigation of childhood adversity and physical illness in midlife in the Adverse Childhood Experience (ACE) studies. Felitti and colleagues researched a very large sample of US health insurance clients in midlife to examine their self-reported childhood experience and their uptake of healthcare (Felitti et al., 1998). Using a simple ACE questionnaire, of ten childhood adversities, including five contextual factors (for example, parental mental illness, parent in prison, partner violence) and five involving maltreatment (emotional neglect, physical neglect, emotional abuse, physical abuse or sexual abuse), they showed the higher the score the greater the likelihood of a range of illnesses such as diabetes, coronary heart disease and early mortality. The same effect held for psychological disorders, such as depression or substance abuse (Merrick et al., 2017). This model has been widely adopted in considering the genesis of midlife ill-health. However, limitations include the oversimplification of the ACE questionnaire, the unequal impacts of the different adversity factors as shown in diverse studies and the lack of identifying mediating factors.

Risk mediation: Although substantial investigation has been made of a range of psychosocial risks and their association with different health outcomes, relatively little is currently known about the process of risk mediation. It is important to note that the origins of a risk factor and mode of mediation on health are not synonymous. Thus, psychosocial risks may be responsible for bringing about certain poor health outcomes but the mediator of risk is often physiological. For example, reasons for smoking are multiple and include personality, cultural factors, social class, deprivation and access to cigarettes. But risk processes linking smoking with cardio-vascular disease and lung cancer concern the physical influences of carbon monoxide and carcinogenic tars on the body. The origin of the risk factor is of critical importance for sociological and psychological study, but on its own is uninformative about the process of risk mediation for illness processes to occur.

There have been three major developments internationally during the last two decades in UK, USA and Canadian research investigations. These developments indicate complex relationships between psychosocial and neurobiological factors affecting health, particularly mental health, with swings in emphasis between them. Whilst complex interactions are involved, observed psychosocial factors once again have a role in driving much of the biological change.

Biological factors and genetics: Psychosocial factors are playing an increasing role in understanding genetic bases of human behaviour in relation to disorder, particularly psychological disorder. Studies have focused on genetic factors in vulnerability for depression, notably the 5-HTTPL serotonin transporter gene (Fisher et al., 2013). Two particular psychosocial risks are implicated – childhood adversity and adult severe life events. However, findings about the gene-environment interaction effect have been inconsistent (Culverhouse et al., 2018). More revolutionary is the epigenetic approach to how environment can actually shape genetic expression, although evidence is still sparse. DNA methylation is an epigenetic event that affects cell function by altering gene expression and is sensitive to environmental conditions. One example is in a study of the effect of childhood maltreatment on a polymorphism of the MAOA gene, associated with violent behaviour only in young adult males who have adverse childhood experience (Caspi, 2002). Another intriguing finding is the 'dandelion/orchid' approach, which identifies the genetic basis of individual sensitivity to the environment. It indicates how for 'orchids' (those who are sensitive), the environment can variously be enriching or depriving depending on whether the circumstances are benign or harsh, thus 'for better or worse' (Bakermans-Kranenburg and van IJzendoorn, 2007). The dandelions are more likely to weather either condition in a similar manner in relation to health.

Attachment theory: Attachment frameworks, devised by John Bowlby, identify a range of social experiences that influence lifetime risk of disorder (both physical and mental). Specifically, early experience of adverse parenting influences subsequent poor ability to relate to others, absence of social support, lack of trust and emotional dysregulation. This theory also fits well with a stress and coping model (Mikulincer and Shaver, 2017). The framework has been effectively adopted internationally, not only for models of childhood care but also for adult psychological disorder. It has been shown that children's early adverse experience of parents (or other responsible adults) leads to changes in their cognitive templates determining trust, which then determine responses to others and the self. Traditionally four styles have been identified: Secure, Anxious-ambivalent, Avoidant and Disorganized. Whereas secure style is adaptive, those insecure styles denoting Anxious or Avoidant or Disorganized characteristics lead to different types of difficulty in relating to others. Insecure styles are known to be associated with a range of psychological disorders but are also investigated in relation to physical illness, such as diabetes and service-use issues (Meng et al., 2015). Attachment style is also shown to be associated with cultural factors, social class, parental adversity and stress showing sociological as well as psychological underpinnings (e.g. Keller, 2018).

Resilience: This concept was first investigated in the 1980s, based on the seminal work of Norman Garmezy and Michael Rutter with colleagues in the USA and UK (see Haggerty et al., 1996). It has now taken a more central role in health research because of important preventative implications. Thus, explanations can be provided for why individuals who have experienced disadvantage do not succumb to disorder. Resilience is usually explained by the presence of positive social and psychological experiences in addition to adversity. Examples include social support, secure attachment style, high IQ, religious belief, but also benign economic environments and even neurobiological status (Wu et al., 2013). Such characteristics can serve to maintain well-being even under adversity.

Challenges for future investigation include improved measurement for investigating multiple factors for different disorders in large samples, identification of causes of time trends in changes in psychosocial risks and their effects, delineation of lifetime liability to poorer health outcomes and understanding individual susceptibility to illness, including genetic influences. Such research needs to incorporate sociological themes that emphasize the importance of socio-economic status, cultural factors and their impact on lifestyle. There is still important research which needs to be done on the role of psychosocial factors in health, including protective mechanisms that can *promote* health. Such research, in turn, could inform health policy critical to mitigating the effects of disadvantage and improving public health.

See also: Geneticization; Life Events; Material and Cultural Factors; Social Class.

REFERENCES

Bakermans-Kranenburg, M.J. and van IJzendoorn, M.H. (2007) 'Research review: genetic vulnerability or differential susceptibility in child development: the case of attachment', *Journal of Child Psychology and Psychiatry*, 48 (12): 1160–1173.

Caspi, A. (2002) 'Role of genotype in the cycle of violence in maltreated children', *Science*, 297 (5582): 851–854.

Culverhouse, R.C., Saccone, N.L., Horton, A.C. et al. (2018) 'Collaborative meta-analysis finds no evidence of a strong interaction between stress and 5-HTTLPR genotype contributing to the development of depression', *Molecular Psychiatry*, 23 (1): 133–142.

Felitti, V.J., Anda, R.F., Nordenberg, D. et al. (1998) 'Relationship of childhood abuse and household dysfunction to many of the leading causes of death in adults. The Adverse Childhood Experiences (ACE) Study', *American Journal of Preventive Medicine*, 14 (4): 245–258.

Fisher, H.L., Cohen-Woods, S., Hosang, G.M. et al. (2013) 'Interaction between specific forms of childhood maltreatment and the serotonin transporter gene (5-HTT) in recurrent depressive disorder', *Journal of Affective Disorders*, 145 (1): 136–141.

Haggerty, R.J., Sherrod, L.R., Garmezy, N. and Rutter, M. (eds) (1996) *Stress, Risk, and Resilience in Children and Adolescents: Processes, Mechanisms, and Interventions*. Cambridge: Cambridge University Press.

Keller, H. (2018) 'Universality claim of attachment theory: children's socioemotional development across cultures', *Proceedings of the National Academy of Sciences*, 115 (45): 11414–11419.

Khayyam-Nekouei, Z., Neshatdoost, H., Yousefy, A. et al. (2013) 'Psychological factors and coronary heart disease', *ARYA Atherosclerosis*, 9 (1): 102–111.

Marmot, M. (2020) 'Health equity in England: the Marmot Review 10 years on', *British Medical Journal*, 368: m693.

Meng, X., D'Arcy, C. and Adams, G.C. (2015) 'Associations between adult attachment style and mental health care utilization: findings from a large-scale national survey', *Psychiatry Research*, 229 (1–2): 454–461.

Merrick, M.T., Ports, K.A., Ford, D.C. et al. (2017) 'Unpacking the impact of adverse childhood experiences on adult mental health', *Child Abuse & Neglect*, 69: 10–19.

Mikulincer, M. and Shaver, P.R. (2017) *Attachment in Adulthood. Structure, Dynamics and Change*, 2nd edn. New York: The Guildford Press.

Wu, G., Feder, A., Cohen, H. et al. (2013) 'Understanding resilience', *Frontiers in Behavioral Neuroscience*, 7 (10): 1–15.

SUGGESTED FURTHER READING

- Belsky, J. (2016) 'The differential susceptibility hypothesis: sensitivity to the environment for better and for worse', *JAMA Pediatrics*, 170 (4): 321–322.

A good overview of the dandelion/orchid genetic approach to susceptibility to psychological disorder.

- Bifulco, A. and Thomas, G. (2012) *Understanding Adult Attachment in Family Relationships: Research, Assessment and Intervention*. London: Routledge.

This work is an overview of research with the Attachment Style Interview in relation to various aspects associated with psychological disorder across the lifecourse and intergenerationally.

- Bifulco, A. and Schimmenti, A. (2019) 'Assessing child abuse: "We need to talk!"', *Child Abuse & Neglect*, 98: 104236.

This paper discusses methodological issues in assessing childhood experience retrospectively with a plea for interview approaches to be utilized as a resource.

- Campbell, J.A., Walker, R.J. and Egede, L.E. (2016) 'Associations between adverse childhood experiences, high-risk behaviors, and morbidity in adulthood', *American Journal of Preventive Medicine*, 50 (3): 344–352.

Further updated discussion of ACE childhood adversity and morbidity.

11

Life Events

Antonia Bifulco

An acute environmental circumstance indicating change and often threat, with an identifiable start and end, and which carries a potential for altering an individual's circumstances and present state of mental or physical well-being.

Life events are the mechanism by which adversity impacts the individual with a direct link to ill-health. In understanding life events, we need to establish their context to gauge the likely meaning for the individual and how life plans or basic psychological needs are challenged. Many events are normative, determining lifecourse changes, such as leaving home, cohabiting or becoming a parent. These events often involve low levels of threat or unpleasantness, and indeed may be highly positive. However, events can at times be threatening when untimely or enforced (for example, unplanned pregnancy, arranged marriage). Additionally, non-normative events are those which are disruptive to the lifecourse, such as conflict with one's partner, untimely bereavement of a child or unexpected material loss. These events are mostly implicated in psychological disorder. *Severe* events are those carrying a high degree of threat or unpleasantness which can provoke onset of illness, notably depression.

Life events can also take the form of national or international crises. Examples include natural disasters (fires, floods, harvesting failures, pandemics) and those more overtly related to the political economy (war and other forms of conflict, forced migration, political repression, economic depression). Such events, constituting what sociologists would regard as a 'critical situation', all impinge on individuals, albeit on a wide scale. Here the coping responses can become communal as well as personal, as exhibited in the COVID-19 pandemic. When experience is particularly extreme, involving threat to life, this can also constitute a trauma event. Examples of trauma events are accidents with serious physical injury, untimely bereavements or violence victimization, affecting the individual involved but also witnesses, including emergency staff. These are known to have increased, for example, with the COVID-19 pandemic. Impacts include depression or anxiety but also post-traumatic stress disorder.

The study of life events has progressed furthest in the field of mental health, their role first identified in schizophrenic relapse, but then explored in more detail in relation to depression and anxiety states and, more recently, bipolar disorder. The research by George Brown, Tirril Harris and colleagues in the 1970s, into social factors in depression, and later physical illness, was responsible for many of the important developments in measurement and conceptualization. An important observation concerning life events is that although disorder (particularly psychological disorder) frequently occurs shortly after the experience of a severe life event, most individuals who suffer severe life events do not become ill. That is, severe life events are a *necessary* but not *sufficient* cause of ill-health. Personal vulnerability, i.e. that which makes an individual susceptible to the impact of life events, has become a substantial area of study and has led to lifecourse investigation of risk going back to childhood and even intergenerationally.

The following aspects are deemed by researchers as important in determining the role of life events in disease processes:

1. Identifying the *characteristics of events*, which might have particular potency for different types of illness, as well as their independence from individual agency and their timing in relation to onset, recovery and relapse from disorder.
2. A *vulnerability model* highlighting the provoking role of life events when interacting with an individual's prior vulnerability and associated with negative coping behaviour in bringing about disorder.
3. The role of life events throughout *the lifecourse*, particularly those in early life, including trauma, increasing risk for event-production and illness in later life.

First, the *characteristics of events* which have most potency for specific disorders have been identified by the Brown and Harris team in the 1990s and since replicated. Characteristics include, for instance, 'loss' for depression and 'danger' for anxiety (Asselmann et al., 2015). In addition, research identifying the match between negative aspects of events and characteristics of the individual experiencing them has sought to improve prediction of impact. Thus, for example, a severe life event in a domain of prior high commitment (such as losing a job in the context of prior sustained work ambition) carries increased risk of affective disorder through the implied disappointment. Another example is a severe event linked to a prior longer-term difficulty – here the event can extinguish any hope previously derived from coping attempts. Events, even those experienced jointly, can incur different impacts. For example, cohabiting couples experiencing a joint severe life event involving children tend to have greater impact on the mother in terms of depression. This is interpreted as due to higher childcare responsibilities, commitments and felt responsibility.

Second, some individuals are more *vulnerable* to life events. Early identification of demographic style vulnerability factors (such as lack of a close confidant, presence of three or more children, loss of a mother in childhood and lack of employment) were argued to reflect underlying loss of self-esteem. This loss was hypothesized as generalizing into hopelessness in the face of a severe life event and thus into depressive illness. Further prospective investigation showed attributes of such roles and relationships to be critical. Thus, negativity in relationships and lack of close support were shown to be associated with low self-esteem and together to interact with a severe life event in creating optimal conditions for depression. Insecure attachment style was subsequently identified as an underlying construct for relational problems and shown to underpin vulnerability to depression (Bifulco and Thomas, 2012). This process involves mistrust, fear or anger toward others and avoidance or dependent behaviour. Insecure individuals also exhibit poorer coping behaviours in response to severe life events and have lower support levels.

Third, debate has centred around the origin of life events over the *lifecourse*. Life events are not evenly distributed, either by individual, gender, family, age, socio–economic group or location. Much can be attributed to social deprivation, resulting in increased numbers of personal stressors and lower resources to reduce their impact. Other explanations have also been sought in terms of individuals creating their own high-risk environments by choices and actions, which generate events increasingly over the lifecourse. The association of life events and difficulties to psychiatric disorder has been shown to hold throughout the lifecourse. This process can have a cumulative effect with childhood and then adult negative events being associated with recurrent disorders. There is a long-term trajectory with childhood adversity relating to greatly increased rates of adult and even older age events, difficulties and depression (Bifulco et al., 2019a).

Certain measurement issues have dogged the study of life events in relation to disease and have required the development of sophisticated measurement, ideally in prospective study designs. These issues include the potential for reporting bias, uncertain timing of an event in relation to the onset of disorder and lack of clarity about the negativity of an event and its likely meaning. Early checklist approaches (for example, the Social Readjustment Scale, by Holmes and Rahe in the 1960s) examined an overall 'degree of change' score based on the sum of event types endorsed. Such checklist questionnaires, while showing a basic association of event score with illness, were unable to address any of the methodological issues such as bias, timing and contextual threat of the event. In contrast, semi-structured interviews, such as the Life Events and Difficulties Schedule developed by Brown and Harris in the 1970s, encouraged narrative accounts of events which, together with extensive probing questions, were able to elicit the full social context of life events and their timing and sequence in relation to disorders such as depression. Characteristics of these events were then assessed by the investigators, aided by manuals of precedent examples and consensus agreement to ensure reliability. This approach showed only one severe event was required to provoke an episode of depression. Those deemed severe were objectively assessed as involving high contextual threat or unpleasantness in the longer-term, to be focused on the individual and independent from the illness itself. The latter is important in avoiding circularity in terms of illness-related events being seen to bring about the disorder (Spence et al., 2015).

Research on life events has been re-invigorated in the last two decades in relation to studies of psychological disorder and the gene environment interaction, particularly by Caspi and colleagues' investigation in the 1990s of the polymorphism of the serotonin producer gene 5-HTTLPR. This relationship has further been refined by specifying a recurrence of depression episodes (Fisher et al., 2012) and by an earlier relationship to childhood trauma (Brown et al., 2014). However, reviews have noted inconsistency of findings (Culverhouse et al., 2018), which has in turn been argued to be influenced by measurement of the environment. There is a plea for more intensive measurement of life events in order to avoid false negatives arising from cursory measurement, but such measures need to be feasible given the large numbers required for genetic investigation. This need for both detailed measurement and large sample sizes has created something of a quandary. One response has been to devise an online measure, which mimics elements of the interview in terms of depth and detail. The Computerised Life Events Assessment Record (CLEAR) is a reliable measure of life events. CLEAR mimics the findings of the LEDS in showing depression related to loss, danger, humiliation and entrapment events, and that positive events increase well-being (Bifulco et al., 2019b).

The importance of studying life events in illness is not purely to understand social causation but also to influence intervention. Help-seeking is an important aspect, with support from close others at the time of life event crisis showing protective effects for both the onset and chronicity of disorders. Befriending interventions, which provide support in dealing with events and ongoing difficulties, have been shown to have a significant effect on recovery from disorder (Harris, 2006). Also, therapeutic approaches, such as Cognitive Behaviour Therapy or Counselling, require formulation of the provoking crises to enable aid with suitable coping responses.

Another aspect to consider in recovery from disorder is that events can be positive and create favourable emotions and entail welcome life change. Positive events are shown to relate to recovery from disorder and increased well-being (Disabato et al., 2017). When measured intensively, positive events are also shown to have dimensions, to aid security (those stabilizing/anchoring) and strengthen identity (those enhancing/fresh starts). Stabilizing/anchoring life events (such as getting a permanent job after unemployment or buying a house after living in poor accommodation) relate specifically to recovery from anxiety disorder and enhancing/fresh start events (such as making a new relationship after a period of isolation) to depression recovery (Brown et al., 1992). More recent research has also shown such events relate to enhanced well-being. However, individuals with vulnerability (for example, low self-esteem or insecure attachment style) are less receptive to the impact of positive change which has less effect on their well-being.

Thus life events continue to be important components in both the disease and recovery process in medical sociology. Recent attention to responses to COVID-19 illustrates how severe events on a national, or even global, scale may provoke a further wave of mental health issues. Related events pertain not only to hospital admissions (of self or significant others) or bereavements but also to the impacts of physical distancing in reducing social exchange, the demands of home schooling, job losses or workplace danger for key workers. The range of negative events is wide and the impacts on those vulnerable is likely to be extensive. Understanding these socio-environmental impacts on health and mental health will be important for researchers and policy-makers to combat such large-scale crisis.

See also: Ageing and the Lifecourse; Geneticization; Social Class.

REFERENCES

Asselmann, E., Wittchen, H., Lieb, R. et al. (2015) 'Danger and loss events and the incidence of anxiety and depressive disorders: a prospective-longitudinal community study of adolescents and young adults', *Psychological Medicine*, 45 (1): 153–163.

Bifulco, A., Jacobs, C., Oskis et al. (2019a) 'Lifetime trauma, adversity and emotional disorder in older age women', *Maltrattamento e abuso all'infanzia*, 21: 29–43.

Bifulco, A., Kagan, L., Spence, R. et al. (2019b) 'Characteristics of severe life events, attachment style and depression – using an online approach', *The British Journal of Clinical Psychology*, 58 (4): 427–439.

Bifulco, A. and Thomas, G. (2012) *Understanding Adult Attachment in Family Relationships: Research, Assessment and Intervention*. London: Routledge.

Brown, G.W., Craig, T.K.J., Harris, T.O. et al. (2014) 'Functional polymorphism in the brain-derived neurotrophic factor gene interacts with stressful life events but not childhood maltreatment in the etiology of depression', *Depression and Anxiety*, 31 (4): 326–334.

Brown, G.W., Lemyre, L. and Bifulco, A. (1992) 'Social factors and recovery from anxiety and depressive disorders: a test of specificity', *British Journal of Psychiatry*, 161 (1): 44–54.

Culverhouse, R.C., Saccone, N.L., Horton, A.C. et al. (2018) 'Collaborative meta-analysis finds no evidence of a strong interaction between stress and 5-HTTLPR genotype contributing to the development of depression', *Molecular Psychiatry*, 23 (1): 133–142.

Disabato, D.J., Kashdan, T.B., Short, J.L. et al. (2017) 'What predicts positive life events that influence the course of depression? A longitudinal examination of gratitude and meaning in life', *Cognitive Therapy Research*, 41 (3): 444–458.

Fisher, H.L., Cohen-Woods, S., Hosang, G.M. et al. (2012) 'Stressful life events and the serotonin transporter gene (5-HTT) in recurrent clinical depression', *Journal of Affective Disorders*, 136 (1–2): 189–193.

Harris, T. (2006) 'Volunteer befriending as an intervention for depression: implications for bereavement care', *Bereavement Care*, 25 (2): 27–30.

Spence, R., Bunn, A., Nunn, S. et al. (2015) 'Measuring life events and their association with clinical disorder: a protocol for development of an online approach', *JMIR Research Protocols*, 4 (3): e83.

SUGGESTED FURTHER READING

- Bifulco, A., Spence, R. and Kagan, L. (2021) *Life Events and Emotional Disorder Revisited: Research and Clinical Applications*. London: Routledge.

This book summarizes a body of research on life events. It ranges from early work by Brown and Harris and colleagues, and updates the literature in terms of the new computerized measurement approach. It also provides a framework linking event characteristics to underlying psychological needs and relevant interventions.

- Harkness, K.L. and Monroe, S.M. (2016) 'The assessment and measurement of adult life stress: basic premises, operational principles, and design requirements', *Journal of Abnormal Psychology*, 125 (5): 727–745.

This paper provides a full and updated discussion of the issues around life event measurement by researchers in the USA.

- van der Kolk, B. (2015) *The Body Keeps the Score: Mind, Brain and Body in the Transformation of Trauma*. London: Penguin.

This book deals with the extreme of life events which denotes trauma. It is an accessible introduction to the biological, psychological and social approaches to trauma experience and resultant disorders.

12

Ageing and the Lifecourse

Paul Higgs

Ageing in humans is primarily a physiological process whereby the body accumulates physical and psychological changes that occur across the lifespan. The lifecourse is a successive sequence of significant biological and socially patterned events, risks and expectations encountered by individuals in particular societies in specific periods.

Ageing, according to bio-gerontologists, is the result of an individual living a long life that goes beyond reproductive fitness and comes close to the limit of the 'natural' human lifespan. Consequently, in this view, ageing connects to limitations in both individual horizons and in older people's capacities. Rather than starting at birth, ageing is demarcated from development. Historically, older models of ageing saw it as the result of a 'fundamental' process of decay. While these have been superseded by more sophisticated and integrated approaches, it is still the case that decline and limitations are inextricably caught up in the understanding of ageing even when considered as a social process. Researchers now accept that multiple complex interacting processes probably account for the changes that take place as and when we grow old. Old age, on the other hand, is a *status* or *social category* marked by a particular chronological age or by a set of physiological signs and/or social markers. Because these terms are often used indiscriminately, it is important to separate ageing from the state or status of old age. It is also important to distinguish between the processes of ageing and those of development. Strehler (1962) defines ageing in terms of four key principles. It must be *universal* across all members of a species, even if it is subject to some variation over timing and impact. It must be *intrinsic* in that the causes must not depend on external factors. It must be *progressive* in that changes due to ageing must occur progressively during the latter part of the lifespan. Finally, ageing must be *deleterious* to the individual's health and survival. Development, like ageing, is also universal, intrinsic and progressive but unlike ageing, it is beneficial rather than deleterious for health and survival. It is, therefore, this last principle that has made ageing so important for its consequences for health.

Over the lifecourse, epidemiological data show us that age is associated with decreasing fitness, as well as a growing risk of illness and disability. Historically, birth and infancy have been more risky than childhood or adolescence. Old age, however defined, has represented greater risk than being young. As long as life expectancy was constrained by high infant mortality rates as well as high attrition rates across the whole of the lifecourse, ageing and old age could be restricted to a minority of the population. In the 19th century this changed in Europe and North America. Improvements in public health and rising living standards led to a decline in infectious diseases across these geographical areas. This pattern has gradually spread to other parts of the world, albeit with considerable regional differences. However, children's declining rates of infectious disease were accompanied by a rise in 'degenerative diseases' mainly affecting older people. This 'epidemiological transition' can be represented graphically as the 'rectangularisation of the survival curve' (Fries, 1980). What Fries meant by this term was that modern populations show less mortality before the onset of adulthood. There is also an increase in morbidity and mortality from middle age. From this point in the lifecourse, morbidity and mortality rise and reach their peak in 'old age'. This has now become the commonest period across the lifecourse for death to occur. However, the average age at which death happens varies between different countries and has increased considerably over the past 50 years in the Global North. Significantly, not only is death compressed into a narrower age range, but survival in later life, even in the presence of morbidity, has also increased. This epidemiological pattern has not necessarily meant that people are 'living longer and sicker' as has been assumed by many thinkers over the centuries; rather, it represents a 'compression of morbidity'. This term describes a situation where, as life grows longer, the proportion of life spent in ill health grows shorter. There has been evidence that disability rates in the United States for older people have been falling. Although this conclusion has been contested (Crimmins and Beltrán-Sánchez, 2011), it suggests that biological ageing is not a simple but inevitable process of decline; rather, it can be thought of as a set of contingent and connected processes linked to the unrepaired accumulation of damage to the body over time. This approach reflects an evolutionary 'selective investment' by the body in those cells that will perpetuate gene inheritance.

Sociological accounts of ageing are generally agnostic on the biological dimensions of ageing and focus much more on the 'social construction of old age'. In doing this, they are much more able to see the various forms in which different societies structure and understand the status of old age. Approaching age from this point of view allows sociologists the advantage of being able to see how the epidemiological and demographic changes are reflected in social and cultural changes. This focus on social change is particularly useful in relation to the changes in the position and status of old age that have occurred in the high-income countries.

Lifecourse studies have been slower to realize the important insight of the social construction of old age and have often naturalized it as a relatively timeless structure. An important development in understanding the contemporary lifecourse, at least in the Global North, has been the introduction of state retirement pensions and the creation of a normative expectation of retirement for the majority of those born in the 20th century. Industrialization and the reliance on wage-labour disadvantaged older workers and created impoverishment in old age. Pensions were instituted (initially for men) to overcome this situation and in doing so established an important aspect of the institutionalization of the modern lifecourse. Retirement was therefore seen as complementing the stages of schooling and work. As can be seen, the contemporary lifecourse has been very much gendered. While work in the formal economy has been considered as central to men's lives, women on the other hand have been seen to be predominantly defined by their role in reproduction and the domestic sphere. This notion of defined gender roles was codified into the very fabric of welfare states established after the Second World War. The cultural transformation of the 1960s that accompanied mass youth culture not only eroded stable occupational identities but also challenged normative assumptions about marriage and the nuclear family. This destabilization also had an impact on old age as cultural norms began to reflect an emphasis on lifestyle and consumption rather than ascription and seniority.

Rising incomes in retirement also meant that from the 1980s the standard of living of retired people rose at a faster rate than that of working people. Similar trends have been visible in the UK, continental Europe and the USA and have led to renewed calls for 'generational equity' to address the advantages that the post-war boomer cohorts appear to have amassed over their lifecourses. In part, 'intergenerational conflict' has also been a reaction to the emergence of a new articulation of old age in the guise of the 'third age'. Popularized by the historian Peter Laslett (1989), the third age was conceived as a liberation from the status of the 'old age pensioner' created by 20th-century social policy. As an alternative, Laslett wanted to accentuate the transformation of later life by the compression of morbidity which could now be represented as a new stage of life. The third age represented opportunities for self-development and was to be separated from the terminal fourth age of decline and dependency. The meaning of the third age has been contested within social gerontology with some arguing that it represents a form of ageing for the better off older population in high-income countries. Others have embraced the idea and see in it both a recognition of the transformation of later life and of the possibilities that post-work lives can now represent. Ideas about 'successful ageing' and 'productive ageing' flow from this perspective.

Whatever the nature of the framing of the third age, what is also occurring is a rewriting of what the lifecourse is supposed to look like. Important figures in the development of both the sociology of ageing and gerontology have been aware that old age is not a singular status and that important implications follow from this. Neugarten's (1974) distinction between what she called the 'young old' and the 'old old' reflects an awareness of the differentiated nature of old age. Similarly, Riley used the age of 85 to demarcate a growing segment of the older population whose health is a key factor in their negative experience of ageing (Suzman and Riley, 1985). Baltes (Baltes and Smith, 2003), who led the Berlin Ageing Study, noted important differences from younger older people among those much older people whose ill health and dependency presaged a terminal phase. While these researchers' approaches diverge on the salient features of such a stage, there is an underlying assumption that some distinction between groups of the older population is necessary. It is noteworthy that Carr and Luth (2019) have also pointed out that death itself now should be identified as a distinct stage in the lifecourse given that it has become for many a protracted and anticipated transition resulting from an incurable chronic illness. Higgs and Gilleard (2015) have proposed that this recognition of the changed nature of old age needs to be understood in terms of both the third and fourth ages where 'real' old age is restricted to a segment of the population understood in terms of their frailty and cognitive decline. The boundaries between these two culturally determined projections of later life increasingly act as the template for understanding later life.

While these may be the analytical constructs for studying later life, it also needs acknowledging that many different inequalities occur across the lifecourse. The most obvious is that of life expectancy itself. As was pointed out above, the belief that most of the population could expect to reach retirement is something that only happened in the Global North or Western nations in the second half of the 20th century. Other areas of the globe have not seen the same pattern and sometimes there have been dramatic falls in life expectancy, as observed among Russian men after the fall of the Soviet Union. We also know that there are social class associated gradients to life expectancy and that illness and disability are maldistributed across the population. These inequalities in health connect to wider social inequalities and the way in which society is structured. Much work examines the way that the lifecourse is impacted by these inequalities. Theories of cumulative disadvantage/advantage have been particularly influential in explaining how disadvantages at particular points in the lifecourse are amplified over the decades to produce outcomes in relation to health.

A noteworthy study illustrating these ideas is Elder's *Children of the Great Depression* (2018), a longitudinal study of the effects of the 1930s economic crisis. Elder has been seen as one of the founders of lifecourse research, integrating the social and biological sciences to examine the multi-generational impact of poverty. While issues of social class and poverty have been staples of this form of research, there have been moves in a number of different disciplines to look at wider forms of inequality that result from other sources such as gender, race, sexuality and disability. Intersectional approaches have sought to bring to light the ways that these different lines of fracture bring about negative consequences for people over the course of their lives. These inequalities are not, however, discrete or isolated processes that can be carefully separated from each other, but rather they intersect with one another in complex and contradictory ways. This realization is at an early point in its development but it is the start of a more finely grained understanding of the connection between the lifecourse and inequality.

In summary, we have seen how ageing and the lifecourse are intrinsically located within the biology of the human species, but we have also shown how old age is fundamentally constructed by human society. The possibilities for growing old and for altering the experience of later life have changed considerably over the last century. It is now a common experience for most people who live in prosperous countries to reach the age of retirement. It is also increasingly true of large parts of the rest of the world. If this situation has been brought about by the impact of industrialization and urbanization which typified early and mid-20th-century modernity, it is also true that the social changes described by Beck (2007) as constituting a 'second' reflexive modernity have transformed many assumptions about ageing and the institutionalized lifecourse. Retirement and old age are no longer interchangeable terms. Later life as a third age is becoming more and more a recognized reality as is the shadow of the fourth age. These transformations continue at pace but, as Jones and Higgs (2010) point out, ideas of what constitutes 'natural ageing', 'normal ageing' or even 'normative ageing' have become highly contested terrains and are likely to remain so. Strehler (1962) will continue to be our guide as to what can be described as ageing, but the nature of what constitutes the lifecourse, and what impact it has on later life, is going to be less circumscribed by the experience of the 20th century and more by the contingencies that the development of 21st-century modernity brings in its wake.

These new contingencies now have to include the impact of the COVID-19 pandemic, which has disproportionately affected the older population. Not only has there been a very strong age-effect in terms of mortality from the virus, with those aged over 70 being particularly vulnerable, but in addition certain categories of older people such as residents of nursing homes have not been protected from the virus in the ways that they should. The impact of this virus on older people, therefore, not only calls into question the long-held assumptions about the epidemiological transition, but also reiterates the connection between age, vulnerability and risk. Furthermore, the treatment of the older residents of nursing homes in many parts of the world raises an additional dimension of an implicit 'fourth ageism'. If old age is to be viewed as a valuable part of the lifecourse, then it is important to recognize that alongside 'successful ageing' we must protect those whose age-related vulnerabilities are also part of the lifecourse. Medical sociological research could inform such concerns, debates and policies and also contribute to exploring the aftermath of the pandemic on young people who appear to have been disproportionately impacted by lockdown measures.

See also: Chronic Illness; Gender; Intersectionality; Life Events; Risk; Social Class.

REFERENCES

Baltes, P.B. and Smith, J. (2003) 'New frontiers in the future of aging: from successful aging of the young old to the dilemmas of the fourth age', *Gerontology*, 49 (2): 123–135.

Beck, U. (2007) 'Beyond class and nation: reframing social inequalities in a globalizing world', *The British Journal of Sociology*, 58 (4): 679–705.

Carr, D. and Luth, E.A. (2019) 'Well-being at the end of life', *Annual Review of Sociology*, 45: 515–534.

Crimmins, E.M. and Beltrán-Sánchez, H. (2011) 'Mortality and morbidity trends: is there compression of morbidity?' *Journals of Gerontology Series B: Psychological Sciences and Social Sciences*, 66 (1): 75–86.

Elder, G.H. (2018) *Children of the Great Depression*. London: Routledge.

Fries, J.F. (1980) 'Aging, natural death and the compression of morbidity', *New England Journal of Medicine*, 303: 130–135.

Higgs, P. and Gilleard, C. (2015) *Rethinking Old Age: Theorising the Fourth Age*. London: Macmillan International Higher Education.

Jones, I.R. and Higgs, P.F. (2010) 'The natural, the normal, and the normative: contested terrains in ageing and old age', *Social Science & Medicine*, 71 (8): 1513–1519.

Laslett, P. (1989) *A Fresh Map of Life*: London: Weidenfeld and Nicholson.

Neugarten, B.L. (1974) 'Age groups in American society and the rise of the young-old', *The Annals of the American Academy of Political and Social Science*, 415 (1): 187–198.

Strehler, B. (1962) *Time, Cells and Aging*. New York: Academic Press.

Suzman, R. and Riley, M.W. (1985) 'Introducing the "oldest old"', *The Milbank Memorial Fund Quarterly. Health and Society*, 63 (2): 175–186.

SUGGESTED FURTHER READING

- Carr, D. (2019) *Golden Years? Social Inequality in Later Life*. New York: Russell Sage Foundation.

This comprehensive and well-documented book looks at the complex ways that socio-economic status, race and gender impact on older peoples' lives. Carr argues that disadvantages accumulate across the lifecourse and can even impact on the nature of death at older ages.

- Dannefer, D. (2003) 'Cumulative advantage/disadvantage and the life course: cross-fertilizing age and social science theory', *The Journals of Gerontology Series B: Psychological Sciences and Social Sciences*, 58 (6): S327–S337.

This paper provides an overview of one of the most interesting research programs linking the lifecourse with long-term processes of disadvantage and advantage.

- Gilleard, C. and Higgs, P. (2020) *Social Divisions and Later Life: Difference, Diversity and Inequality*. Bristol: Policy Press.

This book brings together the different ways that social divisions such as social class, ethnicity, gender and disability intersect with ageing and old age. It explicitly discusses the value of intersectional approaches in addressing the circumstances of contemporary later life.

- Kohli, M. (2007) 'The institutionalization of the life course: looking back to looking ahead', *Research in Human Development*, 4 (3–4): 253–271.

Kohli's paper is an invaluable starting point in understanding the way in which the modern lifecourse has been institutionalized. It is important to understand this debate if the changes to modern old age are to be fully understood.

13

Neoliberalism

Judith Green and Kirsten Bell

Neoliberalism describes processes of global economic restructuring that intensified from the later decades of the 20th century, and the social and cultural ramifications of this, characterized by the increasing marketization and individualization of social relations.

The term 'neoliberalism' came to prominence in the mid-19th century to describe a set of political and economic theories which advocated free trade and the idea of markets as self-regulating and rational, having no need for the intervention of governments. In the later decades of the 20th century, 'neoliberalism' came into common use to describe the resurgence of those ideas in new, globalized forms. From the late 1980s, national governments around the world began to deregulate trade, privatize publicly owned resources and remove capital controls. Economic reforms in Chile under Augusto Pinochet, in the USA under Ronald Reagan, and in the UK under Margaret Thatcher, were particularly associated with political commitments to 'rolling back' the state and moving away from the idea of governments as direct providers of public goods, such as transport, healthcare and welfare. Rotarou and Sakellariou (2017), for instance, argue that neoliberal economic reforms, including the introduction of a marketized health system with private providers and insurers, 'ended the welfare state' (p. 497) in Chile, with long lasting consequences for health inequalities in the country.

Neoliberal economic policy was globalized through transnational organizations such as the International Monetary Fund and the World Bank, which forced 'structural adjustment' policies on countries in the Global South to manage their rising national debts and incentivize trade and production. Structural adjustment typically entailed the privatization of publicly owned resources, and a reorientation of production to goods for export. The resulting reduced barriers to trade intensified the internationalization of capitalism, as corporations shifted production to where labour was cheapest, yet kept investments and profits in states where taxes were low. As state constraints on capitalism reduced, working lives became more fragmented, and capital accumulated within smaller and smaller elites.

Commentators widely suggest that the influence of neoliberalism is felt far beyond the realm of economic policy itself, with markets perceived not only as the rational basis for organizing economies, but also for understanding social life. Values such as freedom of choice, individual responsibility and the primacy of market relations become accepted as taken-for-granted norms, shaping not just how governments do relate to citizens, but how they should. There is considerable debate, however, around how dominant these discourses are, and how far it is theoretically credible to conflate a number of different processes – including commodification, privatization, globalization and marketization – as consequences or facets of neoliberalism, rather than phenomena with their own drivers, trajectories and consequences (Castree, 2006; England and Ward, 2007). Whether these changes are the result of a coherent, right-wing political ideology, and the extent to which they are the variable and ad-hoc results of local responses to economic crises, is also much debated, as are the effects of neoliberalism, and its usefulness as a theoretical concept for sociology and other social sciences.

Although the meaning of 'neoliberalism' is often taken for granted, England and Ward (2007) have identified four distinct ways that the term is employed by social scientists: (1) neoliberalism as an ideological hegemonic project leveraged by global elites; (2) neoliberalism as policy and programme (for example, policies enacted under the banner of privatization, deregulation, liberalization); (3) neoliberalism as state form; and (4) neoliberalism as governmentality – i.e. the ways in which the relations among and between peoples and things are reimagined, reinterpreted and reassembled to effect governing at a distance. Despite these different uses of the term, what is generally agreed is that the changes typically described as 'neoliberal' have had far reaching effects on health and well-being around the world. These changes directly impact on determinants of health, such as the stability of employment and wage levels, and on spending on publicly funded health and welfare services. Bloor (2011), for instance, illustrates the interconnections between an increasingly globalized shipping industry and the health of seafarers themselves, though he does not use the term 'neoliberal' itself. In particular, he highlights the ways in which intensified labour processes, smaller and more international crew, and lack of job security, impact on health in an industry that perhaps typified early neoliberal shifts, as shipping became more globalized, with crewing outsourced as casualized labour.

The social and cultural effects of neoliberal economics, then, flow directly from the operation of liberalized markets, such as the health effects of globalized capital. However, sociologists have also studied the ways in which neoliberal discourses of self-reliance, freedom from the state, and the primacy of economic rationality, have framed social relations, and conceptualizations of agency – in other words, the 'neoliberalism as governmentality' lens. For example, based on interviews with women in the UK, Peacock and colleagues (2014) illustrate the ways in which neoliberal ideas become internalized as part of how people understand their own life trajectories. They suggest that this is characterized through a discourse of 'no legitimate dependency': a pervasive individualistic orientation that disavows the notion that individuals are anything other than self-actualizing, empowered and able to exercise agency. Interviewees thus blamed and criticized themselves for their own vulnerabilities and stigmatized others, thereby marginalizing structural or social accounts of misfortune. The psycho-social processes through which blame and stigma become ways of understanding needs for welfare, or living with long term ill-health, are an indirect means through which neoliberal ideologies come to impact on health and well-being. However, the ways in which these discourses play out are neither universal nor inevitable. In a case study comparing how people managed their diabetes in Bulgaria and the UK, Vassilev and colleagues (2017) note that although UK participants described their struggles as about individual responsibilities, Bulgarian participants were more likely to use structural explanations, focusing on system and resource constraints, which were not linked to their own personal failures. Although there were similar challenges for patients, the specific contexts of each country, including differences in how the health service was funded and managed, and the role of civil society, produced what the authors call different 'articulations of neoliberalism … [in the UK] as a logic of managed choice and [in Bulgaria] as a logic of unmanaged consumerism' (p. 349).

These specificities in how health is conceptualized and suffering attributed (as system failure, or individual responsibility) in neoliberal times suggest some of the problems with the analytical power of neoliberalism as a concept. Empirically, studies of the health consequences of neoliberalism document a diverse range of phenomena in any given domain. Bell and Green (2016), for instance, note that studies of 'neoliberal diets' include those that describe the ways in which contemporary consumers are obliged to manage their health risks through making their own 'healthy' choices in food purchase and consumption – e.g. eating a certain number of fruit and vegetable portions, considering the provenance of food, eating super foods or organic foods, reducing sugars or fat. Conversely, studies also describe neoliberal diets as those characterized by a lack of agency on the part of consumers, who are constrained in their choices by a powerful globalized 'Big Food' industry, producing cheap, unhealthy products (such as sugar-sweetened drinks, or hyper-processed foodstuffs) at the expense of varied local markets, or by the forces of global capital that produce local food deserts and inadequate resources to purchase healthy food.

For some, these apparent contradictions are evidence of the different scales at which neoliberalism operates as a complex political project. Treating obesity as an example of what they term a 'neoliberal epidemic', Schrecker and Bambra (2015) point to its links with growing levels of market liberalization and economic insecurity. Thus, if the lens of neoliberal explanation is directed at the macro-level, the focus is on the impact of neoliberalism on globalized food markets and product availability, and the ways they facilitate high-fat, high-sugar diets. If directed at the micro-level instead, the spotlight shifts as the increased obligations for citizens to be self-empowered consumers, responsible for their own health, come into focus (Schrecker, 2016). The same economic drivers can, then, be theorized as producing very different social and cultural effects. However, such explanatory 'flexibility' is also seen as symptomatic of problems with the concept of neoliberalism itself. Birch (2017), for example, argues that it 'has come to mean whatever anyone wants it to mean, leading to a state of affairs in which almost anything nowadays – from university rankings through to pet food advertising – can be theorized as "neoliberal"' (p. 7).

More fundamentally, some have argued that these differences reflect not just the hybridity and contingency of neoliberal processes, but an inherent weakness in the concept as an abstraction which seeks to conflate so many different processes across time, space, and scale, and which intersects with other social, economic and political changes. Reflecting on these contradictions in the field of geography, Castree (2006) suggests the focus of any neoliberal lens is inevitably 'fuzzy', risking an over-determined role for neoliberalism. He suggests the continuing purchase of the concept for critical scholars is a 'necessary illusion', leveraged in part to make theoretical sense of varied and contingent local manifestations of different processes. There may be diminishing returns from using neoliberalism as a frame for making sense of how the interplay of global systems and local environments impact on disease, health and well-being. Indeed, there is a growing sense in some quarters that the concept of neoliberalism is actively impeding our grasp of recent political events such as Brexit. According to Kapferer and Gold (2017: 31), 'too much is being forced into the frame of neoliberalism, sustaining left/right distinctions of the recent past that are losing their relevance and much of their analytical bite'. The unprecedented social, economic and political crisis engendered by the COVID-19 pandemic will perhaps be the greatest test for neoliberalism – as both an economic policy and academic construct. Are government responses to the pandemic illustrations of neoliberal governance par excellence, with the legitimate introduction of massive state surveillance, and the increasing exercise of biopower? Or do pandemic responses represent its opposite: the frailty and demise of neoliberal governance, as resurgent nation-states rush to control their borders, and instigate command and control economies? Or something else entirely? Only time will tell.

See also: Material and Cultural Factors; Privatization; Social Class; Stigma; Surveillance and Health Promotion.

REFERENCES

Bell, K. and Green, J. (2016) 'On the perils of invoking neoliberalism in public health critique', *Critical Public Health*, 26 (3): 239–243.

Birch, K. (2017) *A Research Agenda for Neoliberalism*. Cheltenham: Edward Elgar Publishing.

Bloor, M. (2011) 'An essay on "health capital" and the Faustian bargains struck by workers in the globalised shipping industry', *Sociology of Health & Illness*, 33 (7): 973–986.

Castree, N. (2006) 'From neoliberalism to neoliberalisation: consolations, confusions, and necessary illusions', *Environment and Planning A*, 38 (1): 1–6.

England, K. and Ward, K. (eds) (2007) *Neoliberalization: States, Network, Peoples*. Malden, MA: Blackwell Publishing.

Kapferer, B. and Gold, M. (2017) 'The cuckoo in the nest: thoughts on neoliberalism, revaluations of capital and the emergence of the corporate state. Part 1', *Arena*, 151: 31–34.

Peacock, M., Bissell, P. and Owen, J. (2014) 'Dependency denied: health inequalities in the neo-liberal era', *Social Science & Medicine*, 118: 173–180.

Rotarou, E.S. and Sakellariou, D. (2017) 'Neoliberal reforms in health systems and the construction of long-lasting inequalities in health care: a case study from Chile', *Health Policy*, 121 (5): 495–503.

Schrecker, T. (2016) '"Neoliberal epidemics" and public health: sometimes the world is less complicated than it appears', *Critical Public Health*, 26 (5): 477–480.

Schrecker, T. and Bambra, C. (2015) *How Politics Makes Us Sick: Neoliberal Epidemics*. Basingstoke: Palgrave Macmillan.

Vassilev, I., Rogers, A., Todorova, E. et al. (2017) 'The articulation of neoliberalism: narratives of experience of chronic illness management in Bulgaria and the UK', *Sociology of Health & Illness*, 39 (3): 349–364.

SUGGESTED FURTHER READING

- Harvey, D. (2007) *A Brief History of Neoliberalism*. Oxford: Oxford University Press.

Harvey's account of neoliberalism describes the global economic changes from the 1970s and various local trajectories, stressing the political dimensions of class relations. He characterizes neoliberalism as a hegemonic discourse and project for consolidating power in a new global elite, made possible via social changes through which the population increasingly understood themselves in individual terms, as having freedoms and individual rights.

- Gatwiri, K., Amboko, J. and Okolla, D. (2020) 'The implications of Neoliberalism on African economies, health outcomes and wellbeing: a conceptual argument', *Social Theory & Health*, 18 (1): 86–101.

This review paper outlines the effects of neoliberal policies on the health of populations in post-colonial economies in sub-Saharan Africa. The authors unpick examples from several countries of consequences of neoliberalism, such as the commercialization of healthcare, the effects of development aid and 'brain drains' of African-trained health professionals. These consequences have eroded access to the determinants of health for many, with resulting poor health an additional barrier for developing sustainable economic growth.

- Keshavjee, S. (2014) *Blind Spot: How Neoliberalism Infiltrated Global Health.* Oakland: University of California Press.

Keshavjee draws on a long experience as a physician and anthropologist in a remote area of Tajikistan to delineate in detail how Western neoliberal ideology is transplanted, often via well-intentioned non-governmental organizations, globally, and becomes constructed as commonsense. As Soviet era conceptualizations of health as a social good, with an emphasis on equity, were replaced with market-driven initiatives, the consequences for health locally were devastating.

14

Social Capital

Orla McDonnell

> *Social capital is generally defined as the social resources that accrue to individuals by virtue of their membership of informal and formal social networks, and which may impact life chances and health.*

Current trends in public health research emphasize the importance of social capital. The concept, however, remains ill-defined and the causal relationship between social capital and health outcomes is inconclusive. Because the concept has different theoretical heritages, social epidemiologists and sociologists disagree about its analytical and explanatory value – they disagree about what is being measured and about the mechanisms that generate social capital and link it to health outcomes. The policy value of public health research rests on the idea that social capital is a feature of communities or whole societies and that by replenishing or building the 'stock' of capital, public health initiatives can reverse or ameliorate negative health outcomes associated with social inequalities. The dominant definition of social capital in public health research is taken from Putnam, a political scientist. He conceives of social capital as a 'civic' property of communities that inheres in 'features of social organization such as networks, norms, and social trust that facilitate action and co-operation for mutual benefit' (Putnam, 1995: 67). Putnam's theory equates the 'stock' of social capital in a given community with levels of civic participation. This is measured by a number of indicators, including: participation in voluntary organizations, democratic engagement (captured by newspaper consumption and voting) and individuals' expressions of interpersonal and institutional trust. These indicators, which are captured in survey data, are understood as the structural and cognitive elements that make up social capital (Rodgers et al., 2019).

Social capital also takes different forms. *Bonding social capital* refers to informal networks such as family ties where members who share the same beliefs are bound together through the norms of trust and reciprocity. This type of social capital functions as both a form of social control and social support. *Bridging social capital* denotes the formal but looser network of ties between different social groups that function to promote community and civic participation (Rodgers et al., 2019). *Linking social capital* refers to the ties that connect social groups across status and power differentials, for example, when people interact with formal institutions to access strategic resources. The manifest function of this type of social capital is to promote institutional trust. As Szreter and Woolcock (2004: 655) explain: 'especially in poor communities, it is the nature and extent (or lack thereof) of respectful and trusting ties to representatives of formal institutions – e.g. banks, law enforcement officers, social workers, health care providers – that has a major bearing on their welfare'. This further conceptual distinction of the different types of social networks was prompted by Putnam's own observation that not all networks promote norms of trust that benefit the community as a whole.

Let us now consider the explanatory theory of social capital in terms of how it may account for health outcomes. According to Putnam (1995), voluntary association and the density of interactions (frequency and intensity) within and between networks of association protect health. The overall stock of the network of ties that binds individuals to each other (and, hence the collective) through relations of reciprocity and mutual trust represents the very foundations of social support. Social support has a direct bearing on health by modulating the psychological impact of social stressors that compromise health. Shared norms within networks also operate as a form of social control and these norms impact on health through the promotion of health-enhancing behaviours. The civic component of social capital is understood to have an indirect impact on population health. The more people are involved in civic organizations and the greater the frequency of the interactions between these organizations across formal and informal networks, the more people are said to engage with political decisions that impact on health and to collectively demand better services (Kawachi et al., 1999).

When the second edition of *Key Concepts in Medical Sociology* was published in 2013 the evidence to support the direct and indirect impact of social capital on health was far from conclusive. Notwithstanding methodological variances and differences in theoretical emphasis (Ehsan et al., 2019), the weight of evidence on the causal role of social capital remains mixed and inconclusive (Rodgers et al., 2019). Despite the growth in public health research on social capital, there have been relatively few published evaluations of public health interventions that seek to foster social capital. In a recent systematic review of journals focused on epidemiology and public health, Villalonga-Olives et al. (2018) identified 17 such studies across the Global North and South. They found that public health interventions tend to focus on individual rather than community-level change, there was a lack of studies taking a 'multi-level perspective' and there was 'an absence of consideration of specific groups that might selectively benefit from social capital interventions' (p. 203).

Given such problems, area-based sociological studies are noteworthy. Some recent literature lends support to the importance of social capital as a contextual feature of communities, which can influence health outcomes, especially for lower socio-economic groups living in areas where there is a spatial clustering of material disadvantage. Garnham (2015) assesses the impact of deindustrialization and austerity on widening area-based inequalities and health inequalities in the UK. Drawing on sociological theories, including Bourdieu's concept of social capital and its relation to other forms of capital such as economic and cultural capital (discussed below), she emphasizes the multiple causal pathways linking social and health inequalities. Over time, deindustrialization and austerity measures have a cascading effect that is detrimental to vulnerable individuals, while community-based social networks and the resources that they make available to support individuals are eroded. Emphasizing political and economic participation as an outcome measure of social capital, Garnham demonstrates how neoliberal policies structure the field of action available to both individuals and communities by undercutting access to important sources of social and other forms of capital.

The aspects of the social environment that are considered most pertinent to health outcomes reflect how the problem of health inequalities and associated policy solutions are framed. For critics such as Portes (1998) and Navarro (2002), social capital was embraced by policy-makers as part of the ascendency of neoliberal ideology because the analysis that it promoted distracted from the structural relationship between social and health inequalities. Globally, neoliberal policies have been shown to increase social insecurity, widen economic inequalities and increase poverty in real terms, all of which have a direct bearing on health outcomes, as well as deepening social anomie. In this respect, the work of Wilkinson and colleagues (Wilkinson, 1996; Wilkinson and Pickett, 2009) is relevant to the debate on social capital and health. Their analysis on the psychosocial pathways that link social and health inequalities clearly points to the policy necessity of addressing income inequality and wealth redistribution – policy issues that are not explicitly addressed in the public health literature on social capital. Wilkinson's (1996) seminal work tackles what increasingly appears as the intractable problem of health inequalities in affluent societies.

Briefly, Wilkinson (1996) demonstrates that there is a threshold beyond which the absolute wealth of a nation ceases to have a direct bearing on population-level health outcomes. Wealthy countries with the greatest health inequalities also have in common the greatest levels of income inequality. These countries, such as the USA, are also marked by the lowest stocks of social capital (at a societal level where the state is a key agent) compared to the Nordic countries, where the social-democratic welfare model underpinning social solidarity is based on income solidarity and a greater proportion of wealth is redistributed from the richest to the poorest in society. This observation leads Dahl and Malmberg-Heimonen (2010) to surmise that community-level social capital may play a more significant role in mediating between socio-economic position and health outcomes in countries such as the USA, where welfare protections are weak and distributive justice is a suspect moral value for guiding social action. Despite the impact of the COVID-19 pandemic in compounding health inequalities (Dorn et al., 2020), the political call for social responsibility and solidarity is likely to be consequential. Indeed, it may well prove to be the moment in the sun for social capital theory that emphasizes community-level influences on behaviour over macro-level social structures that appear to be more directly associated with the spread and impact of the pandemic.

Social determinants literature posits a robust link between material inequalities, educational level and health inequalities. The direction of that research, in general, is on the multifactorial and intergenerational processes linking social and health inequalities. In line with this evidence, Veenstra and Abel (2019) make a strong case for applying Bourdieu's sociological theory to public health research. Bourdieu emphasizes that people have access to different types of social networks depending on their social location or socio-economic status, and the key distinction between networks is the value of the resources that social ties make available to individuals. Hence, this theory challenges the idea that social capital is a universal resource that is neutral in terms of its mechanisms, as Villalonga-Olives and Kawachi (2017) insist, in line with Putnam. Instead, from the perspective of Bourdieu, the amount of social capital that an individual possesses is an outcome of the social reproduction of inequality and privilege. In the context of health some resources are more important than others, depending on what other capitals come into play. Further, the effects that any one form of capital may have on an individual's health vary depending on the amount of other forms of capital they may possess. Therefore, rather than controlling for income (economic capital) and education (cultural capital), as many public health studies do, the focus should be on which form of capital is more likely to mediate the effect of other forms of capital on health (Veenstra and Abel, 2019). Taking their cue from Portes' (1998) original critique, Villalonga-Olives and Kawachi (2017: 106) also appear to be calling for much greater reflexivity within public health research about framing social capital as 'the panacea to solve health related problems'. In this respect, and despite theoretical differences, they are on the same page as Veenstra and Abel (2019).

In light of the evidence, there needs to be a shift away from viewing social capital as universally beneficial to health. More recently, this view is supported by a study examining the role of income inequality and social capital in accounting for cross-national differences in mortality from COVID-19 during the first phase of the pandemic (Elgar et al., 2020). Not surprisingly, the study reports a positive correlation between income inequality and mortality rates. However, the study also found that different forms of social capital varied in their impact and were not consistently beneficial to good health. Whilst civic engagement and confidence in state institutions were associated with fewer deaths, ceteris paribus, the reverse occurred with social trust and group affiliations. This is a timely reminder that social capital is not a panacea for altering the course of a pandemic or the structural inequalities that socially pattern infection and death. While the original research agenda was shaped by a focus on how social capital mediates economic inequalities, current debates point to a shift in focus to how access to and mobilization of specific forms of social capital are linked to power differentials in social relations and social organization. Shiell et al. (2020), for example, point to the need to address social capital as a context-level variable. They make this argument given the contradictory evidence linking social capital to health and the uncertain efficacy of public health interventions intent on building social capital as a way of ameliorating health inequalities. Arguably, Shiell et al.'s thinking could help to reset the research agenda and inform policy. Here the focus would be on how types of social capital are reproduced and mobilized in different social contexts, their 'distributional impacts' and the need to tailor health interventions in order to reduce or avoid negative unintended consequences. In addition, research would need to explore whether specific forms of context-led action can alter the structural dynamics underpinning health inequalities.

See also: Material and Cultural Factors; Neoliberalism; Place; Psychosocial Factors.

REFERENCES

Dahl, E. and Malmberg-Heimonen, I. (2010) 'Social inequality and health: the role of social capital', *Sociology of Health & Illness*, 32 (7): 1102–1119.

Dorn, A.V., Cooney, R.E. and Sabin, M.L. (2020) 'COVID-19 exacerbating inequalities in the US', *Lancet*, 395 (10232): 1243–1244.

Ehsan, A., Klaas, H.S., Bastianen, A. and Spini, D. (2019) 'Social capital and health: a systematic review of systematic reviews', *SSM – Population Health*, 8: 1–18.

Elgar, F.A., Stefaniak, A. and Wohl, M.J.A. (2020) 'The trouble with trust: time-series analysis of social capital, income inequality, and COVID-19 deaths in 84 countries', *Social Science & Medicine*, 263: 113365.

Garnham, L.M. (2015) 'Understanding the impacts of industrial change and area-based deprivation on health inequalities, using Swidler's concepts of cultured capacities and strategies of action', *Social Theory & Health*, 13 (3/4): 308–339.

Kawachi, I., Kennedy, B.P. and Glass, R. (1999) 'Social capital and self-rated health: a contextual analysis', *American Journal of Public Health*, 89 (8): 1187–1193.

Navarro, V. (2002) 'A critique of social capital', *International Journal of Health Services*, 32 (3): 423–432.

Portes, A. (1998) 'Social capital: its origins and applications in modern sociology', *Annual Review of Sociology,* 24 (1): 1–24.

Putnam, R. (1995) 'Bowling alone: America's declining social capital', *Journal of Democracy*, 6 (1): 65–78.

Rodgers, J., Valuev, A.V., Hswen, Y. and Subramanian, S.V. (2019) 'Social capital and physical health: an update review of the literature for 2007–2018', *Social Science & Medicine*, 236: 1–12.

Shiell, A., Hawe, P. and Kavanagh, S. (2020) 'Evidence suggests a need to rethink social capital and social capital interventions', *Social Science & Medicine*, 257: 111930.

Szreter, S. and Woolcock, M. (2004) 'Health by association? Social capital, social theory, and the political economy of public health', *International Journal of Epidemiology*, 33 (4): 650–667.

Veenstra, G. and Abel, T. (2019) 'Capital interplays and social inequalities in health', *Scandinavian Journal of Public Health*, 47: 631–634.

Villalonga-Olives, E. and Kawachi, I. (2017) 'The dark side of social capital: a systematic review of the negative health effects of social capital', *Social Science & Medicine*, 194: 105–127.

Villalonga-Olives, E., Wind, T.R. and Kawachi, I. (2018) 'Social capital interventions in public health: a systematic review', *Social Science & Medicine*, 212: 203–218.

Wilkinson, R.G. (1996) *Unhealthy Societies: The Afflictions of Inequality*. London: Routledge.

Wilkinson, R.G. and Pickett, K. (2009) *The Spirit Level: Why More Equal Societies Almost Always Do Better*. London: Allen Lane.

SUGGESTED FURTHER READING

- Moore, S. and Carpiano, R.M. (2020) 'Introduction to the special issue on "social capital and health: what have we learned in the last 20 years and where do we go from here?"' *Social Science & Medicine*, 257: 113014.

This special issue contains eight articles on social capital, spanning the Global North and South. Themes range from vaccine refusal to power inequalities.

- Bartscher, A.K., Seitz., S., Sieglich, S. et al. (2020) *Social Capital and the Spread of Covid-19: Insights from European Countries*, CESifo Working Paper, No. 8346, Center for Economic Studies and ifo Institute (CESifo), Munich. Online: http://hdl.handle.net/10419/219164

This study compares high and low social capital areas with mobility behaviour from seven European countries. The key policy implications are that investment in social capital is vital to pandemic preparedness and addressing the consequences of the current crisis.

- Borgonovi, F. and Andrieu, E. (2020) 'Bowling together by bowling alone: social capital and COVID-19', *Social Science & Medicine*, 265: 113501.

This article focuses on the association between community-level social capital and behavioural change (reduction in retail and recreational mobility) during the early phase of the pandemic in the USA. It suggests social capital shaped behaviours that helped to reduce the spread and impact of COVID-19. Fostering social capital, via participatory politics and trusting citizens for example, is deemed to be of equal priority to sourcing stocks of facemasks and testing kits.

- Nazroo, J. (2017) 'Class and health inequalities in later life: patterns, mechanisms and implications for policy', *International Journal of Environmental Research and Public Health*, 14: 1533.

By applying Bourdieu's theory of capitals to the English Longitudinal Study of Ageing, Nazroo demonstrates how class mechanisms operate in later life to impact on the resources that individuals can mobilize to protect health and well-being. This mode of analysis has clear policy implications for reforms that seek to increase the state pension age at the same time as privatizing social security and individualizing health risks.

PART 2

EXPERIENCE OF HEALTH AND ILLNESS

15

Medicalization

Jonathan Gabe

Medicalization describes a process by which non-medical problems become defined and treated as medical problems, usually in terms of illnesses or disorders.

Medicalization is now established as a key sociological concept, yet it is difficult to be specific about when it entered the social scientific lexicon. It seems that the process was originally referred to by critics of the growing influence of psychiatry in the 1960s (although these critics did not use the term explicitly), and it increased in popularity in the 1970s when linked with the concept of social control. Since then medicalization has been applied to a variety of putative problems that (at times contentiously) came to be defined as medical, ranging from childbirth and the menopause through to alcoholism and homosexuality.

According to Conrad and Schneider (1980), medicalization can occur on three distinct levels: conceptually, when a medical vocabulary is used to define a problem; institutionally, when organizations adopt a medical approach to treating a problem in which they specialize; and at the level of doctor–patient interaction, when a problem is defined as medical and medical treatment occurs. As these distinctions illustrate, the process often involves physicians and their treatments directly. However, this is not necessarily so, as in the case of alcoholism where the medical profession may be only marginally involved or not involved at all.

Conrad and Schneider's typology can be mapped onto the distinction between macro, meso and micro levels of analysis. Macro level actors include medical researchers and journals, governments and national organizations and the meso level would include local organizations, while doctor–patient interaction concerns mainly micro level actors. Halfmann (2011) argues that medicalization occurs at all three levels. Thus medical discourses can be deployed at the meso level by hospital managers and at the micro level by patients and doctors, as well as at the macro level. He also notes that medicalization at the micro level can involve clinical personnel other than doctors and non-medical actors such as teachers and counsellors. Furthermore, he recognizes that micro level medicalization can occur through the identity construction of various actors, with doctors, for example, fulfilling cultural expectations to varying degrees about what 'being a doctor' involves.

Medicalization is often associated with the control of deviance and the ways in which deviant behaviours that were once defined as immoral, sinful or criminal have been given medical meanings. The process of medicalizing deviant behaviour is not straightforward, however, and can be seen as involving a five-stage sequential process (Conrad and Schneider, 1992). The first stage involves a behaviour being defined as deviant, usually before the emergence of modern medical definitions. For example, chronic drunkenness was held to be highly undesirable before any medical writer defined it as such. The second stage occurs when the medical conception of a deviant behaviour is announced in a professional medical journal. Descriptions of a new diagnosis (for example, hyperactivity) or the proposal of a medical aetiology for a type of deviant behaviour (for example, alcoholism) are used to redefine this as a medical problem. Next comes claims-making by medical and non-medical interest groups. This stage is crucial if a new deviance designation is to emerge. Medical claims-makers are not usually organized specifically to promote a new medical deviance category but involve a loose alliance of people with similar professional interests. The activities of non-medical claims-makers (for example, pharmaceutical companies or self-help groups) may be more overt and involve engaging in publicity campaigns or political lobbying. They often align themselves with medical claims-makers and use these medical champions to lend scientific credibility to their claims. The fourth stage in the process involves the legitimation of a claim. This occurs when claims-makers launch an instrumental, as opposed to merely a rhetorical, challenge to the existing deviance designation. Finally, medicalization occurs when the medical deviance designation is institutionalized. This can be when a deviance designation is codified within a medical classification system, or when a bureaucracy is created to provide institutionalized support for medicalization. The value of this theoretical model is that it suggests that attempts to conceptualize deviance as a medical problem are often hotly disputed and carry uncertain outcomes. Perhaps surprisingly, however, there have been relatively few attempts to evaluate the cost or usefulness of medicalization or to try and develop it as a concept (but see Conrad et al., 2010, and Busfield, 2017).

The logic of this model suggests that the degree to which a condition is medicalized will vary. For some conditions medicalization may be total whereas for others competing definitions may exist and their medicalization will remain incomplete or even minimal. According to Conrad (1992), a number of factors may affect the degree of medicalization. These include the support of the medical profession, the availability of interventions or treatments, the existence of competing definitions and the actions of groups challenging medical definitions.

Nor should it be assumed that medicalization is only a one-way process. It is also possible for demedicalization to occur if a problem ceases to be defined in medical terms and medical treatments are no longer seen as an appropriate solution. Indeed Halfmann (2011) argues that medicalization and demedicalization can occur simultaneously and that even when one of these processes seems to be dominant it is often incomplete.

The most frequently mentioned example of demedicalization is homosexuality in America which, until 1973, was defined by the American Psychiatric Association (APA) as an illness. After protests and picketing by the gay liberation movement and support from some sympathetic psychiatrists, the APA voted to declassify it as an illness, a decision that was later endorsed in the UK. As a result, homosexuality became more widely recognized as a lifestyle choice. With the onset of the AIDS epidemic in the 1980s, however, it became partially remedicalized, although in a different form. Overall, the evidence to date is that medicalization is far more apparent than demedicalization but it remains important to see it as a two-way process.

While there is now some consensus about the nature of medicalization there is no such agreement about its cause. Some have argued that the expansion of medical jurisdiction is primarily a consequence of the medical profession exercising its power to define and control what constitutes health and illness in order to extend its professional dominance. Others have considered medicalization to be the result of broader social processes to which doctors are simply responding. Thus Illich (1976), for example, attributes medicalization to the increasing professionalization and bureaucratization of medical institutions associated with industrialization. For him the expansion of modern medicine has created a dependence on doctors and taken away people's ability to engage in self-care. Zola (1972), too, has argued that medicalization is rooted in the development of an increasingly complex technological and bureaucratic system and a reliance on the expert.

More recently Conrad (2007) has identified a shift in what is driving medicalization, with pharmaceutical and biotech companies, along with consumers, playing an increasingly important role. For Conrad pharmaceutical companies have become the major players, more aggressively promoting their products to doctors as well as to consumers. In the USA and New Zealand drug companies can now advertise prescription medicines directly to the public through direct-to-consumer-advertising on television, thereby creating a market for their products by encouraging consumers to ask doctors to prescribe their particular drugs. Biotechnology companies are becoming increasingly important, with genetic tests for certain diseases, thereby creating the new medicalized status of 'potentially ill', and biomedical enhancements for bodily characteristics and mental and social abilities. And consumers are said to have become major players as health and healthcare have become commodified. The body has become a site for varies types and degrees of 'makeover' with medicine as the vehicle, and patients have been transformed into consumers who are said to have become increasingly vocal about the kind of healthcare they want.

Many writers tend to conceive of medicalization in a negative way, focusing on how the phenomenon has resulted in a form of medical social control that serves particular interests in society. For Marxists such medicalization is best seen as serving the interests of the ruling capitalist class. From this standpoint, the creation and manipulation of consumer dependence on medicine is merely one example of a more general dependence upon consumer goods propagated by that class. For feminists the focus has tended to be on how a male-dominated medical profession has increasingly defined women's experiences or problems in medical terms and advocated medical interventions. Women's experience of childbirth has been a particular focus of attention. Here it has been suggested that doctors' use of obstetric techniques such as foetal monitoring machines, pain-killing drugs, induction and forceps without telling women patients why such techniques are necessary or what the risks are, has resulted in their experiencing childbirth as alienating. Moreover, as it is usually male doctors who control such technology, its coercive utilization is seen as reinforcing existing patriarchal social relations.

In contrast, others emphasize the real clinical and symbolic benefits of medicalization. Redefining a condition as appropriate for medical attention opens up opportunities for the alleviation of symptoms or a cure and also legitimates it, possibly reducing the stigma and censure that may be attached. In the case of chronic fatigue syndrome, for instance, it seems that patients may benefit from a diagnosis simply because it renders an otherwise incoherent and disruptive experience meaningful and opens up possibilities for managing and living with the syndrome. Similarly, those with a drinking problem may benefit from the label of alcoholism as a disease, enabling them to counteract attributions of blame and moral weakness. Medicalization has also meant that they are now less likely to be arrested for being drunk in a public place and more likely to be medically treated in a potentially more humane way than would otherwise be the case.

The medicalization thesis has much to recommend it, including the creation of new understandings of the social processes involved in the development and response to medical diagnosis and treatment and the development of a critical framework for analysing medicine, health and healthcare. However, a number of significant criticisms have also been levelled against it, especially its more negative variant. In particular, it has been criticized for portraying the individual patient and the lay public more generally as essentially passive and uncritical in the face of modern medicine's expanding jurisdiction. For example, Riessman (1989) in her discussion of women's experience of different conditions, ranging from childbirth to premenstrual syndrome, has drawn attention to the way in which women have at times actively participated in the medicalization process to meet their own needs and have not simply been passive victims of medical ascendancy. Williams and Calnan (1996) have developed this critique further by drawing on arguments about 'risk society' and lay re-skilling. They suggest that in late modernity there is a far more critical relationship between medicine and the lay populace and that people's trust in medicine increasingly has to be won and maintained in the face of growing public awareness of the risks as well as benefits of medicine and the limits of medical expertise. Ballard and Elston (2005) agree with this assessment and see the move to a late- or postmodern world as one where there is likely to be more contestation of medicalization and the possibility of its decline.

Others have suggested that the concept has outlived its usefulness and propose that it should be replaced. Thus Clarke et al. (2003) have argued that medicalization should be re-conceptualized in terms of biomedicalization, as this better captures the transformations in the organization and practice of medicine since the 1980s. In particular they assert that much more attention needs to be given to the role of techno-scientific innovations (for example, the computerization of patient medical records) and the increasingly technological and scientific nature of biomedicine (for example, the geneticization of biomedicine and drug design). However, Conrad (2007) argues that biomedicalization is too broad a concept, which emphasizes a more extensive set of changes than is meant by medicalization and as such compromises its focus. And Busfield (2017) suggests that biomedicalization and medicalization cannot be used to refer to specific eras of medicine, as suggested by Clarke et al. (2003), as medicalization is concerned with processes that occur across time and place and not with a particular period in medicine's development.

A further concept that has been introduced is pharmaceuticalization, which it has been argued captures important changes that medicalization does not, namely the growing importance of pharmaceuticals for non-medical as well as medical reasons (for example, the domestic use of pharmaceuticals for aesthetic purposes such as building muscle mass). Conrad (2013) claims that pharmaceuticalization is merely a subset of medicalization, and Busfield (2017) agrees, suggesting that we do not need to treat them as parallel terms and that it has little analytical value beyond what medicalization already offers. Others, such as Williams et al. (2017) and Abraham (2010), argue that there are significant differences between them and that they need to be treated as analytically distinct, even if they may overlap and can be difficult to disentangle.

While many of the criticisms of medicalization are well made, it remains a useful multi-dimensional concept for sociologists of health and illness. Indeed, its continuing relevance can be seen in the context of COVID-19 where vaccinations have been turned to as the main way to end 'lockdown' by reducing the prevalence of disease. There is, however, a need to go beyond the accumulation of different cases of medicalization in order to try and develop a more integrated theory of the process of medicalization, its causes and consequences and to relate these to recent changes in medical organization, knowledge and the growing challenge to medical authority. Clarifying the link between medicalization and globalization is also important, as the COVID pandemic illustrates.

See also: Consumerism; Geneticization; Medical Autonomy, Dominance and Decline; Pharmaceuticalization; Reproduction; Risk; The Medical Model.

REFERENCES

Abraham, J. (2010) 'Pharmaceuticalization of society in context: theoretical, empirical and health dimensions', *Sociology*, 44 (4): 603–622.

Ballard, K. and Elston, M.A. (2005) 'Medicalization: a multi-dimensional concept', *Social Theory & Health*, 3 (3): 228–241.

Busfield, J. (2017) 'The concept of medicalisation reassessed', *Sociology of Health & Illness*, 39 (5): 759–774.

Clarke, A., Mamo, L., Fishman, J.R. et al. (2003) 'Biomedicalization: technoscientific transformations of health, illness and biomedicine', *American Sociological Review*, 68: 161–194.

Conrad, P. (1992) 'Medicalization and social control', *Annual Review of Sociology*, 18: 209–232.

Conrad, P. (2007) *The Medicalization of Society*. Baltimore: The Johns Hopkins University Press.

Conrad, P. (2013) 'Medicalization: changing contours, characteristics and contexts', in W. Cockerham (ed.), *Medical Sociology on the Move*. New York: Springer.

Conrad, P. and Schneider, J.W. (1980) 'Looking at levels of medicalization: a comment on Strong's critique of the thesis of medical imperialism', *Social Science & Medicine*, 14A: 75–79.

Conrad, P. and Schneider, J.W. (1992) *Deviance and Medicalization. From Badness to Sickness*, 3rd edn. Philadelphia: Temple University Press.

Conrad, P., Mackie, T. and Mehrotra, A. (2010) 'Estimating the costs of medicalization', *Social Science & Medicine*, 70 (12): 1943–1947.

Halfmann, D. (2011) 'Recognizing medicalization and demedicalization: discourses, practices and identities', *Health*, 16 (2): 186–207.

Illich, I. (1976) *Medical Nemesis*. London: Calder and Boyars.

Riessman, C.K. (1989) 'Women and medicalisation: a new perspective', in P. Brown (ed.), *Perspectives in Medical Sociology*. Belmont, CA: Wadsworth.

Williams, S.J. and Calnan, M. (1996) 'The "limits" of medicalisation? Modern medicine and the lay populace', *Social Science & Medicine*, 42 (12): 1609–1620.

Williams, S.J., Coveney, C. and Gabe, J. (2017) 'The concept of medicalisation reassessed: a response to Joan Busfield', *Sociology of Health & Illness*, 39 (5) 775–780.

Zola, I. (1972) 'Medicine as an institution of social control', *Sociological Review*, 20 (4): 487–504.

SUGGESTED FURTHER READING

- Strong, P.M. (1979) 'Sociological imperialism and the profession of medicine: a critical examination of the thesis of medical imperialism', *Social Science & Medicine*, 13A: 199–215.

Strong provides a still relevant critique of sociology's employment of the medicalization concept. While noting that the negative portrayals of medical expansion often found in the medicalization thesis contain important insights, he argues that they are in certain respects exaggerated and self-serving. Medical sociologists' failure to be self-conscious about their own vested interests has resulted, he suggests, in a tendency to exaggerate the degree of medical power and ignore constraints on medicalization, such as state control.

- Williams, S. and Gabe, J. (2015) 'Peter Conrad: the medicalisation of society', in F. Collyer (ed.), *The Palgrave Handbook of Social Theory in Health, Illness and Medicine*. Basingstoke: Palgrave Macmillan.

A broad ranging assessment of Conrad's contribution to the developments and debates regarding the 'medicalisation of society'. Conrad is viewed as the leading sociological exponent of medicalization.

- Bell, A.V. (2017) 'The gas that fuels the engine: individuals' motivations for medicalisation', *Sociology of Health & Illness*, 39 (8): 1480–1495.

An interesting study of lesbian reproduction in the USA, exploring the claim that individual patients/consumers are pushing the process of medicalization forward rather than macro processes of institutional prestige and control. It is argued that while individual patients may be propelling this process forward, often their motivation for doing so resides in the prestige and control of medicine, thus revealing the interplay between micro and macro. The data come from in-depth interviews with same-sex couples seeking to benefit from assisted reproductive technology.

16

Pharmaceuticalization

Jonathan Gabe

Pharmaceuticalization is a multi-dimensional process that involves 'the translation or transformation of human conditions, capabilities and capacities into opportunities for pharmaceutical intervention' (Williams et al., 2011a: 711).

Sociologists have studied pharmaceutical medicines, designed to treat illness, since the 1970s. However, interest in pharmaceuticals has grown significantly in recent years in recognition of their increasing role in people's lives and the expanding power and profitability of the companies that manufacture them. Some sociologists have argued that the escalating reach of such companies and their products can be incorporated under the concept 'medicalization' (Conrad, 2007); that is a process by which non-medical issues become defined and treated as medical problems, usually in terms of illnesses or disorders. Others have suggested that a new concept, pharmaceuticalization, is needed to understand fully the contemporary importance of pharmaceuticals and their manufacturers (Abraham, 2010; Williams et al., 2011a). Below we consider the argument in favour of this new concept, the factors which distinguish it from medicalization and the dimensions that mark it out. We conclude by considering some of the debates about the concept's utility.

According to Williams et al. (2011a: 711), pharmaceuticalization is part of a 'pharmaceutical regime' made up of networks of institutions, organizations, actors and artefacts, as well as the cognitive structures associated with the creation, production and use of new therapeutics. It is a complex, dynamic socio-technical process that involves the discovery, use and governance of pharmaceutical products centred on a chemically-based technology. One of the important benefits of defining the concept in this way is that it encompasses *non-medical* uses of pharmaceuticals for lifestyle enhancement by 'healthy' people. Such substances may be bought over the internet without any direct involvement by a medical practitioner. As this suggests, one can therefore have pharmaceuticalization without any significant medicalization.

Like some advocates of medicalization, Williams et al. see pharmaceuticalization as a value-neutral, descriptive term which involves both gains and losses for society. The extent to which the process has occurred is also seen as an empirical question to be established on a case-by-case basis. It is thus possible to envisage the process as both partial and incomplete. Like medicalization it can also be conceptualized as involving different levels (macro processes such as drug testing and regulation through to micro level processes concerned with the meaning and use of medicines) and as being bi-directional (allowing for de-pharmaceuticalization as well as pharmaceuticalization). It is also possible that some people may seek to resist pharmaceuticalization while others may campaign for increased access to particular medicines.

Williams et al. (2011a) identify six interrelated and overlapping dimensions of pharmaceuticalization, which have been developed as a heuristic: selling sickness; changing forms of governance; the role of the mass media; the actions of patients and consumer groups; drugs for non-medical purposes; and pharmaceutical futures in the making. These will be briefly summarized below, also drawing from the work of others.

The first dimension, *selling sickness*, is concerned with the way in which health problems are redefined as having a pharmaceutical solution. It can be broken down into two aspects. One way in which this can be seen is through the massive growth of drug markets, especially in the USA and Europe. As a result, drug solutions to defined health problems have become much more widespread. The pharmaceutical industry is one of the most profitable in the world, enjoying profits of 25 per cent for most of the 1990s and with worldwide yearly spending on medicines reaching $1.25 trillion in 2019 (up from $887 billion in 2010) (Mikulic, 2020). Sales in middle-income countries such as China and India have been increasing at a faster rate than in the West, but from a lower base. Pharmaceutical industry profits are likely to grow further from COVID vaccine development and distribution, especially in the Global North, although drug companies in countries like China and India are also likely to benefit. Another way in which sickness has been sold is through the marketing, if not manufacture of disorders. Moynihan (2002) has claimed that pharmaceutical companies have been involved in 'disease mongering' by which he means that drug companies have widened the boundaries of treatable illness in order to expand the market for their products. This has involved turning ordinary ailments into medical problems such as 'restless leg syndrome'. While the arguments underpinning 'disease mongering' are of potential interest Williams et al. (2011a) argue that this concept's analytic value is restricted because it contains an inbuilt element of normative judgement.

The second dimension, *changing forms of governance*, concerns reforms that have reduced the regulatory hurdle while increasing regulators' dependence on the pharmaceutical industry. This is illustrated by the work of Abraham and colleagues, involving detailed empirical case studies of the regulation of medicines for diseases such as cancer and diabetes (e.g. Davis and Abraham, 2013). These studies have provided evidence of corporate bias and privileged access of pharmaceutical companies to regulatory bodies such as the Food and Drug Administration (FDA) in the USA and the Medicine and Health Care Regulatory Agency in the UK. At the same time the relationship between these companies and regulators is getting closer as the former now have to pay most of the cost of funding the latter in return for a significant reduction in review times for new drugs. And fast tracking has been introduced for the approval of drugs for life-threatening conditions, with companies now required to provide less data than usual to demonstrate efficacy. As a result, regulators have become increasingly vulnerable to market pressures, with agencies competing with each other.

A third dimension concerns *the mass media*, which is clearly involved in the process of pharmaceuticalization as a conveyor or amplifier rather than as a catalyst. The best example of this process can be found in Direct to Consumer Advertising (DCA) in the USA and New Zealand, where media advertising of prescription only products is commonplace. Techniques used in DCA include the voices of experts and patients, celebrity endorsements and offering symptom-based self testing. Such self testing provides diagnostic validity to the condition and proposes a pharmaceutical solution. At the same time mass media are not puppets of the drug companies. Media coverage can be contradictory or condemnatory, oscillating between extremes, and proclaiming the benefits of a medication or demonizing its users (Seale, 2002). Media coverage of new drugs is largely uncritical or even celebratory; however, if unwanted side effects appear, negative or critical portrayals follow. Abraham (2011) has suggested that the shift in media coverage, from an enthusiastic welcome to subsequent criticism may simply be a consequence of the media reporting new clinical evidence after the drug has come to market. However, the evidence to date about media coverage of a range of pharmaceuticals suggests that such reporting is not dependent on the novelty of medicine but is a result of the nature of media reporting. Journalists constantly need to come up with a new angle or newsworthy story (Williams et al., 2011b). While the discussion so far has been about traditional media (newspapers, television and magazines) we also need to consider new media in the form of the internet. The latter is particularly important because it provides the opportunity for people to buy pharmaceuticals online, thus bypassing the doctor–patient relationship. According to Fox and Ward (2009), the pharmaceuticalization of daily life via the internet involves two broad processes. First there is the domestication of pharmaceutical consumption, as computer-mediated access to and use of these products usually occurs at home. Second is the pharmaceuticalization of daily life, as pharmaceuticals are presented as 'magic bullets' for a range of day-to-day problems. Like other media, however, these processes are not straightforward as the internet offers both new opportunities for pharmaceuticalization and new spaces for challenging these processes. We can see this process in play with regard to vaccines for COVID-19.

The internet has provided opportunities for advocates of vaccination to proclaim these as a way out of lockdown, while others have questioned their efficacy and the risks of side effects, such as blood clots.

A fourth dimension involves *patient and consumer groups*. Much has been written in recent years about the increasingly active, if not critical, role that patients and consumers play in their own healthcare. This is particularly true with regard to studies of users of medicines, who are often portrayed as knowledgeable, reflexive actors, assessing the risks and benefits of the medicines offered and making informed choices about which ones to consume (Stevenson et al., 2002). And these developments have been reinforced by current health policy in many countries in the Global North which construct patients as experts and partners with clinicians in their own healthcare. The rise of the articulate, information rich consumer offers contrasting opportunities. On the one hand, it suggests the potential for various challenges or forms of resistance to pharmaceuticalization, as we have seen in response to COVID-19 vaccinations. On the other hand, it may fuel further pharmaceuticalization through patient-driven demands for medicines, with or without DCA. At the same time it seems that professional expertise is still valued when it comes to people making decisions about medicines. Patients continue to ask general practitioners and pharmacists for advice. Moreover, patients may have a collective voice as members of self-help groups or patient advocacy organizations. Furthermore, some of these groups may receive financial support from pharmaceutical companies to press for early access to an as yet unlicensed drug, while others may demand that companies remove what they feel to be unsafe drugs from the market.

The fifth dimension involves the *use of medications for non-medical purposes*: the shift from treatment to enhancement. The desire to improve ourselves in one way or another is as old as human history. What has changed are the means of doing so. Enhancement itself is however a contested term as it is frequently used to indicate going beyond treatment or health to become better than well. Conrad (2007) discusses three main types of biomedical enhancement: a) normalization, where biomedical enhancements are used to bring the body into line with what doctors or patients consider is normal or socially expected; b) repair, in which biomedical interventions are used to restore the body to its previous condition; and c) augmentation, to boost performance in order to give someone a competitive edge. Context is of course important, so the notion of enhancement relates to when or how it is used more than the type of intervention per se. It is also clear that not all forms of enhancement are for non-medical purposes: medical professionals perform cosmetic surgery and prescribe medicines, such as human growth hormone, for medical reasons. Pharmaceuticalization may nonetheless occur in the absence of any medical involvement, for example when healthy people use pharmaceuticals for non-medical reasons to enhance their performance and/or appearance. One example which illustrates this point about performance well is the use of cognitive enhancement medications to improve alertness and memory (Coveney et al., 2019a). Given the lack of knowledge about the medical or social risks of using these drugs for non-medical reasons we need to be cautious when evaluating their use. What is clear is that any attempt by pharmaceutical companies to reconstruct the use of these drugs for enhancement represents another case of creating new drug markets involving a relationship with consumers, outside the control of the medical profession.

The sixth and final dimension of pharmaceuticalization is termed *pharmaceutical futures in the making*. Work in Science and Technology Studies on the sociology of expectations has drawn attention to the key role of the future in shaping the present (Gardner et al., 2015). In particular, it highlights the dynamic role that expectations play in attracting support and investors and building communities of hope for those who have life-threatening conditions. Take, for example, the field of pharmacogenetics – the use of genetic knowledge to predict drug reactions. Pharmacogenetics has generated much speculation about the dawn of a new era of personalized medicine, where tailor-made treatments are geared to an individual's genetic profile. This in turn holds out the promise of more effective drugs that have far fewer adverse reactions than is the case currently with 'one size fits all' treatments. As a result, alternative futures are crowded out and the search for new medicines is seen as the best way to improve human health. At the same time, despite much talk of a pharmacogenetic revolution, progress has been slow and there is currently little evidence of the widespread benefits envisaged by these expectations. As such, one might well ask why the belief in the biotechnology revolution remains so influential? The answer is, in part at least, the power of expectations. Claims about the biotechnology revolution act as rhetorical devices to generate the necessary political, social and financial capital to allow the perceived promise to emerge.

Having considered the arguments in favour of pharmaceuticalization, the factors which distinguish it from medicalization and the dimensions that mark it out, we now turn to some of the debates about its use and value. One is to do with how expansive the definition of pharmaceuticalization should be. Abraham (2011) has argued that Williams et al.'s (2011a) definition is too expansive as it could include taking heroin or cocaine or overdosing to commit suicide. Williams et al. have defended their position and suggested that the definition needs to be expansive in order to include the use of medicines outside of medical authority. However, they argued that the illicit use of heroin or cocaine for 'lifestyle purposes' is excluded because these drugs are not produced by pharmaceutical companies. Another concern relates to the amount of emphasis given to de-pharmaceuticalization. Abraham (2011) has suggested that Williams et al. (2011a) have underplayed the possibility of de-pharmaceuticalization. The latter have responded by suggesting that pharmaceuticalization has so far outstripped de-pharmaceuticalization and that there are few if any areas of life which, once pharmaceuticalized, have subsequently become fully de-pharmaceuticalized. Their underplaying of de-pharmaceuticalization was therefore intentional. A further argument revolves around whether pharmaceuticalization is better understood as a postmodern or modern development. For Bell and Figert (2012), medicalization, the forerunner to pharmaceuticalization, is grounded in the modern world, which focuses on progress, mass production and consumption, whereas pharmaceuticalization is best understood in terms of postmodern characteristics such as contingency, fragmentation and volatility. Others have questioned the assumption that only a postmodern standpoint can take account of contingency and complexity (Williams et al., 2012). Finally some (e.g. Busfield, 2017) have suggested that pharmaceuticalization has little analytical value beyond what medicalization already offers. Those advocating pharmaceuticalization, such as Coveney et al. (2019b), have suggested that pharmaceuticalization can intertwine with medicalization in complex ways which should not be conflated or collapsed into one another. Coveney et al. demonstrate this complexity in their study of the medical management of sleeplessness as insomnia. For example, they report that sleep experts seemed to want to have greater medicalization of sleeplessness as insomnia without necessarily more pharmaceuticalization, given the availability of other non-pharmaceutical alternatives.

To conclude, it has been argued that pharmaceuticalization is a complex and dynamic process involving the development of a pharmaceutical regime. This regime comprises a range of actors, from clinicians, patients and consumers to regulators and pharmaceutical companies. The extent to which these actors can be seen to be involved in pharmaceuticalization is context-specific and depends on the interplay between them at any one time. The six dimensions discussed above have a number of common features: the expansion of drug markets outside traditional areas (new medical indications and conditions, new applications in healthy individuals); the increasing dominance of state regulators; moves to bypass the medical profession and create more direct relations with patients and consumers; and the colonization of daily life by pharmaceutical solutions. Taken together they reflect a process that is distinct from medicalization in important respects. As we have seen, there have been a number of critical assessments of pharmaceuticalization as a concept since it was first introduced. Further research is necessary to continue to assess and develop this concept as a means of exploring the dynamic interactions between the pharmaceutical industry, regulators, the medical profession, the media, patients, publics more generally and the shaping of health and illness. The COVID-19 pandemic provides a particularly useful case study of such interactions, with vaccines offering an example of both the risks and benefits of pharmaceuticalization. Indeed, debates about the safety of particular vaccines and the actions of regulators in (temporarily) halting vaccination programmes while the latest data on side effects are assessed and the risk benefit ratio re-calibrated are ripe for sociological research. Lay and professional understandings of such risks and the situated nature of their rationality also need to be considered. Finally, what about unequal access to vaccines, especially in the Global South, and attempts to challenge what some call 'vaccine apartheid'?

See also: Consumerism; Geneticization; Medicalization; Medicines Regulation; Risk; The Medical Model; Trust in Medicine.

REFERENCES

Abraham, J. (2010) 'Pharmaceuticalization of society in context: theoretical, empirical and health dimensions', *Sociology*, 44 (4): 603–622.

Abraham, J. (2011) 'Evolving sociological analyses of pharmaceuticalisation: a response to Williams, Martin and Gabe', *Sociology of Health & Illness*, 33 (5): 726–728.

Bell, S. and Figert, A. (2012) 'Medicalization and pharmaceuticalization at the intersections: looking backwards, forwards and sideways', *Social Science & Medicine*, 75 (5): 775–783.

Busfield, J. (2017) 'The concept of medicalisation re-assessed', *Sociology of Health & Illness*, 39 (5): 759–774.

Conrad, P. (2007) *The Medicalization of Society*. Baltimore: Johns Hopkins University Press.

Coveney, C., Williams, S.J. and Gabe, J. (2019a) 'Cognitive enhancing drugs: re-imagining the drug user in drugs policy', *Drugs: Education, Prevention and Policy*, 26 (4): 319–328.

Coveney, C., Williams, S.J. and Gabe, J. (2019b) 'Medicalisation, pharmaceuticalisation or both? Exploring medical management of sleeplessness as insomnia', *Sociology of Health & Illness*, 41 (2): 266–286.

Davis, C. and Abraham, J. (2013) *Unhealthy Pharmaceutical Regulation*. Basingstoke: Palgrave Macmillan.

Fox, N.J. and Ward, K.J. (2009) 'Pharma in the bedroom... and in the kitchen ... The pharmaceuticalisation of daily life', in S.J. Williams, J. Gabe and P. Davis (eds), *Pharmaceuticals and Society: Critical Discourses and Debates*. Oxford: Blackwell.

Gardner, J., Samuel, G. and Williams, C. (2015) 'Sociology of low expectations: recalibration as innovation work in biomedicine', *Science, Technology, & Human Values*, 40 (6): 998–1021.

Mikulic, M. (2020) *'Global spending on medicines 2010–2024'*. Online: www.statista.com/statistics/280572/medicine-spending-worldwide/

Moynihan, R. (2002) 'Disease mongering: how doctors, drug companies, and insurers are making you feel sick', *British Medical Journal*, 324 (7342): 923.

Seale, C. (2002) *Media and Health*. London: SAGE.

Stevenson, F., Britten, N., Barry, C. and Barber, N. (2002) 'Perceptions of legitimacy: the influence of medicine taking and prescribing', *Health*, 6 (1): 85–104.

Williams, S.J., Gabe, J. and Martin, P. (2012) 'Medicalization and pharmaceuticalization at the intersections: a commentary on Bell and Figert', *Social Science & Medicine*, 75 (12): 2129–2130.

Williams, S.J., Martin, P. and Gabe, J. (2011a) 'The pharmaceuticalisation of society? A framework for analysis', *Sociology of Health & Illness*, 33 (5): 710–725.

Williams, S.J., Martin, P. and Gabe, J. (2011b) 'Evolving sociological analyses of pharmaceuticalisation: a response to Abraham', *Sociology of Health & Illness*, 33 (5): 729–730.

SUGGESTED FURTHER READING

- Gabe, J., Williams, S., Martin, P. and Coveney, C. (eds) (2015) 'Pharmaceuticalization: problems and prospects', *Social Science & Medicine (Special Issue)*, 131: 193–330.

A useful compilation of papers covering issues ranging from the overuse of medicines to clinical trials and contract research organizations and the non-medical use of prescription stimulants. Case studies cover both the Global North and Global South.

- Dew, K. (2019) *Public Health, Personal Health and Pills. Drug Entanglements and Pharmaceuticalised Governance*. London: Routledge.

Building on both the medicalization and pharmaceuticalization literatures this book explores the processes and effects of the increasing governance of our lives through pharmaceuticals. It combines macro considerations of pharmaceutical consumption, regulation and policy, micro considerations of the negotiation of medicine use in homes and clinics and institutional analysis of the role of drug monitoring agencies, drug trial methodologies and the media.

- Johnson, E. with Sjogren, E. and Asberg, C. (2016) *Glocal Pharma*. Abingdon: Routledge.

Engaging with debates about pharmaceuticalization, the authors consider how global pharmaceutical products are localized, or become glocal. The book explores the tensions that exist between a global pharmaceutical market and the locally bounded discourses and regulations encountered as markets are created for new drugs in particular contexts. The emergence, representation and regulation of Viagra in Sweden is used as a case study to explore these issues.

17

Illness and Health Behaviours

Lee F. Monaghan

Illness behaviour refers to how people interpret and define their symptoms and their actions when coping with or accommodating their ills. Health behaviour, especially in biomedical research, typically refers to lifestyle 'choices' associated with an increased mortality risk and which are deemed amenable to change.

Medical sociologists increasingly debate the value of 'behaviour' as a concept, with terms such as 'action' or 'practice' instead gaining traction. However, ideas about behaviour have not disappeared within the sub-discipline and the concept is prominent in major interdisciplinary writings on health, illness and society (Cockerham et al., 2014). Illness behaviour refers to people's experiences and interpretations of the symptoms of illness/disease/injury etc., and their interactions with various social networks as they try to cope with or accommodate these symptoms. Illness behaviour is a long-standing topic within medical sociology (e.g. Zola, 1973). Medical sociologists also have a critical interest in health behaviour. Examples include modifying one's diet and physical activity in response to public health discourses about obesity or observing good hygiene, as with COVID-19, in order to avoid sickness and spreading infection to vulnerable others. The major causes of mortality tend to be framed in behavioural terms, with health promoters often seeking to tackle 'lifestyle choices' that are deemed 'problematic' (costly, risky, burdensome). Qualitative methods typically inform research on illness behaviour whilst quantitative methods tend to be used when researching health behaviour, though this distinction is not absolute (Young, 2004).

This entry in the second edition of *Key Concepts in Medical Sociology* began with four caveats, ranging from socio-historical to terminological considerations. These caveats are worth reiterating albeit with an eye on subsequent literature that suggests a need to go 'beyond behaviour' (Will, 2018). In her editorial for a virtual special issue of *Sociology of Health & Illness*, Will observes that medical sociology usefully locates health 'problems' (such as antimicrobial resistance, antibiotic prescription and use) within institutions, interactions and inequalities, thus serving as an important resource that otherwise tends to be ignored within politically influential behavioural approaches. One message here is that more needs to be understood about embedded routines and logics including, somewhat presciently, the meanings of various infections. I will briefly revisit the aforementioned caveats within this context, before turning to illness and then health behaviours.

First, according to Armstrong (2009), the focus on illness and health behaviours reflects post-Second World War concerns about 'the problem of behaviour' in the larger population, with their antecedents in moralized public health efforts to target child hygiene alongside biologists' reductionist foci on the individual. Accordingly, questions such as the following, which retain relevance following the outbreak of COVID-19, should be borne in mind: 'Whose morality?', 'What conception of the body is being formulated?' and 'Whose interests does this conception reflect and serve?' Such questions demand sociological consideration, especially in view of what Dingwall, in his entry on 'Pandemics and Epidemics' in this volume, calls 'patrician policy-making', wherein practitioners display limited understanding of the conditions under which many people live and act. Second, in a related vein, past and present sociological writing on the illness behaviours of the poor and powerless in (state) funded research should not detract critical attention from the socially structured illness-producing behaviours of the rich and powerful. In his polemically-named Greedy Bastards Hypothesis (GBH), Scambler (2012) considers how the strategic 'illness behaviours' of global capitalists may (unintentionally) amplify health inequalities through, for example, changing pension plans and outsourcing work. Third, the reference to 'health' in the study of 'health behaviours' is arguably a misnomer: health is negatively defined in contrast to the positive meanings often ascribed to health and well-being in everyday life. For example, smoking, obesity and unsafe sex are defined as health-related behaviours that necessitate interventions in order to help tackle major causes of death. Fourth, from an interpretivist sociological perspective, the term 'action' or 'conduct' is preferable to 'behaviour'. Although widely used in the policy field, 'behaviour' connotes notions of stimulus and response that are outside of human interpretation, intentionality, projection and planning. In contrast, 'action' (social actions, interactions, conduct) implies meanings and definitions, the very stuff of socially constructed life worlds. Other medical sociologists, who question the uncritical acceptance of dominant public health frames, are also instructive here when favouring the concept of 'social practice' – a concept that denotes tacit, practical knowledge and shared ways of being within broader fields of embedded and embodied action (see, for example, Nettleton and Green, 2014).

Although the above points need to be borne in mind, sociological writings on 'illness behaviour' from the mid-20th century onwards do provide a useful point of reference for subsequent work on how people experience and respond to various ills. Following on from and also critiquing Parsons' structural functionalist writing on illness as a form of behavioural deviance, sociologists have provided empirical and theoretically informed insights on the human world of sickness, pain and suffering, alongside people's varied and contingent efforts to cope with and attenuate their symptoms with or without medical help. Medical sociologists have explored, for example, the 'lay referral system' or how people typically talk with others in their social networks before consulting medical professionals. Rogers et al. (1999), for instance, document the contingent nature of these networks vis-à-vis people's uptake of formal healthcare amidst changing familial and other social relations. An emphasis on social networks is also evidenced in Pescosolido's (1992) influential work, a 'social organization strategy framework', where illness behaviour is understood as a fundamentally social action. Indeed, for Pescosolido, the patterns and pathways to care cannot be understood without fully appreciating people's connections to diverse networks and, in turn, institutions.

Young (2004) presents a selective review and synthesis of the social scientific literature on illness behaviour. He explains that the 'illness behaviour' concept can be traced back to the 1920s, though its salience was elaborated after Parsons in the 1950s. Besides critically reviewing research on the economic, geographical, socio-demographic and psychosocial dimensions of illness behaviour and service (under) utilization, Young considers micro-sociological writings on medical consultations 'in the Western world' (p. 15). One key argument is that the asymmetrical and hierarchical relationship between the paternalistic doctor and supplicant patient, as posited in Parsons' heuristic, has been challenged. Increasing lay knowledge, for instance, has reduced the power that clinicians exercise over their patients and there has been an institutionalization of a more egalitarian, contractual and consultative type relationship. Such trends are important not least given the proliferation of information sources, exemplified by the internet and digital health, which are also co-opted by formal health services. Observing complex interactions beyond the doctor–patient relationship are increasingly at play, Young asserts that diverse 'social networks, institutions and government and world systems [now] comprise the broad view of the problem of illness behaviour' (p. 10).

An exhaustive review of the literature on illness behaviour is beyond the scope of this entry, though some seminal and classic sociological literature should be flagged. Writings here include Mechanic and Volkart (1960), who, in the opening volume of the *Journal of Health and Human Behavior*, 'described the problem of patients' failure (sic) to consult with health services in terms of "illness behavior"' (Armstrong, 2009: 919). For Mechanic and Volkart, 'illness behaviour' included 'the ways in which given symptoms may be differentially perceived, evaluated, and acted (or not acted) upon by different kinds of persons' (1960: 87). Underscoring the responses of these 'different kinds of persons', they suggested that social factors (for example, education, religion and social class) shape illness behaviour.

Subsequent sociological research substantiated these claims. Zola (1973) described how different ethnic groups in New York responded to illness, with social factors or 'triggers' ultimately resulting in the decision to consult (for example, sanctioning from another person or disruption to work roles). The import of social factors is also illustrated by the contrasting orientations of Irish and Italian respondents to illness. On the intersections of gender and class, Blaxter and Paterson (1982) explored Scottish working-class mothers' understandings and accommodation of health problems. Amidst demanding gendered role obligations, illness was deemed a normal part of daily life and women seldom accessed the sick role even when experiencing symptoms (for example, backache). This observation corresponds more generally with research on class-related understandings of health, with the working class typically expressing functional definitions that reflect the need to continue working in order to secure their hard-earned lives.

Moving to 'health behaviour', public health and policy prioritize strategies that are intended to promote health maintenance through lifestyle changes. Despite the disappointing results of intervention studies and the limited role of lifestyle factors in explaining the social gradient in ill-health, health behaviours are typically framed as changeable habits that are conducive to health, or are key to reducing risk. Sociologists have engaged such concerns in relation to what is called 'the health role' (Frank, 1991), where the prevention of illness and maximization of productive capacity are prioritized and even promoted via social marketing. Supporting the health role, health professionals typically expect people to monitor/change their everyday behaviours as part of a 'responsible' and ultimately individualized qua entrepreneurial project of self-control or governance. This expectation is rearticulated via the notion of 'nudging' (seeking to change behaviour through 'unobtrusive influences'), though that concept has been criticized as vague, based on limited evidence and potentially harmful (Bonnell et al., 2011).

Whilst the idea of 'nudging' is problematic, medical sociologists are interested in cultural/behavioural factors as explained in Part 1 of this book. Sociological research explores, for example, ethnic differences in health-related behaviours, including nutritional behaviour as a possible explanatory variable in health inequalities research (Riley Bahr, 2007). However, such research is tentative and there is an ongoing tendency to reproduce pathologizing biomedical categories and interventions uncritically, ignoring arguably implicit eugenicist logics. Consider, for example, the framing of family dynamics as a 'huge barrier to health behaviour change' vis-à-vis young children and 'emerging obesity issues' (Hoeeg et al., 2020: 1243). In short, whilst the promotion of health behaviours may appeal to various groups (for example, paternalistic governments seeking to 'nudge' populations and cut costs), such calls cannot be taken at face value. Aside from the body being a very crude proxy for health behaviours together with ethical and technical concerns about ineffective 'solutions' (O'Hara and Taylor, 2018), 'choices' are shaped and constrained by the inequitable material conditions of existence. By way of example, contrast public health advice in the Global South regularly to wash one's hands, to prevent the spread of COVID-19, with the absence of clean running water in various regions in that part of the world.

Critically reviewing 'health behaviours' research, to return to Armstrong (2009), cited above, is not limited to a structuralist type of analysis. Using post-structuralism, Armstrong explains how the idea of 'health-related behaviour' proliferated in medicine in recent decades. He considers the genealogy of this concept using Foucauldian theory. His discussion is noteworthy when considering the *experience* of illness. After all, it is within the idiom of a widely recycled 'behavioural' discourse that (potentially) sick people risk being positioned as culpable for their actual or anticipated ills, rendering them open to various forms of opprobrium or stigma, meddlesome advice and 'encouragement' (nudging) etc. Arguably, such positioning is the consequence of surveillance or anticipatory medicine where people are increasingly labelled 'diseased', 'ill', or 'at risk' of (spreading) illness without necessarily feeling ill or accepting the biomedical definitions that constitute them as (potentially) sick. The archetype of such framing today is, of course, the asymptomatic carrier of SARS-CoV-2 (the virus that causes COVID-19). The maximization of self- and social responsibility is also noteworthy here in relation to what has been called 'the bio-citizen' (Rose, 1999). This concept is suggestive of emergent modes of subjectivity, with people charged with becoming 'active agent[s] in the maintenance of health … exercising a reflexive scrutiny of personal' conduct in the putative interests of the common good (p. 228).

The rise of molecular science and the marketing of pharmaceutical 'solutions' for myriad 'ills', ranging from mental health problems to severe illness from viral infection, gives added impetus to bio-citizenship where biological and social bodies are mutually implicated in health outcomes and risk. For Rose (2007: 9) this framing reproduces 'a culture of prevention and precaution', comprising 'technologies of life' (future oriented assemblages that aim to optimize vital action, health and life chances) and the embodiment of 'responsibility, foresight and prudence'. Framing health outcomes in behavioural terms is thus far from innocent. Armstrong (2009: 919) asserts that the dominant behavioural focus is individualizing, positioning social agents as 'autonomous' in their 'choice' of 'whether to act in response to illness (illness behaviour) or to maintain their health (health behaviour)'. The possible consequences of this biopolitical framing include the relative neglect of formal healthcare provision in favour of individual behaviours – or, in line with marketization, 'consumer choices'. Yet, it is also the case, especially within health behaviour research, that recent studies seek to take a 'multi-dimensional approach' that incorporates the broader context (structures, social determinants, place, the lifecourse etc.) or '"extra-individual" social factors' (Short and Mollborn, 2015: 78). Unfortunately, though, as seen in the context of obesity discourse, there is the recurrence of what Popay et al. (2010) term 'lifestyle drift' (cited by Monaghan et al., 2022). This 'drift' means that public health policies, which begin with a recognition of 'upstream' social determinants of health, ultimately favour 'downstream' lifestyle interventions that aim to change the behaviours of errant/deviant/pitiable/risky/sick individuals.

In sum, the concepts of illness and health behaviour continue to be used within sociology and other health-related disciplines and discourses. Caveats are necessary and limitations exist in this research, with medical sociologists recently suggesting a need to go beyond behaviour in favour of concepts such as social practices. Yet, important studies, which use 'behaviour' as a referent, are identifiable. Classic interactionist research on illness behaviour, in particular, elucidates the meanings and experiences of diverse groups as they make sense of, and cope with, symptoms with or without medical assistance. Increasingly, in the context of an anticipatory medicine, the focus has also shifted towards so-called health or health-related behaviour (for example, in the context of nutrition and viral infection) and medical sociologists have vital contributions to make here. However, the task and promise of a critical sociology is to evaluate widely endorsed approaches to health and illness behaviours. Possible topics for future research might include exploring how COVID-19 lockdown restrictions provided the conditions under which different groups negotiated, and even rejected, various fear-based public health injunctions to behave responsibly. Another topic might include the ways in which pathways to the doctor, for different illnesses, may have been impacted by the pandemic and government calls to 'stay home, save lives' and 'protect' public health systems.

See also: Lay Knowledge; Material and Cultural Factors; Risk; Social Class; Surveillance and Health Promotion; The Sick Role.

REFERENCES

Armstrong, D. (2009) 'Origins of the problem of health-related behaviours: a genealogical study', *Social Studies of Science*, 39 (6): 909–926.

Blaxter, M. and Paterson, E. (1982) *Mothers and Daughters: A Three Generation Study of Health Attitudes and Behaviour*. London: Heinemann Educational Books.

Bonnell, C., McKee, M., Fletcher, A. et al. (2011) 'One nudge forward, two steps back', *British Medical Journal*, 342: d401.

Cockerham, W.C., Dingwall, R. and Quah, S. (eds) (2014) *The Wiley Blackwell Encyclopedia of Health, Illness, Behavior, and Society*, 5 volumes. Oxford: Wiley-Blackwell.

Frank, A. (1991) 'From sick role to health role: deconstructing Parsons', in R. Robertson and B.S. Turner (eds), *Talcott Parsons*. London: SAGE.

Hoeeg, D., Christensen, U. and Grabowski, D. (2020) 'Intra-familial health polarisation: how diverse health concerns become barriers to health behaviour change in families with preschool children and emerging obesity', *Sociology of Health & Illness*, 42 (6): 1243–1258.

Mechanic, D. and Volkart, E.H. (1960) 'Illness behaviour and medical diagnoses', *Journal of Health and Human Behaviour*, 1: 86–94.

Monaghan, L.F., Rich, E. and Bombak, A.E. (2022) *Rethinking Obesity: Critical Perspectives in Crisis Times*. London: Routledge.

Nettleton, S. and Green, J. (2014) 'Thinking about changing mobility practices: how a social practice approach can help', *Sociology of Health & Illness*, 36 (2): 239–251.

O'Hara, L. and Taylor, J. (2018) 'What's wrong with the "war on obesity?" A narrative review of the weight-centered health paradigm and the development of the 3C framework to build critical competency for a paradigm shift', *SAGE Open*, 8 (2): https://doi.org/10.1177/2158244018772888

Pescosolido, B. (1992) 'Beyond rational choice: the social dynamics of how people seek help', *American Journal of Sociology*, 97 (4): 1096–1138.

Riley Bahr, P. (2007) 'Race and nutrition: an investigation of Black–White differences in health-related nutritional behaviours', *Sociology of Health & Illness*, 29 (6): 831–856.

Rogers, A., Hassell, K. and Nicolaas, G. (1999) *Demanding Patients? Analysing the Use of Primary Care*. Buckingham: Open University Press.

Rose, N. (1999) *Powers of Freedom: Reframing Political Thought*. Cambridge: Cambridge University Press.

Rose, N. (2007) 'Molecular biopolitics, somatic ethics and the spirit of biocapital', *Social Theory & Health*, 5 (1): 3–29.

Scambler, G. (2012) 'Health inequalities', *Sociology of Health & Illness*, 34 (1): 130–146.

Short, S.E. and Mollborn, S. (2015) 'Social determinants and health behaviors: conceptual frames and empirical advances', *Current Opinion in Psychology*, 5: 78–84.

Will, C.M. (2018) 'Editorial: beyond behaviour? Institutions, interactions and inequalities in the response to antimicrobial resistance', *Sociology of Health & Illness*, 40 (3): E1–E9.

Young, J.T. (2004) 'Illness behaviour: a selective review and synthesis', *Sociology of Health & Illness*, 26 (1): 1–31.

Zola, K. (1973) 'Pathways to the doctor: from person to patient', *Social Science & Medicine*, 7 (9): 677–689.

SUGGESTED FURTHER READING

- Cohn, S. (2014) 'From health behaviours to health practices: an introduction', *Sociology of Health & Illness*, 36 (2): 157–162.

Cohn introduces a special issue that advances critical perspectives in this field. Besides Nettleton and Green's article, cited above, which draws from Bourdieu on 'social practice' the special issue features work on, inter alia: the inadequacy of behavioural forms of health promotion, advancing the constructive use of 'context' in behaviour change interventions and critiquing the health behaviour concept with reference to alcohol consumption.

- Elias, T. and Lowton, K. (2014) 'Do those over 80 years of age seek more or less medical help? A qualitative study of health and illness beliefs and behaviour of the oldest old', *Sociology of Health & Illness*, 36 (7): 970–985.

This article redresses a gap in the literature on how 'the oldest old' decide to seek help in response to symptoms. Age is an important factor in mediating how problems might be demedicalized and possible resistances to 'the sick role', as older people seek to maintain a sense of control amidst 'uncertain health' and possible 'functional dependence'.

- Cooper Stoll, L. and Egner, J. (2021) 'We must do better: fatphobia and ableism in sociology', *Sociology Compass*, 15 (4): e12869.

Based on a review of articles in several leading sociology and health journals, the authors challenge representations of disability and fatness that reproduce oppression, eugenical language and logics. Behavioural concerns run though this critique, with Cooper Stoll and Egner urging sociologists to avoid reproducing taken-for-granted designations that imply deviance, deficiency and the need for individuals to make better choices.

18

Stigma

Lee F. Monaghan and Simon J. Williams

Stigma commonly refers to a negatively defined condition, attribute, trait or behaviour conferring 'deviant' status, which is socially, culturally and historically variable. It is a political process, entwined with macro-social issues such as structured power relations, discrimination and the distribution of resources in society.

The term stigma has a long lineage. The ancient Greeks originated the term to refer to bodily signs, cut or burnt onto the flesh, designed to expose the bearer as a slave, a criminal or a social outcast. Stigma was thus a political phenomenon from the outset, intimately related to citizenship and (lack of) entitlement to community membership. Today, stigma still entails exclusionary practices though the term is applied more widely to any condition, attribute, trait or behaviour that symbolically marks the bearer out as 'culturally unacceptable' or 'inferior' and has, as its subjective referent, the notion of shame or disgrace (Goffman, 1968 [1963]). Blame may also emerge, with the stigmatized being held culpable when illnesses, disease or injury are cast as (self-inflicted or perpetuated) deviance. Scambler (2020) characterizes this 'heaping of blame upon shame' as 'the weaponising of stigma' in fractured societies.

Seminal work on stigma was undertaken in the mid-20th century within the interactionist tradition of American sociology, exploring the structure of face-to-face encounters and issues pertaining to identity and selfhood. Whilst recent sociological research on health-related stigma revisits and deepens such thinking in order to underscore the role of macro-social structures and power, attention should first be drawn to Goffman's (1968 [1963]) pioneering study, *Stigma: Notes on the Management of Spoiled Identity*. Part and parcel of his own inimitable dramaturgical perspective on the vicissitudes of self-presentation in everyday life, Goffman's book explores the maintenance and integrity of the self, or perhaps more correctly in this case, the presentation of a 'discredited' or 'discreditable' self. Taking such a stance, in other words, provides a 'special application of the art of impression management' (p. 155), revealing through its potential disruption much about the taken-for-granted ways in which people organize their lives and everyday encounters.

Goffman identifies three types of stigma, pertaining to: (1) the body (such as blemishes or deformities); (2) character (for example, the mentally ill or the criminal); and (3) social collectivities ('racial' or tribal). When defining stigma, Goffman distinguishes between 'virtual social identity' – normative expectations of what the person *ought* to be – and 'actual social identity' – the category or attributes the individual *actually* possesses (p. 12). The stigmatized, from this perspective, possess an unwanted *discrepancy* between virtual and actual social identity vis-à-vis those 'normals' for whom no such discrepancy occurs. A stigma, then, 'is really a special kind of relationship between attribute and stereotype' (p. 14) – a meaning imposed on an attribute via negative images, stereotypes and attitudes that potentially discredits members of a particular social category. Furthermore, as touched on above, Goffman differentiates between the *discredited* and the *discreditable*: with the former, stigma is evident or 'known about' whilst the latter refers to the opposite situation (p. 14). For the discredited the prime dramaturgical task is one of 'managing tension', for the discreditable it is one of 'managing information' – 'to tell or not to tell', to reveal or conceal, that is the question (p. 57). Few people are totally without discrediting attributes; indeed, 'stigma involves not so much a set of concrete individuals who can be separated into two piles, the stigmatized and the normal, as a pervasive two-role social process in which every individual participates in both roles ... the normal and stigmatized are not persons but rather perspectives' (pp. 163–164). Hence, rather than 'deviant', the stigmatized individual might be regarded as a 'normal deviant' (p. 155).

As explained in the second edition of *Key Concepts in Medical Sociology*, these ideas have translated more or less readily into sociological studies of the meaning and experience of illness, both mental and physical, over the years. Our 2013 entry on stigma in *Key Concepts* referred, for example, to early British research on epilepsy (Scambler, 1989) and the uptake, review and revision of these insights in subsequent theoretically informed and empirically grounded studies of other conditions, notably HIV in India (Steward et al., 2008). On the latter topic, recent research usefully locates different types of HIV-related stigma (anticipated, internalized and enacted) within Iranian society (Akbari and Safari, 2020). Other recent research, again indebted to Goffmanesque sociology and *critical theory* (discussed further below), includes Monaghan and Gabe's (2019) qualitative study in Ireland on young people with asthma. Drawing from interviews with participants from a middle-class community and Irish Travellers, the article utilizes Goffman's insights on managing discreditable stigma in response to real, imagined and anticipated negative social reactions. The study also considers how stigma is inseparable from macro-social structures (class, gender and ethnicity) and the layering of stigma (for example, how racism may further spoil identity). Rather than rejecting Goffman's (1968) seminal work, therefore, and, indeed, negating his own awareness of how the wider society matters, a case is made for including but also going beyond micro-level analysis.

The above literature aims to complement and deepen interactionist analyses by underscoring issues that were largely (though not entirely) neglected by Goffman, notably macro-social structural forces and conditions that pattern stigma and reproduce inequality. This revised approach seems ever more vital in a changed and changing society, with more recent critical sociological attention directed at how stigma is but one 'ingredient' of disadvantage in neoliberal societies comprising many faces of oppression (Scambler, 2009: 450). As explained further by Scambler (2020), myriad groups risk being defined as 'superfluous, undesirable or threatening' (p. 3) in what he calls 'the fractured society' (the UK and kindred societies that have been negatively impacted by financial capitalism and austerity policies), resulting in 'the weaponising of stigma' (p. 7) or its intensified use for political ends. Scambler's 'post-individualistic' reasoning, which might usefully be read alongside Tyler (2020) on 'the machinery of inequality' and stigma, not only seeks to engage with large scale political economic changes that have occurred since Goffman was writing but also conflict theory and disability studies. Themes such as oppression, discrimination, power and calls to learn from earlier exchanges between medical sociologists and disability activists all point to the need to move beyond what have been called 'personal tragedy' approaches to stigma (Scambler, 2009, 2018).

Such reasoning fits well with other writings, such as Link and Phelan (2014) on 'stigma power' in the context of mental illness, Monaghan (2017) on what underlies weight-related stigma and Reidpath et al. (2005) on stigma, social value and exclusion. Briefly, Link and Phelan (2014) explicate hidden, or misrecognized, mechanisms that serve the interests of those seeking to keep the mentally ill 'down, in or away' (p. 24); Monaghan (2017) considers how those labelled obese are, for example, scapegoated in trying economic times; and, Reidpath et al. (2005) refer to how stigma in general is tied to social investment and the marking of groups as 'unworthy' amidst finite resources and expectations of reciprocity. Such literature throws light on how the stigmatized are defined as a drain on society and excluded given their perceived lack of social function, productivity or fitness. Under such conditions, stigma may adversely impact health in various ways. Problems range from psychological stress and discrimination in healthcare settings (for example, as reported by women labelled 'morbidly obese') (see Bombak et al., 2016), to 'disinvesting from general social infrastructure' (for example, due to racism, which has a boomerang effect on the broader population) (Reidpath et al., 2005: 469). Whilst Reidpath et al. do not explicitly critique notions of individual culpability for illness and related neoliberal ideologies, they do draw attention to poverty and social justice. These are recurrent themes within medical sociology. For example, research in Northeast England reveals that '[c]laiming welfare, *even* for a cancer-related illness, is stigmatising' and that 'structural forces are hugely implicated' (Moffatt and Noble, 2015: 1203, emphasis in original).

The above literature considers or implies a need for broader stigma reduction strategies. The implication of Moffatt and Noble's (2015) research is that there is a need to dismantle welfare to work policies, which are premised on the assumption that recipients should be incentivized to return to the labour market (an impracticality for many older cancer patients). For Reidpath et al. (2005), strategies should comprise efforts to include those who are stigmatized and increase their perceived social value through 'social investment' (p. 472). Whilst they cite the appropriateness of 'socio-structural changes' (p. 483) – for example, in terms of the built and communicative environments – such interventions might be limited in view of Moffatt and Noble's (2015) research and critiques of 'the fractured society' (Scambler, 2020) wherein money is able to 'buy' policies that are antithetical to public health. Critically, Monaghan (2017) and Monaghan and Gabe (2019) assert that stigma reduction strategies necessitate political action to change inequitable macro-social structures, which are 'upstream' and beyond the direct control of clinicians. In all of this, clinicians should not only become 'wise' or sensitive to the plight of the stigmatized (Goffman, 1968 [1963]) but also understand broader structural matters. As described by Metzl and Hansen (2014), there are shifts in US medical education to ensure future physicians are 'structurally competent'. This concept refers, *inter alia*, to an awareness of how socio-economic forces are implicated in stigma and inequality. Structural competency necessitates responses ranging from humility to grass-roots advocacy for social justice, though the effectiveness of medical education interventions has also been questioned by Reidpath et al. (2005) with reference to HIV-stigma in the Global South.

In sum, there is a rich body of conceptual and empirical sociological literature on illness-related stigma, drawing critical attention to micro- and macro-social processes. This literature is also entering a new phase of development amidst dialogue and debate involving contributors from within and outside of medical sociology (for example, disability theorists and activists, medical educators advocating for structural competency). Certainly, much still remains to be done in terms of not only synthesizing modes of analysis, methodologies and research but also advancing stigma reduction strategies that are more ambitious than well-meaning attempts to change public attitudes. Future stigma research on the COVID-19 pandemic response, within and outside of healthcare, would also be important. Are previous lines of stigma research discussed above relevant here, with the current pandemic in mind? If so, in what ways, for whom and with what implications? However, what is encouraging, as seen in recent writings that seek to re-frame 'personal tragedy' types of analysis, is an attempt to offer more politicized and ambitious conceptualizations that incorporate conflict as well as interactionist sociology (Scambler, 2018). Such writings usefully draw attention to larger structural forces and challenge the uncritical acceptance of hitherto dominant social or medicalized framings of stigma, which, we would stress, are consequential for health, well-being and equity.

See also: Chronic Illness; Citizenship and Health; Disability; Illness and Health Behaviours; Social Constructionism.

REFERENCES

Akbari, H. and Safari, S. (2020) 'Conditions of experienced stigma in people living with HIV in Iran: a qualitative comparative analysis', *Sociology of Health & Illness*, 42 (5): 1060–1076.

Bombak, A.E., McPhail, D. and Ward, P. (2016) 'Reproducing stigma: interpreting "overweight" and "obese" women's experiences of weight-based discrimination in reproductive healthcare', *Social Science & Medicine*, 166: 94–101.

Goffman, E. (1968 [1963]) *Stigma: Notes on the Management of Spoiled Identity*. Harmondsworth: Pelican Books.

Link, B.G. and Phelan, J. (2014) 'Stigma power', *Social Science & Medicine*, 103: 24–32.

Metzl, J.M. and Hansen, H. (2014) 'Structural competency: theorizing a new medical engagement with stigma and inequality', *Social Science & Medicine*, 103: 126–133.

Moffatt, S. and Noble, E. (2015) 'Work or welfare after cancer? Explorations of identity and stigma', *Sociology of Health & Illness*, 37 (8): 1191–1205.

Monaghan, L.F. (2017) 'Re-framing weight-related stigma: from spoiled identity to macro-social structures', *Social Theory & Health*, 15 (2): 182–205.

Monaghan, L.F. and Gabe, J. (2019) 'Managing stigma: young people, asthma, and the politics of chronic illness', *Qualitative Health Research*, 29 (13): 1877–1889.

Reidpath, D.D., Chan, K.Y., Gifford, S.M. and Allotey, P. (2005) '"He hath the French pox": stigma, social value and social exclusion', *Sociology of Health & Illness*, 27 (4): 468–489.

Scambler, G. (1989) *Epilepsy*. London: Routledge.

Scambler, G. (2009) 'Health-related stigma', *Sociology of Health & Illness*, 31 (3): 441–455.

Scambler, G. (2018) 'Heaping blame on shame: "weaponising stigma" for neoliberal times', *The Sociological Review*, 66 (4): 766–782.

Scambler, G. (2020) 'The fractured society: structures, mechanisms, tendencies', *Journal of Critical Realism*, 19 (1): 1–13.

Steward, W., Herek, G., Ramakrishna, J. et al. (2008) 'HIV-related stigma: adapting a theoretical framework for use in India', *Social Science & Medicine*, 67 (8): 1225–1235.

Tyler, I. (2020) *Stigma: The Machinery of Inequality*. London: Zed Books.

SUGGESTED FURTHER READING

- Tyler, I. and Slater, T. (2018) 'Rethinking the sociology of stigma', *The Sociological Review: The Sociology of Stigma*, 66 (4): 721–743.

The above reference introduces a special issue of *The Sociological Review*, featuring 11 articles that seek to rethink the sociology of stigma. Themes in the issue include:

historicizing Goffman with reference to Black Americans' civil rights struggles, the political economy of stigma in neoliberal times, living with stigma and the stigma of place. Health-related themes include: ageing and dementia; disability policy and practice; and the fatal consequences of austerity, poverty and inequality with reference to the Grenfell Tower fire in 2017.

- Rocca, C., Samari, G., Foster, D.G. et al. (2020) 'Emotions and decision rightness over five years following an abortion: an examination of decision difficulty and abortion stigma', *Social Science & Medicine*, 248: 112704.

This article on 'abortion stigma' in the USA is one of the most downloaded articles from *Social Science & Medicine* in the first quarter of 2020, illustrating the value of longitudinal quantitative research plus the ways in which personal and social context are more significant for women's emotional lives than the actual abortion procedure.

- Hatzenbuehler, M.L. and Link, B.G. (2014) 'Introduction to the special issue on structural stigma and health', *Social Science & Medicine*, 103: 1–6.

Scholars from a range of disciplines have sought to conceptualize stigma as a social determinant of population health. Hatzenbuehler and Link's editorial, in building upon critiques of individualized approaches, introduces 14 articles on structural stigma and population health. The special issue is organized into four sections: conceptualizing structural stigma, measuring and modelling structural stigma as a risk indicator for poor health, linking micro and macro, and reducing structural stigma.

- Pescosolido, B.A. and Martin, J.K. (2015) 'The stigma complex', *Annual Review of Sociology*, 41: 87–116.

After summarizing 14 years of *Annual Review* articles on stigma (including mental illness, sexuality, HIV/AIDS etc.) and related concepts (for example, prejudice, discrimination), the authors seek to provide clarity and 'theoretical architecture' for the next generation of stigma research. Drawing from complex and systems science, this article proposes a multilevel, transdisciplinary approach that also has relevance for health policy.

19

Embodiment

Simon J. Williams and Lee F. Monaghan

Embodiment cannot be reduced to dualisms of the mind–body, biology–society kind, but instead refers to the lived, experiential, expressive body and the bodily basis of our being-in-the-world, in sickness and in health.

There is now a vast 'corpus' of writing on bodily matters in sociology and the social sciences and humanities more generally. Indeed, there has been a proliferation of writings on any and all aspects of our bodies from a variety of different angles and theoretical vantage points. Claims of a neglect of the body as something of an 'absent-presence' in past sociological work have now therefore been well and truly remedied in these ways, including a corporeal or embodied re-reading of classical writings (Shilling, 2012; Turner, 2008).

A key approach, which has gained considerable traction in this broader corpus, draws on *phenomenology* to explore the *lived* body and the embodied nature of our being-in-the-world. This perspective goes beyond social constructionist approaches to bodies (of the discursive, linguistic or symbolic kind), by foregrounding the *embodied* nature of human experiences (Turner, 2008). Inspired by the philosopher Merleau-Ponty (1962), who grounds perception in our embodied being-in-the-world, such an approach takes us beyond the duality of mind and body found in Cartesianism and its associated legacies in biomedical thought and practice. Leder (1990), for example, provides a fascinating phenomenological exploration of these embodied issues, including the distinction between *Körper* (physical body) and *Lieb* (lived body), how recourse to the latter 'subverts' Cartesian dualisms of the mind–body kind, and the way in which the lived body opens out onto the world in a deliberative fashion – what Leder terms *ecstasis*. Embodiment, in these ways, not only provides the practical basis for engaging and acting in the world, it is also integral to our sense of self and identity.

Medical sociology has provided rich soil to explore further these embodied themes and concerns, including experiences of pain and suffering and associated issues to do with relations between the body, self and identity in sickness and in health. Pain typically calls into question people's habitual, taken-for-granted relationship to their bodies and the world: a transition, in Leder's (1990) terms, from our usual modes of corporeal 'disappearance' whereby we remain largely unaware of our bodies, to the '*dys*-appearance' of our bodies in problematic fashion as a thematic object of attention. Pain, after all, hurts; it demands attention, however unpleasant, unwelcome and unwanted this might be. The existentially charged and emotionally laden nature of such events, including the gendering of these embodied experiences and expressions (Bendelow, 2000), is all too apparent here. Whilst pain, moreover, can destroy or shatter our world, the symbolic search for meaning through narratives enables people to make sense of suffering and their place in society. Of course, more positive renderings of pain are also possible. Pain is defined as constructive, creative and productive in relation to childbirth, for instance (Bendelow, 2000), or exercise as per the populist 'no pain, no gain' mantra. Pain then, as this suggests, throws into critical relief the material and emotional dimensions of mindful embodiment and their inextricable intertwining across culture, time and place. In these ways the biological body is not so much lost sight of but placed within a broader embodied, non-reductionist perspective that is grounded in our being-in-the-world in all its richness and complexity – what Turner (2008: 229) terms the 'stuffness' of human existence.

The second edition of *Key Concepts in Medical Sociology* referred to qualitative research, undertaken in the 1990s, on bodybuilding and the embodiment of health. Such work drew from Watson's (2000) useful 'male body schema', which is attuned to different modalities of embodiment, including: the *normative* (body size, shape, weight, appearance), the *experiential* (for example, the sense of well-being), the *pragmatic* (relating to gendered role requirements in everyday life), and the *visceral* (the hidden biological processes that may be medically visualized or glimpsed during exercise). Subsequent extensions of this framework, synthesized with literature on embodying health identities, is noteworthy, especially in the midst of reinvigorated concerns about a putative global obesity crisis. Drawing from research with Canadian women identifying as (formerly) obese, Bombak and Monaghan (2017) explore orientations to bodily change and weight-loss trajectories, incorporating themes such as: attractiveness/acceptability, well-being, stigma, disordered eating, projected health (risk) and physical (in)activity through the lifecourse.

As evidenced in the aforementioned study, the pursuit of health (identities) is unfolding with the aid of new mobile digital technologies to track, monitor, manage and quantify any and all aspects of our bodies and selves. Such practices mean people are becoming 'digital cyborgs' – another example of the blurring of human–machine boundaries – with these technologies acting both as 'prostheses' and 'interpreters' of our bodies through generated metrics (Lupton, 2012). Extending her earlier work on the implications of digital technologies for our bodies and health (practices), Lupton (2018) discusses 'digitized self-monitoring' with reference to, among other things, public health campaigns, websites, apps, public pedagogy and the enactment of 'new assemblages of digitized biopolitics' (pp. 43–45). Lupton also raises ethical issues here with reference to 'governing fat bodies' (inspired by Foucauldian scholarship), such as 'overtly authoritarian' tendencies that 'reduce the achievement of defined body capacities to specific norms' (p. 45). To the extent, moreover, that the body is 'worked at' in these new digital ways 'as part of an individual's self-identity', this amounts to another example of what Shilling terms 'body projects' (2012: 6) within broader dynamics of (gendered) power.

Bodies are also *rhythmic* of course: a point of no small importance for the sociology of health and medicine, body studies and the social sciences and humanities in general (see for example Lefebvre, 2013 [1992]; Henriques et al., 2014). It is not simply a case of bodies in time on this count, nor even simply of bodies dominated by social clock time, important as that is, but of time itself, or timing (*Kairos*) to be precise, *embodied* in these rhythmic ways (Adam, 1990). We *are* time in other words, with time and health *mutually implicated* in these rhythmic ways too (Adam, 1992). All our vital life processes display rhythmic variations, including heart rate, blood pressure, temperature, respiration, hormone production, organ function, cell division and reproduction. These rhythms, in turn, are attuned to the rhythms of daylight and darkness, lunar rhythms, tidal rhythms and rhythms of a seasonal kind as the earth spins on its axis. Whilst these biological rhythms largely remain unconscious to us – the sleep–wake cycle and the menstrual cycle being obvious exceptions here – the rise of chronobiology (the science of these rhythms of life) is now resulting in an increasing number of calls for us to wake up and wise up to these 'body clocks' and biological rhythms of ours. Such calls might not (easily) be heeded in the context of busy or distracted lives and myriad inequalities. However, they appear to resonate with contemporary middle-class sensibilities and values given their importance not simply for health and well-being, but for productivity, performance and the optimisation of all we do. Moreover, insofar as people live *out of sync* with these 'body clocks' – *qua* organizers and orchestrators of these rhythms of life – they are likely to be suffering what chronobiologists term 'social jet lag' – the social equivalent of jet lag without stepping on a plane (Roenneberg, 2012). Such thinking underpins calls for more 'biocompatible' forms of school and work, and the popularization of these ideas in contemporary culture, including invitations to find out which 'chronotype' you are and thereby know on this basis the 'best' or 'optimal' time to do everything. In short, rhythmic bodies, and the circadian forms of governance/optimization they are now becoming entangled with in these desynchronized times of ours, add another *vital* dimension to the picture, quite literally, in sickness and in health (Williams et al., 2021).

Another example, with these embodied matters in mind, returns us squarely to debates on social inequalities and health. Social divisions and inequalities, including class, gender and ethnic inequalities, all impact human bodies as socially located, lived and experienced: impacts which the COVID-19 pandemic has further exposed. Social inequalities in these ways are *embodied* (Krieger and Davey Smith, 2004), including the biological effects of socio-economic conditions and social disadvantage (Vineis et al., 2020). Moreover, it is not simply a case of the material and structural effects of these inequalities on the health and illness of our bodies, but of the psychosocial or emotional and expressive effects too (Freund, 1980), including impacts of a neurohormonal kind. In these ways then, embodiment provides a 'missing link' between the micro and the macro levels of sociological analysis.

Whilst a sociology *of* the body then furnishes us with many valuable insights, approaches which focus on *lived* embodiment provide the basis for a more fully *embodied sociology*, including the embodiment of sociologists themselves. As for attempts to develop a more comprehensive framework for analysing these body and society relations, Shilling (2012) provides one promising way forward, which builds on critical realism, through his notion of 'corporeal realism'. This is an approach, as Shilling states, which allows us to analyse how 'societal and cultural transmission, people's lived experiences, and the actual embodied outcomes in terms of propensities towards the re-creation of society resulting from these processes, *interact* and *alter* over time' (p. 252, emphasis in original). Viewed in this way, the body, and the embodied experiences and practices it engenders, becomes the 'multi-dimension medium for the constitution of society' (p. 252). Such theorizations demand further attention in a field committed to knowledge of sickness and health, including the embodiment of inequalities and the embodied 'doing' of sociology itself as a craft, a practice and a vocation.

As for future lines of research, clearly there are many, as the above examples and the links to other entries in this volume suggest (see below). Perhaps the most pressing and obvious thing to mention here, however, is a need for further research on the embodied aspects of the COVID-19 pandemic and its aftermath. Promising lines of investigation include research on the embodied experiences of having and recovering from the disease, including the possible long-term effects on the body. A second, closely related, issue concerns the mental health impacts of the pandemic and mass lockdowns, which themselves of course are embodied. Further research is also needed on the embodied inequalities associated with this crisis, particularly research which takes an *intersectional* approach. The temporal and rhythmic dimensions of our embodiment during the pandemic provide another vitally important topic for further research, including the impacts on our sleep, our health and our well-being during and following lockdowns. There is, then, more to do with these embodied matters in mind, within and beyond these pandemic times of ours.

See also: Chronic Illness; Digital Health; Disability; Emotions; Illness Narratives; Intersectionality; Sexuality; Social Class.

REFERENCES

Adam, B. (1990) *Time and Social Theory.* Cambridge: Polity.

Adam, B. (1992) 'Time and health implicated: a conceptual critique', in R. Frankenberg (ed.), *Time, Health and Medicine.* London: SAGE.

Bendelow, G. (2000) *Pain and Gender.* Harlow: Prentice-Hall.

Bombak, A.E. and Monaghan, L.F. (2017) 'Obesity, bodily change and health identities: a qualitative study of Canadian women', *Sociology of Health & Illness*, 39 (6): 923–940.

Freund, P.E.S. (1980) 'The expressive body: a common ground for the sociology of emotions and health and illness', *Sociology of Health & Illness*, 12 (4): 452–477.

Henriques, J., Tiainen, M. and Väliaho, P. (2014) 'Rhythm returns: movement and cultural theory', *Body & Society*, 20 (3–4): 3–29.

Krieger, N. and Davey Smith, G. (2004) 'Bodies count and body counts: social epidemiology and embodying inequalities', *Epidemiological Reviews*, 26 (1): 92–103.

Leder, D. (1990) *The Absent Body.* Chicago, IL: University of Chicago Press.

Lefebvre, H (2013 [1992]) *Rhythmanalysis: Space, Time and Everyday Life.* London: Bloomsbury Academic.

Lupton, D. (2012) 'M-health and health promotion: the digital cyborg and surveillance society', *Social Theory & Health*, 10 (3): 229–244.

Lupton, D. (2018) *Fat*, 2nd edn. New York: Routledge.

Merleau-Ponty, M. (1962 [1945]) *The Phenomenology of Perception.* London: Routledge.

Roenneberg, T. (2012) *Internal Time: Chronotypes, Social Jet Lag, and Why You're So Tired.* Cambridge, MA: Harvard University Press.

Shilling, C. (2012) *The Body and Social Theory*, 3rd edn. London: SAGE.

Turner, B.S. (2008) *The Body and Society*, 3rd edn. London: SAGE.

Vineis, P., Delpierre, C., Castagné, R. et al. (2020) 'Health inequalities: embodied evidence across biological layers', *Social Science & Medicine*, 246: 112781.

Watson, J. (2000) *Male Bodies: Health, Culture and Identity.* Buckingham: Open University Press.

Williams, S.J., Meadows, R. and Coveney, C. (2021) 'Desynchronised times? Chronobiology, (bio)medicalisation and the rhythms of life itself', *Sociology of Health & Illness*, 43 (6): 1501–1517.

SUGGESTED FURTHER READING

- Engman, A. (2019) 'Embodiment and the foundation of biographical disruption', *Social Science & Medicine*, 225: 120–127.

This article explores the embodied dimensions of biographical disruption using the experiences of organ transplant recipients to shed further light on these issues.

- Twigg, J., Wolkowitz, C., Cohen, R.L. and Nettleton, S. (2011) 'Conceptualising body work in health and social care', *Sociology of Health & Illness: Special Issue: Body Work in Health and Social Care: Critical Themes, New Agendas*, 33 (2): 171–188.

Body work entails paid labour on other people's bodies and it is a key feature of health and social care. Twigg and colleagues introduce a special issue of *Sociology of Health & Illness* on body work, containing 10 contributions. Themes include, among others: 'body work in complementary and alternative medicine', 'the embodiment of trust by health-care professionals in gynae-oncology' and 'managing the body work of home care'.

• Meadows, M. (2005) 'The "negotiated night": an embodied conceptual framework for the sociological study of sleep', *The Sociological Review*, 53 (2): 240–254.

A useful exploration of Watson's (2000) four dimensions of embodiment with sleep matters in mind, illustrated through a case study of sleep negotiation between a couple.

• Monaghan, L.F. and Gabe, J. (2016) 'Embodying health identities: a study of young people with asthma', *Social Science & Medicine*, 160: 1–8.

Illustrates the importance of the lived body when negotiating health amongst young people with mild to moderate asthma.

20

Emotions

Gillian Bendelow and Iain Wilkinson

> Often defined as the part of consciousness that involves bodily 'feeling', emotions
> provide the crucial link between mind, body and society. Sociological theory and
> research on emotions are of particular relevance when understanding stress, mental
> health and chronic illness.

Whilst it is possible to recognize an interest in emotions within the classical texts of sociology, for most of the 19th and 20th centuries they were not addressed as an obvious or significant matter of sociological concern. By contrast, in the 21st century, the sociology of emotions is an established, wide-ranging and influential field of study. There is now a widely shared cross-disciplinary understanding that emotional experiences and responses are not only products of human physiology and bodily process, but also of social conditions and cultural circumstances (Bericat, 2016). In this way, a sociologically informed conceptualization of emotion is an essential component of the complexity in researching health, medicine and illness.

For example, Hochschild's ground-breaking social theory of emotion, first published in 1983, acknowledged that whilst emotions undoubtedly have a biological substratum, they are socially shaped and managed along with the various social divisions such as class, ethnicity, gender, age and sexuality. Restated, emotions emerge and may be subject to manipulation within a network of social relations, meanings and practices that include the demands imposed by formal employment and commercial (for profit) interests. Accordingly, the lower one's status is in the social hierarchy and division of labour, the more one may have to conform to social expectations. The concepts of *emotion management, emotion work* and *emotional labour* subsequently developed by Hochschild and her followers (for example, Drach-Zavery et al., 2017) combine both internal subjective states and bodily displays in the development of *status shields,* i.e. the socially distributed resources that people have for protecting their sense of self in various social situations. This interactionist approach sees emotions through the notion of the 'mindful body' as the nexus of phenomenological experience and the body in its social context. Emotions, in this model, are the link not just between mind and body, but also between mind, body and society (Hochschild, 2003).

Distinctions might be drawn between 'primary' or global emotional states and responses and 'secondary' or specified types and sets of feelings. Whereas the former are shared across societies and cultures, the latter are more heavily subject to processes of social and cultural conditioning in context (Ahmed, 2004). Contexts of social interaction have become more conceptually elaborated. Understandings of the contrasting ways in which emotions are acquired, moderated and exchanged have been analytically refined via a focus on the temporal and spatial differences of the worlds in which emotions are experienced but also the worlds that they shape. Emotions have histories that are moderated by societal contexts (Stearns, 2019), and it is also the case that emotions are significant components of prevailing social conditions and their propensities to change (Rosenwein and Cristiani, 2017), both as products and markers of social and health inequalities.

Ultimately, in the 21st century, emotions can be seen as crucial, both as intrinsic components of health and illness, but also as aspects of the conditions that either enable or inhibit effective medical treatment and healthcare. The types of *emotional labour* carried out by health professionals are further recognized as holding pivotal importance for the achievement of 'clinical outcomes' and for the delivery of effective healthcare (Theodosius, 2008). The social components and conditions of emotions are not only of increased concern within the practice of medicine, but also for health policy, as witnessed following the outbreak of the COVID-19 pandemic (Monaghan, 2020). The sociology of emotions is of particular relevance in unravelling the complex phenomena of mental health and stress (including the role of suffering), as well as chronic illness, pain and *contested conditions* or medically unexplained symptoms (MUS). We focus on these in turn below.

In challenging the unhelpful mind/body polarization between mental and physical health, it is widely recognized that many aspects of human health are adversely impacted and are significantly moderated by the extent to which people are made vulnerable to distressing circumstances and stressful life events. A vast amount of research now points to the fact that emotional distress (or in everyday terms '*stress*') is not merely a trait of personality or a result of how an individual is self-oriented to cope with life's difficulties, but rather, an embodied consequence of socio-economic status. Accordingly, a focus is brought to the ways in which those living within the most economically deprived and institutionally under-privileged sections of society are made to suffer the highest rates and intensities of negative emotions associated with increased rates of psychiatric morbidity (Wilkinson and Pickett, 2017). A considerable amount of sociological interest has congregated around the components, conditions and incidence of emotions connected with experiences of distress and suffering (Wilkinson, 2006). Critical and analytical attention to the extent to which definitions of pain, both medical and non-medical, are entwined with the incidence of social suffering (i.e. social processes and conditions that operate to place people in harm's way and which frequently involve considerable amounts of damage being done to their health), has also emerged. Notably, holistic and interdisciplinary attention to the moderating role of emotions within the physiology of pain has revolutionized and improved the understanding and treatment of chronic pain (Denny, 2017). Where for many years medical science was more preoccupied with purely sensory aspects of pain, the emotional aspects of the experience tended to be treated as secondary phenomena that were not necessarily or directly connected to the feeling and intensity of pain itself. Sociologists have been highly visible in the movement to expose the extent to which the experience of pain takes place as a product of 'the intersection of bodies, minds and cultures' (Morris, 1991: 3), that is, as a process constituted by our embodied experience of society and culture.

Consequently the person-centred focus on an emotional body, rather than on diagnosis, has served to highlight the ways in which many chronic illness and pain conditions are manifested through MUS. The acronym MUS signifies illnesses or syndromes which cannot be defined in terms of organic pathology and are thus seen as abnormal and lowly placed in the medicalized 'illness hierarchy' (Nettleton et al., 2004). Likewise, the term *contested conditions* is used to signify illnesses that have a controversial scientific status (for example, chronic fatigue syndrome/CFS/ME or fibromyalgia), but which may include distressing physical symptoms such as impaired mobility or coordination, intermittent paralysis, fitting, pain and fatigue alongside anxiety and/or depression. Once again, however, there is usually an absence of physical signs, clinical explanations or medical diagnoses. The limitations of modern biomedicine have been especially highlighted in connection with the most complex and difficult to treat types of *idiopathic* pain – that is, pain for which there is no established physical pathology – often termed *chronic pain syndrome*.

Social science, and in particular the sociological literature on chronic illness, offers a framework for understanding the emotional experiences and consequences of contested chronic illness conditions and chronic pain by focusing on the *person* rather than the pain per se. Concepts such as biographical disruption, narrative reconstruction and illness adjustment (Bury, 1991) are particularly valuable, and the theoretical and methodological explosion of interest in illness narratives has helped to convey the highly emotional and phenomenological experience of illness, pain and suffering at the global level.

The development of narrative medicine and medical humanities has also highlighted the importance of embodied knowledge and lay expertise. 'Expert patients' have since gained much currency in medical as well as social science research (Maguire and Britten, 2018) and health policy, for example, the emphasis on *self-management*. Using models from the recovery movement in mental health, self-management is a reflexive holistic approach. It combines an individual's emotional literacy (defined as the ability to understand and/or name emotions being experienced which may impact on their general health) with lay expertise of a condition or medical diagnosis in order to develop autonomy and self-determination in health maintenance and illness prevention. The term *emotional health* is gaining popularity, much in the way that *sexual health* became an umbrella category for service provision which encompasses emotional, cultural and lifestyle factors as well as medical aspects (Bendelow, 2010). However, scepticism is needed to ensure it is not simply a strategy to shift the responsibility for health entirely onto the individual and relocate the economic burden associated with chronic illness from the welfare state and public health services to private consumers of healthcare.

In conclusion, addressing the role of emotions in health and illness – as with an embodied approach to sociology more generally – is crucially important. It helps to challenge dualistic legacies within Western philosophy and biomedicine that operate with a crudely mechanistic approach to the body and which often fail to acknowledge the psychological and inherently social components of our health. These theoretical and methodological insights also enable the development of integrated and holistic models of health, medicine and illness. They promote deeper understandings of the more socially constructed or contested aspects of diagnosis and the phenomenological experience of chronic illness, stress and pain. In turn, this sociologically informed knowledge enables more sophisticated understandings of the relationship between social structure, agency and health. Writing in the midst of responses to the global COVID-19 pandemic and potentially its aftermath, the implications of the social distribution of suffering have rarely been so visibly paramount.

See also: Chronic Illness; Embodiment; Emotional Labour; Illness Narratives.

REFERENCES

Ahmed, S. (2004) *The Cultural Politics of Emotion*. Edinburgh: Edinburgh University Press.

Bendelow, G. (2010) 'Emotional health: challenging biomedicine or increasing health surveillance?' *Critical Public Health*, 20 (4): 465–474.

Bericat, E. (2016) 'The sociology of emotions: four decades of progress', *Current Sociology*, 64 (3): 491–513.

Bury, M. (1991) 'The sociology of chronic illness: a review of research and prospects', *Sociology of Health & Illness*, 13 (4): 451–468.

Denny, E. (2017) *Pain: A Sociological Introduction*. Oxford: Blackwell.

Drach-Zavery, A., Yagil, D. and Cohen, I. (2017) 'Social model of emotional labour and client satisfaction: exploring inter- and intrapersonal characteristics of the client–provider encounter', *Work & Stress*, 31 (2): 182–208.

Hochschild, A. (2003 [1983]) *The Managed Heart: The Commercialization of Human Feeling*. Berkeley: University of California Press.

Maguire, K. and Britten, N. (2018) '"You're there because you are unprofessional": patient and public involvement as liminal knowledge spaces', *Sociology of Health & Illness*, 40 (3): 463–477.

Morris, D. (1991) *The Culture of Pain*. Berkeley: University of California Press.

Monaghan, L.F. (2020) 'Coronavirus (COVID-19), pandemic psychology and the fractured society: a sociological case for critique, foresight and action', *Sociology of Health & Illness*, 42 (8): 1982–1995.

Nettleton, S., O'Malley, L., Watt, I. and Duffy, P. (2004) 'Enigmatic illness: narratives of patients who live with medically unexplained symptoms', *Social Theory & Health*, 2 (1): 47–67.

Rosenwein, B.H. and Cristiani, R. (2017) *What is the History of Emotions?* New York: John Wiley & Sons.

Stearns, P.N. (2019) 'Periods in emotion history: a next step?' *Emotions and Society*, 1 (1): 67–82.

Theodosius, C. (2008) *Emotional Labour in Health Care: The Unmanaged Heart of Nursing*. New York: Routledge.

Wilkinson, I. (2006) 'Health, risk and "social suffering"', *Health, Risk & Society*, 8 (1): 1–8.

Wilkinson, R.G. and Pickett, K.E. (2017) 'The enemy between us: the psychological and social costs of inequality', *European Journal of Social Psychology*, 47 (1): 11–24.

SUGGESTED FURTHER READING

- Stets, J.E. and Turner, J.H. (eds) (2014) *Handbook of the Sociology of Emotions*. Boston, MA: Springer.

Overview of theoretical perspectives and social arenas within the sociology of emotions, includes 'Mental health and emotions' by R. Simon, which addresses identity and affect control theory. There is also a chapter in the 2008 edition by L.E. Francis on 'Emotions and health'.

- Bendelow, G. (2009) *Health, Emotion and the Body*. Cambridge: Polity Press.

Building on Hochschild's social theory of emotion and applying it to health, illness and stress, this volume examines the interplay between mind/body/society across a wide range of illness conditions and healthcare settings. In particular, the significant challenge to biomedicine by the complexities of chronic illness and mental health conditions is addressed in order to develop holistic and integrative approaches to contemporary healthcare.

- Fraser, S., Maher, J.M. and Wright, J. (2010) 'Between bodies and collectivities: articulating the action of emotion in obesity epidemic discourse', *Social Theory & Health*, 8 (2): 192–209.

This paper articulates the role of emotions in a sophisticated account of power, agency and corporeality in the debates around obesity. It also develops a critique of conventional tendencies to individualize and psychologize emotional states and dynamics and to exclude emotion from public debate.

- Drajoljvic, A. and Broom, A. (2017) *Bodies and Suffering: Emotions and Relations of Care.* London: Routledge.

This volume draws on theories of emotion, embodiment, the phenomenology of illness and moralities of care to explore the 'lived experience of suffering'. Using case studies and empirical research, the authors explore the idea of the suffering body across different cultures and contexts.

21

Chronic Illness

Lee F. Monaghan and Mike Bury

Chronic illness commonly refers to those forms of long-term health disorders that interfere with social interaction and role performance. It is often disruptive of people's lives, though responses can and do vary depending on context.

Medical sociologists have long been interested in studying chronic illness. The public health and demographic reasons for this are easily appreciated. In the latter half of the 20th century many nations in the Global North, and increasingly thereafter in the Global South, experienced a 'demographic transition'. The decline in mortality at all ages, but especially in infancy and early adulthood, led to an increase in average life expectancy from birth and (in the presence of low fertility rates) an ageing population. Whilst increasing life expectancy is never guaranteed, even in high-income nations (Marmot et al., 2020), most people can still expect to live into old age and, consequently, may be more likely to experience disorders associated with adult and later life. Many of these conditions are chronic disorders, such as arthritis, stroke, dementia, Parkinson's disease and some forms of heart disease and cancer.

Sociological interest in chronic illness has, in part, stemmed from the limitations of medical treatment for chronic disorders. Whilst some forms of treatment are very effective, for example, hip replacement and cataract surgery, many disorders can only be treated palliatively, to relieve pain and to help physical functioning. The long-term implications of chronic illness inevitably bring social and psychological factors to the fore and many physicians have looked to wider forms of collaboration with medical sociologists in order to understand the issues as they are experienced and managed by lay people. A perusal of a key medical sociology journal, *Sociology of Health & Illness*, makes clear that these issues are not only many and varied but also highly topical; for instance, the role of partners in the management of chronic illness (Hudson et al., 2020) and the long-term observance of hygiene measures among those vulnerable to infection (Brown et al., 2020). Whilst the latter study was conducted among people with cystic fibrosis before COVID-19 erupted, as explained by Will (2020: 967), when reflecting on 'the sociology of health and illness in COVID-19 time', it offers 'a window on the lives of people for whom sensitivity to infection is nothing new, and who have lived with physical distancing and special hygiene measures for years'.

Sociological interest in chronic illness stemmed from key work carried out in the 1960s and 1970s, especially in the USA. Initially, research focused on the social patterning of chronic illness and whether this differed from life-threatening conditions that produced high mortality. Conover (1973) reviewed and re-analysed data that had been the subject of a debate between two sociologists, Kadushin and Mechanic, and concluded that the occurrence of chronic illness was, indeed, related to social class and poverty. Critically, whilst such a finding suggests that more should have been written on the political economy of chronic illness, most sociological research has been micro-interactionist in approach. Indeed, much research has explored the meanings and consequences of chronic illness, and the steps taken to mitigate the effects of chronic conditions as experienced by sufferers themselves in a micro-social context (for example, in relation to family, friends and carers).

In contrast to the 'systems' perspective formulated in Parsons' writing on 'the sick role', sociological research on chronic illness has largely focused on people's experiences within the context of their everyday lives. Whilst Lawton (2003) reviews some of this literature, focusing specifically on articles published in *Sociology of Health & Illness* during the previous 25 years, there are important antecedents. Perhaps the most significant publication in the 1970s, in this regard, was Strauss and Glaser's book, *Chronic Illness and the Quality of Life* (1975). Although it begins by noting the healthcare implications of chronic illness, especially the need for professionals to widen their horizons from their preoccupation with acute conditions, subsequent chapters are strongly interactionist in tone. From this viewpoint, chronic illness is not just a given biological entity, patterned by social conditions, but is itself a 'negotiated reality'. Chronic illness and its outcomes are shaped by the decisions, tactics and organization of 'work' carried out by patients and others, over the 'trajectory' of the illness. The contingent nature of this process is part of a general view of society as the product of interaction and negotiation, amenable to qualitative analysis.

In Britain, Bury (1982) developed this position when undertaking research among people recently diagnosed with rheumatoid arthritis (for related research on 'seasoned' sufferers see Williams, 1984). Bury (1982: 169) took Giddens' notion of a 'critical situation' that might be applied to 'major events such as war' and extended it to the illness experience as a 'biographically located event'. Bury conceptualized chronic illness as 'biographical disruption' that disturbs 'the structures of everyday life and the forms of knowledge which underpin them' (p. 169). Bury's concept is worth focusing on since, as Williams (2000: 45) explains, it has been an 'abiding theme within the sociology of chronic illness since the early 1980s'. Indeed, its formal and international relevance persists as demonstrated in research in the Global South (for a recent study in Thailand on breast cancer diagnosis as biographical disruption, see Liamputtong and Suwankhong, 2015). For Bury's (1982) research participants, arthritis was seen to threaten their taken-for-granted world. Modern medical categories, the medical understanding of disease and the treatment it could offer might be appropriated by patients, and employed in legitimating and explaining their altered condition to family and friends. At the same time, the diagnosis and its implications for the future might confirm the fact that the individual is suffering from a progressively disabling condition from which there is no escape. Without a medical cure, individuals must negotiate and manage their altered state with what support they can muster. Thereafter Bury (1991) distinguished between three dimensions of this process: *coping* (cognitive dimensions), *strategy* (managing the condition and its impact on interaction and life chances) and *styles of adjustment* (for example, deciding on how much should be disclosed or disguised about the condition). Such responses could include withdrawal from all but essential interaction or 'normalization', where the disorder is integrated into an altered public identity. Biographical disruption may not, therefore, be the only outcome.

Much research and debate has since been published on the variable meanings and consequences of chronic illness and people's different responses in relational context. Here lay perspectives, voices and relations are given due weight, rather than remaining hidden behind closed doors and eclipsed by a biomedical remit that has traditionally emphasized cure over care and acute over chronic illness. Interestingly, contrary findings have emerged during empirical research, serving to complicate the picture as well as confirm aspects of Bury's (1991) later writings, such as the significance of people's expectations. Our entry on chronic illness in the second edition of *Key Concepts in Medical Sociology* illustrated that point with reference to Pound et al.'s (1998) research on stroke among elderly respondents in the East End of London. Socio-economic context and age mediated the experience and rendered it, relatively speaking, 'not that bad' as respondents bore witness to continued or worsening hardship in their hard-earned lives. Subsequent research on other conditions adds to this knowledge. Note, for example, Kerr et al.'s (2018) review of literature published in the previous decade on the sociology of cancer, particularly studies focusing on 'identity and subjectivity' (p. 555).

Mounting evidence and theoretical appraisal makes clear that the biographical disruption concept cannot be viewed in mechanistic or universalistic terms (which, it should be stressed, was never Bury's intention). What has been unfolding in the field in recent years tallies well with Williams' (2000) efforts to stimulate further empirical research whilst reflecting on questions such as: 'Does a focus on "disruption" mask as much as it reveals?' (p. 41). After defending the biographical disruption concept against postmodernist and disability theorists' critiques, where bodies and pain are dissolved into discourse and social oppression, Williams makes several germane points about this concept and the 'future direction of sociological research in this and other related domains' (p. 41). For example, alongside the possible role of biographical disruption in the aetiology of disease he cites research on people's circumscribed expectations of health and illness amidst 'normal crises', highlighting the largely underresearched implications of social inequalities for people's embodied experiences of chronic illness. Williams also maintains that the common focus on biographical disruption remains *adult-centric*. It obscures the realities of chronic illness among children who may have congenital conditions, that is, when illness has always been part of the embodied self and thus where 'continuity rather than change remains the guiding principle' (p. 50). With the lifecourse and other structural considerations in mind, Monaghan and Gabe (2015) subsequently explored how young people in Ireland (boys and girls from a middle-class and a minority ethnic group) presented mild-to-moderate asthma as 'biographically contingent' – that is, 'an "only sometimes" problem' that varies in terms of its 'symptoms, meanings and consequences' (p. 1236). Besides foregrounding the varied experiences of asthma, the authors question the uses and limitations of 'biographical contingency' as a concept alongside others when researching chronic illness (for instance, biographical disruption, reinforcement and anticipation).

There has been a recurrent tension in discussions on chronic illness. This tension, also evidenced in studies focusing on health-related stigma, comprises a broader dynamic pertaining to ways of seeing, reading or experiencing chronic illness. More specifically, there are discrepancies between a 'problems' or 'personal tragedy' perspective, in which the difficulties people face are documented and brought into view, and one in which chronic illness can be approached in a positive, if not always an overtly political, light. Calls to move beyond a largely 'reformist' position on the one hand and a 'radical' position on the other – positions attributed respectively to medical sociologists and disability activists – have been complicated by an emphasis on a postmodern culture of illness and disability. Charmaz (2000), for example, suggests that sociology needs to go further than document the 'patient's perspective' and the normalization processes that 'contain' the effects of illness and disability on everyday life, important though these are. Significantly, she adds that 'chronic illness can mean embarking on an odyssey ... to integrate the self on a different level ... facing such losses moves them [the chronically ill] towards transcending loss' (p. 287). As with other sociologists, especially in North America, the dividing lines between chronic illness, disability and health appear to become blurred in such arguments. Here a form of 'biographical reinvention' may be seen, whether among disability activists, patients' groups or others, in what Frank (1997) calls the 'remission society' wherein many people may be experiencing or recovering from various ills. What in the earlier literature was seen to be a process of stabilization and normalization by the chronically ill now becomes a ceaseless and nomadic journey with no clear end point (see Williams, 2001, for a critique). The links between body, self and society, from this viewpoint, are not simply the outcome of interactional difficulties or 'social oppression', but constitute a shifting terrain, on which individuals and groups attempt to construct new identities and new realities. As seen in recent studies of cancer, medical sociologists have continued to engage with such matters, with some challenging the sort of theorizations associated with Frank and 'the search for alternative meanings in the post-modern age' (Kerr et al., 2018: 555).

None of the above means bridges cannot be or are not currently being built between different approaches. In the context of what has been described as a 'transitional phase' in this field (see Suggested Further Reading) and in the spirit of advancing the sociology of chronic illness, we will finish with six propositions and related questions for future research.

First, medical sociologists in conversation with others (for example, disability theorists and patient advocacy groups) are well placed to synthesize perspectives in a theoretically, empirically and critically informed manner. In so doing, issues of impairment, bodily change or the persistence of distressing symptoms may be explored in a sociologically robust manner, highlighting the active responses made in everyday settings. Second, besides drawing from the interactionist tradition in sociology, research could reconnect with earlier disciplinary concerns about the political economy, class and poverty thereby linking micro and macro foci and qualitative and quantitative methodologies. What might we say, for instance, about the continuing if not deepening impact of austerity and debt on the illness experience as well as the patterning of morbidity? Third, such questions could be addressed with a view to informing efforts to redress inequitable structures, processes and practices as evidenced in critical realist scholarship and policy debates. Fourth, there is a need to test many of the ideas that have grown in the past decade, especially in the (post) COVID society. For instance, what does Sanderson et al.'s (2011) study of different types of normalization mean in *collectively disrupted times* wherein multiple domains, including formal health and social care, appear to be in a critical situation? Might exogenous shocks and crises suddenly render a potentially manageable chronic illness terminal, bringing the spectre of death to the forefront of consciousness? Fifth, when researching possible yet currently unknown long-term health consequences of COVID-19, especially among structurally disadvantaged groups with pre-existing conditions, it will be important to mine what is already known within the sociology of chronic illness. For instance, Brown et al.'s (2020) research could proffer lessons at a time when governments, public health authorities and mass media have elevated and dramatized concerns about airborne infection, hygiene and 'social distancing' (sic). Finally, researching the relations between non-communicable and communicable disease (how they become layered or entwined) during and in the aftermath of the pandemic could also help to integrate disparate and asymmetrical fields of study within medical sociology.

See also: Disability; Embodiment; Emotions; Illness Narratives; Medicalization; Stigma.

REFERENCES

Brown, N., Buse, C., Lewis, A. et al. (2020) 'Air care: an "aerography" of breath, buildings and bugs in the cystic fibrosis clinic', *Sociology of Health & Illness*, 4 (5): 972–986.

Bury, M. (1982) 'Chronic illness as biographical disruption', *Sociology of Health & Illness*, 4 (2): 167–182.

Bury, M. (1991) 'The sociology of chronic illness: a review of research and prospects', *Sociology of Health & Illness*, 13 (4): 451–468.

Charmaz, K. (2000) 'Experiencing chronic illness', in G.L. Albrecht, R. Fitzpatrick and S.C. Scrimshaw (eds), *The Handbook of Social Studies in Health and Medicine*. London: SAGE.

Conover, P. (1973) 'Social class and chronic illness', *International Journal of Health Services*, 3 (3): 357–368.

Frank, A. (1997) *The Wounded Story Teller: Body, Illness and Ethics*. Chicago: University of Chicago Press.

Hudson, N., Law, C., Culley, L. et al. (2020) 'Men, chronic illness and healthwork: accounts from male partners of women with endometriosis', *Sociology of Health & Illness*, 42 (7): 1532–1547.

Kerr, A., Ross, E., Jacques, G. and Cunningham-Burley, S. (2018) 'The sociology of cancer: a decade of research', *Sociology of Health & Illness*, 40 (3): 552–576.

Lawton, J. (2003) 'Lay experience of health and illness: past research and future agendas', *Sociology of Health & Illness*, 25 (3): 23–40.

Liamputtong, P. and Suwankhong, D. (2015) 'Breast cancer diagnosis: biographical disruption, emotional experiences and strategic management in Thai women with breast cancer', *Sociology of Health & Illness*, 37 (7): 1086–1101.

Marmot, M., Allen, J., Boyce, T. et al. (2020) *Health Equity in England: The Marmot Review 10 Years On*. London: Institute of Health Equity.

Monaghan, L.F. and Gabe, J. (2015) 'Chronic illness as biographical contingency? Young people's experiences of asthma', *Sociology of Health & Illness*, 37 (8): 1236–1253.

Pound, P., Gompertz, P. and Ebrahim, E. (1998) 'Illness in the context of older age: the case of stroke', *Sociology of Health & Illness*, 20 (4): 489–506.

Sanderson, T., Calnan, M., Morris, M. et al. (2011) 'Shifting normalities: interactions of changing conceptions of a normal life and the normalisation of symptoms in rheumatoid arthritis', *Sociology of Health & Illness*, 33 (4): 616–633.

Strauss, A. and Glaser, B. (1975) *Chronic Illness and the Quality of Life*. St Louis, MO: Mosby.

Will, C.M. (2020) '"And breathe..."? The sociology of health and illness in COVID-19 time', *Sociology of Health & Illness*, 42 (5): 967–971.

Williams, G. (1984) 'The genesis of chronic illness: narrative reconstruction', *Sociology of Health & Illness*, 6 (2): 175–200.

Williams, G. (2001) 'Theorizing disability', in G.L. Albrecht, K.D. Seelman and M. Bury (eds), *Handbook of Disability Studies*. London: SAGE.

Williams, S.J. (2000) 'Chronic illness as biographical disruption or biographical disruption as chronic illness? Reflections on a core concept', *Sociology of Health & Illness*, 22 (1): 40–67.

SUGGESTED FURTHER READING

- Williams, G.H. and Jones, I.R. (2017) 'Editorial. Making sense: further studies of living with chronic illness', *Sociology of Health & Illness*, 39 (5): 653–658.

Introducing a special themed section on chronic illness, Williams and Jones foreground the importance of sense-making and medical sociology. Acknowledging Bury's early classic on chronic illness as biographical disruption and the research and questioning it prompted, the editorial introduces five articles that explore the variable disruptions associated with inflammatory bowel disease, myalgic encephalomyelitis or chronic fatigue syndrome, insomnia, HIV and Meniere's disease. The editors also suggest ways forward, underscoring narrative, imagination, meaning-making and difference in relational context.

- Locock, L. and Ziebland, S. (2015) 'Mike Bury: biographical disruption and long-term and other health conditions', in F. Collyer (ed.), *The Palgrave Handbook of Social Theory in Health, Illness and Medicine*. New York: Palgrave Macmillan.

Collyer's large edited collection contains many useful chapters, with Locock and Ziebland's contribution focusing specifically on Bury's highly influential work on chronic illness.

- Scambler, G. and Scambler, S. (eds) (2010) *New Directions in the Sociology of Chronic and Disabling Conditions: Assaults on the Lifeworld*. London: Palgrave Macmillan.

This collection aims to facilitate rapprochement between medical sociologists and disability theorists during a 'transitional phase' in the study of chronic and disabling conditions. Despite historical divisions, space is promoted among scholars who view such conditions as 'assaults on the lifeworld' with this book furthering 'a range of different theorizations and interpretations of the interrelations of the biological, psychological and social' (p. 1).

- Rosqvist, H.B., Katsui, H. and McLaughlin, J. (2017) '(Dis)abling practices and theories?: Exploring chronic illness in disability studies', *Scandinavian Journal of Disability Research*, 19 (1): 1–6.

Rosqvist and colleagues introduce a special issue on chronic illness and disability, underscoring the value of working across boundaries between disability studies and medical sociology.

22

Disability

Janice McLaughlin

> *Disability emerges in the interaction between impaired bodies and social structures and processes. This means that it is not primarily a medical issue; instead it is a social problem created by the way society is organized. Therefore, it is important that sociological research on disability both understands and addresses this problematic.*

The most authoritative report on the prevalence of disability across the globe remains the WHO *World Health Survey*, undertaken between 2002 and 2004 (see WHO, 2011). It states that there are approximately 785 million people aged 15 years and older living with a disability. The survey also highlights that the rate of disability is higher in lower income countries and that people living in poverty are more likely to be disabled. The data contained in the report also capture some of the many social problems and barriers disabled people face, including lower employment rates, limited access to education, lower levels of social participation and citizenship rights. It also notes that trends towards greater numbers of people living longer, often with chronic health conditions, mean that disability is and will continue to increase across the globe. The survey generates two important implications for thinking about disability and its presence in medical sociology:

1. There is an overlap between disability and ill health, although they are not the same. Some health conditions bring with them impairments that affect people's lives, while others do not. Likewise, disability can be associated with health issues, but not always.
2. Disability is associated with a range of social problems that affect disabled people's lives.

There have been ongoing debates and disputes between medical sociology and disability studies, tensions which began in the 1970s with the emergence of the latter field. How we understand the relationships between health, impairment and disability lies at the heart of these debates, which have at times been quite fraught. This controversy in itself speaks to the political aspects of both the concepts and the issues explored in both fields. In this entry, I will outline the nature of differences in perspective, before indicating points of overlap, which show where there are opportunities for productive working across the different approaches.

When disability studies emerged in the UK (and elsewhere) in the 1970s, it was rooted in the Disability Movement and strongly influenced by Marxist ideas (Oliver, 1990). From its inception, disability studies positioned itself in opposition to both medicine and existing sociological approaches to studying medicine and disability; in particular, it rejected understandings of disability that focused on limitations within the body. The argument was, and is, that this way of framing disability positions disabled people as tragic figures either to be cured by medicine or locked away from society in oppressive institutions. Key disability writers from this period saw medical sociology and influential ideas such as Goffman's model of stigma and deviance, Parsons' concept of 'the sick role' and Bury's argument that chronic illness generates 'biographical disruption' as complicit in the problems disabled people face. They challenged medical sociology for not scrutinizing important aspects of medical approaches to disability and for being uninterested in the socio-economic hardships experienced by disabled people. In 1976 UPIAS (Union of Physically Impaired Against Segregation) proposed *The Fundamental Principles of Disability* as an alternative understanding of disability, one which it called the 'social model'. The document makes a crucial distinction between impairment and disability: impairment refers to the aspects of the body that are limited in their functionality, while disability pertains to the creation of social disadvantage due to the inability of society to adapt to those limitations:

> [I]t is society which disables physically impaired people. Disability is something imposed on top of our impairments, by the way we are unnecessarily isolated and excluded from full participation in society. (UPIAS, 1976: 4)

A straightforward way to understand this is that someone who uses a wheelchair is not disabled by the fact that they need a wheelchair to be mobile; they are disabled by the presence of stairs and doors that do not open easily. Social model advocates are not saying impairments do not matter; what they assert is that the most important thing to study, if you want to improve disabled people's lives, is disability. This understanding also explains why British disability studies use the terminology of 'disabled people' rather than 'people with disabilities'. While the latter is preferred in disability politics in other countries (for example the USA), the British movement argues the language of 'with' still positions disability as in the person rather than in the social environment.

Disability studies writers argue that medical sociology examines disability through an approach that primarily is concerned with questions of health and ill health, ignoring key issues about social structure and marginalization. For a variety of disability writers, a focus on an individual's health also ignores those who are disabled but not ill – the healthy disabled. Ignoring those whose health is not an issue means that the conceptual tools of medical sociology are not fit for purpose for both researching disability and seeking to create social change. Advocates of the social model have asserted that medical sociology's emphasis on experiences of living with illness and interactions with medicine ignores the broader dynamics of imposed oppression and marginalization. For example, Barnes (1998), in a polemical critique, argues that medical sociology has not questioned why disabled people have medical treatments which may help someone who is unwell but are not helpful, or are even harmful, to healthy disabled people. In response medical sociologists did counter some of these arguments. Bury (1996) emphasized the field's evident interest in oppressive societal dynamics, while Williams (1999) stressed that medical sociology research was cognizant of the role of structures and inequalities in mediating people's experiences of both ill-health and impairment. Nevertheless, doubt over medical sociology's capacity to explore disability has remained in some areas of disability studies. Notably, Thomas (2007) has argued that sociological work on stigma and disability has failed to recognize the structural factors that lead to stigma, and instead treated it as an understandable response to people who do not match the norm.

The social model is an important intervention in understanding disability and in shaping policy and legislative responses. Some of its arguments are present in the WHO *International Classification of Functioning, Disability and Health,* which acknowledges that disability is, in part, a result of the interaction between individuals with a health condition or impairment and natural, societal or built environments. Many countries now have legislation geared to tackling discrimination and structural barriers against disabled people. In the UK the Equality Act 2010, which incorporates and enhances the provisions made in the Disability Discrimination Act (DDA) 1995, provides some protection from discrimination based on disability and requires organizations to make 'reasonable adjustments' to ensure greater accessibility. Since the DDA we have seen changes in the accessibility of buildings, educational provision, the built environment and other areas of social life. However, disability organizations argue that much remains to be done and that issues such as welfare austerity have undermined some of the progress that has been made.

Given the social model has been around for some time, criticisms of it have grown; these criticisms, alongside changes in medical sociology, mean there is more scope now for these different approaches to overlap and work together. One key criticism of the social model is that because it emphasizes social structures and asserts that not all disabled people experience ill-health, it ignores impairment and difficulties that are associated with health problems. For example, it does not explore the implications of living with pain and fatigue due to chronic illness, something many disabled people do experience. Critics have suggested that disability studies deliberately avoids particular issues that complicate the impairment/disability distinction and the sole focus on disability. For example, people who have life-limiting and degenerative conditions and actively seek medical intervention and improvements in treatment are sidelined by a desire to reject medical practices (Shakespeare, 2006). Feminist disability writers and activists, such as Crow and Morris, have been particularly important in their advocacy of bringing impairment into consideration (Morris, 1996). Examining impairment involves bringing the body back as an object of inquiry, and a variety of disability studies writers are now doing so. Hughes and Paterson (1997) have influentially argued that the body disappeared in disability studies and that sociological approaches, such as phenomenology, are needed to ensure it is not just medicine that studies it. Williams (1999), from within medical sociology, has likewise argued that critical realism is an approach that can bring illness and disability together. Researchers who are influential in the emergence of critical disability studies (e.g. Shildrick and Garland-Thomson) draw from Queer, post-structural and psychoanalytic approaches to examine the social construction of 'the normal body' as a fictional figure against whom others are judged (see Goodley, 2011). Other disability studies work is re-engaging with stigma, particularly research on the experiences of families with disabled members. This work uses Goffmanesque concepts, such as 'courtesy stigma' or stigma by association, but with a greater emphasis on the political and inequality dimensions of these dynamics rather than the capacity of disabled people to manage them (Ryan, 2005).

What these areas of disability work point to is a useful shared interest with medical sociology; in particular, with ways of understanding lived experience and placing such experiences in the broader social, cultural and economic contexts that inform them. Nevertheless, while Thomas (2007) agrees such shared interests exist, she argues that it would be better for disability research within sociology to be seen as a distinct sub-discipline associated with sociological work on equality and diversity, rather than medical sociology (which, in contrast, she argues is better suited to study impairment effects). This positioning situates disability alongside other areas of inequality such as gender, class and race and ethnicity, as well as the intersections between them. Emphasizing disability as primarily a dynamic of inequality also helps stress that understanding disabled people's lives, including of health and ill-health, cannot be divorced from their socio-economic location and the implications that has for oppression and discrimination. Across usefully blurred lines between disability studies, medical sociology and sociologies of equality and diversity much work now exists drawing out these connections in powerful and insightful ways. For example, research undertaken in Northeast England, looking at the impacts of welfare austerity and the emergence of Universal Credit, has captured crucial impacts on disabled people and those with chronic health conditions (Moffatt and Noble, 2015). Scambler's (2020) critical realist work on the politics of disability, shame and blame, is also noteworthy in that regard, building on his structurally minded efforts to go beyond Goffmanesque micro-sociology.

The COVID-19 pandemic brings into sharp relief the argument that socio-economic factors need to remain at the heart of sociological work on disability. Across the globe, it is clear that disabled people are particularly vulnerable both to the virus and to the implications of how governments respond to it. In the UK, the different government advice given to people with 'underlying health conditions' covers both non-disabled people, with health conditions, and people with impairments due to their health conditions. Disability groups are at the forefront in arguing that the different advice to people with underlying health conditions on self-isolation and self-shielding are discriminatory. For example, guidance on restrictions to using public space has not considered differential impacts on disabled people, leading to successful legal challenges because they have not made the reasonable adjustments required by the Equality Act (2010). There are also significant concerns that people with 'underlying health conditions' and disabled people generally risk having less access to life-saving treatments. As the virus has progressed in multiple countries, residential care homes have been a key site of infection, affecting both the people who live there, and those who work within them. While much of the media debate has focused on the impact of this on older people, disability groups have highlighted this is not just an issue of age, but also of disability, given the numbers of disabled people also living in residential, or supported living, contexts. Finally, disability activists have argued that the use of the phrase 'underlying conditions' in government figures on death rates has created a distinction between those whose death is less important (people ill already) and those who are more important (healthy people) in a way that echoes and reinforces the marginalization of ill and disabled people in society as expendable (Abrams and Abbott, 2020). It will require close collaboration across medical sociology and disability studies to explore and understand the societal impacts and implications of COVID-19 for disabled people and those living with chronic health-conditions.

See also: Chronic Illness; Medicalization; Social Movements and Health; Stigma.

REFERENCES

Abrams, T. and Abbott, D. (2020) 'Disability, deadly discourse, and collectivity amid Coronavirus (COVID-19)', *Scandinavian Journal of Disability Research*, 22 (1): 168–174.

Barnes, C. (1998) 'The social model of disability: a sociological phenomenon ignored by sociologists', in T. Shakespeare (ed.), *The Disability Reader: Social Science Perspectives*. London: Continuum International Publishing Group.

Bury, M. (1996) 'Disability and the myth of the independent researcher: a reply', *Disability & Society*, 11 (1): 112–115.

Goodley, D. (2011) *Critical Disability Studies: Expanding Debates and Interdisciplinary Engagements*. London: SAGE.

Hughes, B. and Paterson, K. (1997) 'The social model of disability and the disappearing body: towards a sociology of impairment', *Disability & Society*, 12: 325–340.

Moffatt, S. and Noble, E. (2015) 'Work or welfare after cancer? Explorations of identity and stigma', *Sociology of Health & Illness*, 37 (8): 1191–1205.

Morris, J. (ed.) (1996) *Encounters with Strangers: Feminism and Disability*. London: The Women's Press.

Oliver, M. (1990) *The Politics of Disablement*. Basingstoke: Macmillan.

Ryan, S. (2005) 'Busy behaviour in the land of the golden M: going out with learning disabled children in public places', *Journal of Applied Research in Intellectual Disabilities*, 18 (1): 65–74.

Scambler, G. (2020) *A Sociology of Shame and Blame: Insiders Versus Outsiders*. Cham: Palgrave Pivot.

Shakespeare, T. (2006) *Disability Rights and Wrongs*. London: Routledge.

Thomas, C. (2007) *Sociologies of Disability and Illness. Contested Ideas in Disability Studies and Medical Sociology*. Basingstoke: Palgrave.

UPIAS (1976) *Fundamental Principles of Disability*. London: Union of the Physically Impaired Against Segregation.

WHO (2011) *World Report on Disability*. Geneva: World Health Organization.

Williams, S.J. (1999) 'Is anybody there? Critical realism, chronic illness and the disability debate', *Sociology of Health & Illness*, 21 (6): 797–819.

SUGGESTED FURTHER READING

- Barnes, C., Mercer, G. and Shakespeare, T. (1999) *Exploring Disability: A Sociological Introduction*. Cambridge: Polity Press.

Although published in 1999, this remains an important text that uses the social model (critically) to make the case that sociology needs to think differently about disability. The authors advocate that disability studies is better placed to produce research on disability that is socially and politically useful.

- Goodley, D. (2017) *Disability Studies: An Interdisciplinary Introduction*. London: SAGE.

This is a very accessible introduction to disability studies. It charts the development of different approaches to disability studies which have emerged in different geographical and disciplinary locations. It also makes the case for the importance of critical disability studies.

- Watson, N. and Vehmas, S. (eds) (2019) *Routledge Handbook of Disability Studies*, 2nd edn. London: Routledge.

This reader incorporates the broad scope of work within disability studies. Across 35 chapters, from established and new voices in disability studies, it explores many issues that have strong relevance for medical sociology.

23

Illness Narratives

Lee F. Monaghan and Mike Bury

Illness narratives refer to the storytelling and accounting practices that occur in the face of illness. Narrative analysis addresses the 'plot' of the account given and its motivational and social dimensions, including identity construction, embodied experiences, power and the situations wherein stories generate biographical value.

Human cultures are reproduced through narratives, that is, in the construction and telling of stories. Narratives provide the opportunity for using metaphors and other linguistic devices to convey and produce shared meanings and construct social identities, especially in difficult or threatening circumstances. Interestingly, whilst scholars in fields such as climate change are beginning to recognize the significance of narratives and storytelling (Moezzi et al., 2017), medical sociologists and anthropologists have long understood their relevance in the experiential world of illness, pain, suffering, vulnerability and uncertainty.

Those interested in illness narratives typically seek to understand and analyse the meanings produced in one cultural setting and communicate this knowledge to an audience in another setting, often in the hope of informing policy and practice. The idea that patients' narratives can inform clinical practice has gained ground in the USA, the UK and other countries. At a time when 'evidence-based' practice has become the watchword in many medical systems, analysts argued that the 'patient's view' is likely to be downplayed in favour of scientifically based and statistically oriented 'evidence'. However, attending to illness narratives may be just as important as evidence-based guidelines, notably in general practice that typically entails close contact with patients' everyday lives and the meanings attached to symptoms. Attending to such meanings is termed 'narrative-based medicine' and is intended to help clinicians make better decisions (Greenhalgh and Hurvitz, 1999) – a sentiment echoed in emerging health services research on patients' narratives on what has been called 'long Covid' (Ladds et al., 2020).

Sociologists and anthropologists have adopted a somewhat wider perspective, to include the multi-layered character of illness narratives, as well as their possible practical usage. Whilst empirical research on narratives is accumulating on various topics and among diverse groups – such as stories of embodiment and space in the case of limb amputation or HIV-infected children's accounts in the Global South (see Suggested Further Reading) – classic writings should first be acknowledged. For instance, we would be remiss if we did not highlight Williams' (1984) early study on 'narrative reconstruction', a process of continuous accounting whereby sufferers seek to align their biographically disrupted body, self and society. At the time Williams was writing he noted that, as a concept, 'narrative' was not well established in sociology but, as with other British medical sociologists during this period, his research on rheumatoid arthritis set a high standard for others to emulate.

Outside of sociology, Kleinman (1988), an anthropologist and clinician, is perhaps the best-known advocate of illness narratives. For Kleinman, listening to and interpreting the illness experience is an essential art form that has often been obscured during biomedical training. Yet illness narratives have relevance within and outside of clinical practice. For clinicians, such narratives are important because, firstly, patients with chronic disorders need a 'witness to suffering' and, secondly, heeding them may assist in the practical management of the condition. Outside of the clinic, illness narratives also enable sufferers to grapple with questions that the medical model often finds difficult to answer: Why me? Why now? And, 'What can be done? – the question of order and control' (p. 29). Through various examples, Kleinman explains how narratives connect the 'internal' reality of illness with other areas of life. Narratives are more than a 'reporting' of illness; they are efforts to integrate or reintegrate individuals into their social worlds. As with Williams' (1984) earlier work, there is in many such cases a 'narrative reconstruction' occurring as sufferers seek to make sense of their disrupted lives and address fundamental questions about their illness experience.

Illness narratives inevitably take particular forms as well as having specific contents. Each narrative will be fashioned by individuals in unique ways and to some extent in unique circumstances. Yet the sociological study of chronic illness has shown that narratives may involve one of a limited number of formal properties. These forms may exist prior to the construction or the telling of the story. They are 'accessed' through membership of a culture, where common understandings allow, indeed, constrain meanings to be fashioned in specific ways. The forms that illness narratives take will also be shaped by underlying psychological needs and motivations concerning the presentation of the self to others in particular contexts – for example in an interview setting, as similarly noted in recent literature on 'nonfatal suicidal behaviour' (Banjes and Swartz, 2019) that also draws from Goffman's sociology.

Subsuming some aspects of schemes developed by other authors, Bury (2001) elucidates three main illness narrative forms: contingent, moral and

core. *Contingent narratives* describe the events surrounding the onset and early
course of a disorder. They may address 'life events' such as bereavement, or the
'external' circumstances of difficult work situations. They may also assimilate
medical explanations for the disorder and how these relate to life experiences.
Contingent narratives deal with proximate causes and effects, often outlining
the steps taken to deal with the illness and strategies to manage it. Such narratives tend to be practical and descriptive; they foreground unfolding events
and the immediate impact these have on the relationship between the self, body
and others. In dealing with 'biographical reconstruction' individuals will often
feel the need (not always consciously) to present themselves as culturally competent, thus expressing *moral narratives*. This second form is evaluative. Moral
narratives not only order experience but also express the 'dynamic relations'
between the self and others. These narratives may include social apologia in
which the person tries to close the gap between their previous self-image and
what they perceive or experience as failures in self-presentation or role performance. Moral narratives may also be a means to portray the self as active and
socially engaged. The third form, *core narratives*, include 'genres of expression'
through which the narrator 'emplots' herself in a more or less dramatic fashion;
such narratives may be epic or heroic, tragic, comic or didactic (p. 278). Core
narratives may also convey the underlying illness trajectory; for instance, stable, progressive or regressive (Robinson, 1990). Progressive narratives, in particular, convey a positive and more engaging response. Such narratives chime
with a late- or post-modern culture surrounding illness, one where 'restitution'
and the search for a more positive identity through suffering may be found
(Frank, 1995).

Analysing illness narratives is associated with the interpretative wing of
sociology. Clearly, the eliciting and recording of illness narratives requires the
employment of qualitative methods, especially extended interviews and life histories. Researchers often use such methods to elicit *individuals'* narratives, that
is, 'first-person accounts by respondents of their experience' (Riessman, 1993:
1). However, there is growing recognition of the importance of co-constructed
talk, as per Radcliffe et al.'s (2013) research with older stroke survivors and
their spouses – a study that consisted of 'joint biographical narrative interviews'
in order to explore the 'shared creation of meanings' and the 'co-presentation
of identity' (p. 993). In general, narrative analysis differs from other qualitative
methods in its stress on the need to examine long sequences of text and whole
accounts rather than breaking the text up, as in thematic analysis. Whole narratives across a sample of respondents can then be compared for their similarities and differences. Though such narratives may take on the properties of one
of the forms outlined above, it is likely that they will combine more than one
element.

Whilst recent research underscores the need to explore the content and
style of co-constructed narratives via joint interviews, other methodological
and epistemological issues have been subject to deliberation over the years.
As Riessman (1993: 2) explains, the employment of interpretative methods in

analysing illness narratives involves tackling 'the inevitable gap between the experience ... and any communication about it'. This cautions against sociological approaches to narratives that regard them as a move in reclaiming illness from a dominant medical model as well as a 'colonial' medical practice. For example, illness narratives are, according to Frank (1995), 'stories that are their own truth'; frameworks of analysis are, from this viewpoint, merely devices to 'heighten attention' to these truths (p. 24). Whilst, in one sense, it must be the case that individuals have a unique insight on their own experience, Riessman's (1993) methodological considerations suggest the need to proceed with care.

If illness narratives are treated as a 'revealed truth', then all claims take on equal weight. Yet the gap between experience and communication discussed by Riessman leads the researcher to ask 'why was the story told that way?' (1993: 2). This question may reveal, in the analysis, contradictions and ambiguities in expression and in the relationship between the accounting procedures and the motivations for presenting matters in one way and not another. Motivational elements suggest that illness narratives need to be interpreted and not taken as given. The ethic of the sociologist must be governed by the recognition that the teller 'has the first word on which the interpretation depends' (Riessman, 1993: 52), but also illness narratives are 'always edited versions of reality, not impartial or objective descriptions of it' (Riessman, 1990: 1197).

Medical sociologists have continued to reflect upon such matters. Thomas (2010) offers a useful account of an ongoing debate between influential writers in this field (including Atkinson, Frank, Kleinman and others), where '[m]atters of theoretical perspective, methodology, ethics, and personal politics are found to be at stake' (p. 647). Thomas summarizes various claims and counter-claims when explicating Atkinson's critique of Frank, for instance. She explains that Atkinson takes Frank to task for romantically 'privileging' illness narratives as a source of authenticity, that is, 'special' or 'valid' accounts about people's illness experiences. Summarizing a debate that began in the 1990s, Thomas states that whereas Atkinson argues for an analytic approach to narratives as 'speech-acts' (p. 649), Frank and those with post-modern leanings tend to mix politics and advocacy in their interpretations.

Thomas (2010) locates such discussions in wider sociological context. What underpins the crux of the debate, for her, is the type of sociology (implicitly) being practised. She uses Burawoy's influential schema on sociology's division of labour to make sense of this. Some contributors may be more interested in producing public knowledge for extra-academic audiences (patient advocacy groups, for example) rather than analytic accounts for their peers. Reflecting these tensions between public and professional sociologies, alongside the interplay of critical and policy lines of analysis, Thomas sympathizes with both sides of the debate. She endorses aspects of Atkinson's reasoning; notably, the importance of systematic research and formal analysis over sentimentality and romanticism. Various points raised by Frank and Kleinman are also credited where ethics and personal standpoint have dialogical significance, furthering what Thomas sees as the 'emancipatory' potential for communities of ill people.

Thomas arrives at such a position with reference to her personal experiences and research on illness narratives among people with cancer and their informal carers. She writes: 'I believe that qualitative social scientific research of the type referred to here can, if carefully disseminated, assist in making cancer and palliative care services more responsive to the needs and interests of patients, carers, and other service users' (p. 657).

Whatever the reader's position might be in these debates, the concept of illness narratives continues to stimulate sociological research, discussion and conceptual development. For instance, Sanderson et al. (2015) seek to redress what they describe as the 'neglected' focus on 'the moral component' of illness narratives with reference to Punjabi women living with rheumatoid arthritis in the UK. In another study, Vassilev et al. (2017) explore how different articulations of neoliberalism in the UK and Bulgaria shape narratives of chronic illness management. They observed that respondents with type 2 diabetes offered different accounts depending upon the logics of the broader social environments of these two countries. Mazanderani et al. (2013) also offer an interesting contribution. They provide a 'theoretical toolbox' in order to analyse how illness narratives are situationally commodified, again highlighting how broader contextual or 'socio-political factors' matter (pp. 892–893). Drawing from secondary data on a range of conditions in the UK and analyses of the 'bioeconomy' that blur economic and ethical considerations, Mazanderani et al. advance calls to explore how illness narratives attain value not only in a research interview but also through various media (television, books, websites). Potentially relevant considerations in the generation of value include: the sharing of embodied experiences that are deemed 'authentic', the role of celebrities diagnosed with a condition in raising awareness and attracting research funding, and a desire to help other sufferers and charities. These are important considerations, one might suggest, given the proliferation of illness narratives and how they obtain 'biographical value' within 'contemporary healthcare and its social environment' (p. 891). This conceptualization seems especially apt today given how, for instance, the health service research on 'long Covid' (Ladds et al., 2020), cited above, was facilitated via popular social media platforms (such as Facebook) that not only distribute but also monetize users' 'data', thus generating shareholder value. These are not Ladds et al.'s (2020) or Mazanderani et al.'s (2013) concerns. Arguably, though, they warrant further investigation as ever more aspects of our lives, in sickness and in health, move online and generate commodifiable data within an international 'narrative economy' (for more on the latter concept, in relation to AIDS activism in the Global South, see Burchardt, 2016).

In sum, medical sociologists must carefully engage the rich and complex stories recounted by people, whilst also being reflexive about their own aims when interpreting and analysing illness narratives for different audiences. Furthermore, as with moves to analyse how narratives are socially situated and commodified there is plenty of scope for medical sociologists to undertake critical studies on the conditions under which people share stories about their illness experiences and the different interests such storytelling serves in ways that may not be intended or realized by narrators themselves. Narrative forms and structures are crucial topics of analysis but so too are broader dynamics within (digitized, embodied, globalized) fields of power that constitute not only micro but also organizational and macro levels of society.

See also: Chronic Illness; Digital Health; Disability; Embodiment; The Medical Model.

REFERENCES

Banjes, J. and Swartz, L. (2019) '"What can we learn from first-person narratives?" The case of nonfatal suicidal behaviour', *Qualitative Health Research*, 29 (10): 1497–1507.

Burchardt, M. (2016) 'The self as capital in the narrative economy: how biographical testimonies move activism in the Global South', *Sociology of Health & Illness*, 38 (4): 592–609.

Bury, M. (2001) 'Illness narratives, fact or fiction?' *Sociology of Health & Illness*, 23 (1): 263–285.

Frank, A. (1995) *The Wounded Storyteller: Body, Illness, and Ethics*. Chicago, IL: University of Chicago Press.

Greenhalgh, T. and Hurwitz, B. (1999) 'Why study narrative?' *British Medical Journal*, 318: 48–50.

Kleinman, A. (1988) *The Illness Narratives: Suffering, Healing and the Human Condition*. New York: Basic Books.

Ladds, E., Rushforth, A., Wieringa, S. et al. (2020) 'Persistent symptoms after Covid-19: qualitative study of 114 "long Covid" patients and draft quality principles for services', *BMC Health Services Research*, 20: 1144.

Mazanderani, F., Locock, L. and Powell, J. (2013) 'Biographical value: towards a conceptualisation of the commodification of illness narratives in contemporary healthcare', *Sociology of Health & Illness*, 35 (6): 891–905.

Moezzi, M., Janda, K.B. and Rotmann, S. (2017) 'Using stories, narratives and storytelling in energy and climate change research', *Energy, Research & Social Science*, 31: 1–10.

Radcliffe, E., Lowton, K. and Morgan, M. (2013) 'Co-construction of chronic illness narratives by older stroke survivors and their spouses', *Sociology of Health & Illness*, 35 (7): 993–1007.

Riessman, C.K. (1990) 'Strategic use of narratives in the presentation of self and illness: a research note', *Social Science & Medicine*, 30 (11): 1195–2000.

Riessman, C.K. (1993) *Narrative Analysis*. Newbury Park, CA: SAGE.

Robinson, I. (1990) 'Personal narratives, social careers and medical course: analysing life trajectories in autobiographies of people with multiple sclerosis', *Social Science & Medicine*, 30 (11): 1173–1186.

Sanderson, T., Calnan, M. and Kumar, K. (2015) 'The moral experience of illness and its impact on normalisation: examples from narratives with Punjabi women living with rheumatoid arthritis in the UK', *Sociology of Health & Illness*, 37 (8): 1218–1235.

Thomas, C. (2010) 'Negotiating the contested terrain of narrative methods in illness contexts', *Sociology of Health & Illness*, 32 (4): 647–660.

Vassilev, I., Rogers, A., Todorova, E. et al. (2017) 'The articulation of neoliberalism: narratives of experience of chronic illness management in Bulgaria and the UK', *Sociology of Health & Illness*, 39 (3): 349–364.

Williams, G. (1984) 'The genesis of chronic illness: narrative reconstruction', *Sociology of Health & Illness*, 6 (2): 175–200.

SUGGESTED FURTHER READING

- Heavey, E. (2018) '"If I can walk *that* far": space and embodiment in stories of illness and recovery', *Sociology of Health & Illness*, 40 (6): 1005–1018.

Drawing from a case study of a woman in England who underwent a lower-limb amputation, Heavey develops a framework for analysing the intersections of embodied experience, space and narrative identity construction. In so doing, she centres the phenomenological and material body, the socio-symbolic relevance of space and its symbiotic relation to time.

- Caddick, N., Smith, B. and Phoenix, C. (2015) 'Male combat veterans' narratives of PTSD, masculinity, and health', *Sociology of Health & Illness*, 37 (1): 97–111.

Caddick et al. link illness narratives and masculinities scholarship when studying stories about post-traumatic stress disorder primarily among former British army combat veterans. The article reveals the tensions at play in men's narratives, with militarized masculine performances not simply constituting a danger but also a resource for their health and well-being.

- Hillman, A., Jones, I.R., Quinn, C. et al. (2018) 'Dualities of dementia illness narratives and their role in a narrative economy', *Sociology of Health & Illness*, 40 (5): 874–891.

Drawing conceptually from Burchardt's work on 'the self as capital in the narrative economy', cited above, Hillman et al. explore dementia illness narratives. Their analysis is attuned to how narratives emerge within exchange relationships, constituting currency that may facilitate access to resources as well as generating meaning and purpose for narrators.

- Bernays, S., Seeley, J., Rhodes, T. and Mupambireyi, Z. (2015) 'What am I "living" with?: Growing up with HIV in Uganda and Zimbabwe', *Sociology of Health & Illness*, 37 (2): 270–283.

Research among HIV-infected children, their carers and healthcare workers in Africa reveals how, even when receiving anti-retroviral treatment, the medicalized language of sickness results in a 'narrow narrative' rather than narratives of readjustment and restoration. These observations are interpreted in a relational context consisting of uncertainty, power and silencing that shape children's illness narratives and undermine 'a quest for ordinariness'.

24

Risk

Jonathan Gabe

Risk involves exposure to a given danger or hazard.

The language of risk is now frequently used in both popular and expert discourse, especially when it comes to discussing health issues. This has not always been the case. In pre-Renaissance times the dominant popular discourse was that of 'fate' – in which personal misfortune and disaster were explained in terms of chance, destiny and the will of the gods. In this period dangers such as floods and epidemics were perceived as natural events rather than as man-made and the idea of human fault or responsibility was not considered. With the emergence of modernity in the 17th century a new materialistic and deterministic discourse was established, premised on the belief that the social and natural world followed causal laws. From this standpoint risks were the products of such determinism and the vagaries of nature. Subsequently, risk was scientized as a result of the growing influence of mathematical explanations relating to probability. During the 19th century it became possible to measure the risk of an event by calculating its statistical probability, thereby taming chance. Risk also came to be located in human beings as well as in nature and unintended outcomes were acknowledged as being a possible consequence of human action. According to Lupton (1999), modernist notions of risk also recognized that risk could be either 'good' or 'bad', involving gain or loss and could thus be seen in neutral terms. Since the 19th century, however, the meaning of risk has been transformed and it has mainly come to be seen as involving only negative outcomes. Risk now typically means danger, and the greater the risk the greater the danger. Against this dominant discourse there has however developed a counter discourse which sees risk-taking more positively as involving emotionally charged dangerous activities which give pleasure, for example sky-diving or bungee-jumping, described by Lyng (1990) as 'edgework'.

Traditionally research on risk has been the preserve of the risk industry, drawing primarily on disciplines such as engineering, toxicology, biostatistics and actuarial science. Assessing public health risks has also become a major issue for epidemiologists who aim to calculate the 'relative risk' or numerical odds of a population developing an illness when exposed to a risk factor, compared with a similar population that has not suffered such exposure. It is on the basis of these risk assessments that governments have conducted health education campaigns, for example about AIDS, to warn the public about the dangers of 'risky behaviour'. Likewise, governments have more recently been running campaigns in the media warning people about the risks of catching or transmitting COVID-19 if they do not maintain 'social distance' (or, more accurately, physical distance), wash their hands regularly and wear masks in public settings. It is expected that the provision of such information about how to minimize risk will lead to the reduction of disease, though there is debate on such matters in the context of scientific uncertainty as discussed among critical public health scholars (Martin et al., 2020; see also Brown, 2020, below).

Since the 1990s a concerted effort has been made to develop social analyses of risk. In what follows a variety of such analyses will be discussed starting with the cultural approach, inspired by the anthropologist Mary Douglas. Douglas was one of the first to draw attention to the need for an analysis that challenged the status of risk as an objective measure, as argued by members of the risk industry. Instead she took a weak constructionist view, like many others after her, and considered that objective hazards were inevitably mediated by cultural processes and could only be known in relation to these processes. She was interested in why some dangers were selected as risks while others were not, the importance of ritual in understanding our pre-occupation with particular risks and how risk acts as a symbolic boundary between groups. For her what was of significance was that groups of people identify different risk attributes and even types of risk as a result of their particular form of social organization and interaction in the wider culture. In her view the way in which such collectivities respond to risk is functional for the maintenance of their form of social organization. The argument was formalized in an analytic scheme that has come to be known as grid/group analysis. For Douglas the degree of collectivism found in groups and the degree of internal difference within groups impact on perceptions of risk. Collectivism, whether strong or weak, is defined in terms of 'group', while the degree of difference is defined in terms of 'grid'. By linking grid and group, Douglas, along with her colleague Wildavsky (1982), identified four distinct world views which justified different ways of behaving towards a hazard. These were named hierarchist (high grid/high group), egalitarian (low grid/high group), fatalist (high grid, low group) and individualist (low grid, low group). Hierarchists, for example, were considered to be well-integrated (group axis) and to accept externally imposed risk assessment by experts (grid axis) while egalitarians, although being well-integrated too, tended to challenge the experts' assessments on the grounds that these experts' calculations threatened their group's way of life (grid axis). Douglas and Wildavsky also believed that when people feel they are at risk they tend to blame outsiders rather than focus on dangers from within their own community. In the health field grid/group analysis has been applied to studying differences in response to hazards in contexts ranging from hospitals to transport.

Recently Douglas' work has been employed by Brown (2020) to help us understand institutional and social responses to the risks of COVID-19. He notes how different governments' responses to COVID risk can be seen as cultural–organizational in origin and are reflected in different institutional processes of risk management. He also discusses the symbolic and emotional significance of material objects like bodies and face masks to understand the development of practices to minimize risk. He suggests that COVID is being seen as a threat to 'pure bodies' from bodies from 'outside' which are viewed as dirty, or in Douglas' words as 'matter out of place'. Ritualized practices such as mask wearing can also generate heightened emotions and, we might speculate, reinforce differences between a sense of 'us' (those wearing masks to minimize risk) and 'them' (non mask wearers). These ritualized practices might also involve 'magical', that is non rational, elements designed to make a particular future more likely. Thus handling uncertainty might be said to combine rational and non-rational/magical elements. Moreover, epidemiological research which categorizes the over 70s as more at risk can be seen as shaping people's cultural understandings of risk, with the implicit othering of these older people in comparison to mainstream 'normals'. While the grid/group approach in particular has been criticized for being too static and for failing to explain how organizations and individuals can change their perception of risk over time, Douglas' general theory nonetheless offers a way of exploring how conflicts over risk can be understood in terms of plural constructions of meaning that are culturally framed.

Other more sociological work on risk perception has adopted an interpretivist approach and generally concentrated on two broad areas: (1) perceptions of risk and risk behaviour and (2) the relationship between lay and expert knowledge of risk. The first of these has emphasized the role of contextual factors in risk perception. For example, Webster (2020) examined the risk perceptions of children and family members to the diagnosis of epilepsy. This diagnosis provides parents and their children with a new framework to evaluate risks posed by the physical environment. An explicit language of risk was regularly employed by parents when discussing the dangers from water, roads and falling from a height if their child had a seizure. It is argued that the parents' focus on physical risks reflects their view of children as a particularly vulnerable group. The parents also acknowledged that they had reconceptualized everyday environments and activities as more risky as a result of their child's diagnosis. In other words the diagnosis had shaped their perception of risk. Children's concerns did not always align with those of their parents. For while the parents focused on new and reconceptualized physical risks, children were primarily concerned with being stigmatized by their peers because their epilepsy made them feel different, reflecting the importance of childhood culture. Others have focused on the relationship between lay and expert perceptions of risk. For instance, Armstrong and Murphy (2008) have explored the extent to which lay understandings of cervical cancer risk incorporate medical professionals' understandings. They found that women's engagement with such expert understandings was complex. Where expert-defined risk factors were incorporated they were transformed and woven into a coherent whole within the context of the women's prior understandings, experiences and other socially situated factors. However this process was hampered because of incomplete medical information about the link between behavioural risk factors such as sexual behaviour and smoking and cervical cancer.

In addition to this interpretivist work on group risk perceptions and behaviour, there have also been more macro level studies about the role of social institutions and structures in the framing of risk. One key institution involved in shaping risk perception is the mass media, as discussed by Tulloch and Zinn (2011). They review the literature on media and health risks and show how the media reproduce and amplify expert risk assessment yet also create limited opportunities for counter definitions to emerge. They also note how media frame health risks so that audiences may see health risks in one particular way and not another and how audiences may act as critical consumers, questioning the media messages in terms of their own values. More recently Zinn (2020) has shown how the growing social prominence of health and well-being has acted as a driver of risk language in the print media. Such language now not only appears in the news section but in the features and opinion sections which have grown over time and helped fuel the frequency of 'at risk' constructs.

The importance of the media as an institution is reflected in the way that the media frame health risks about obesity and the role of scientists in this process. Holland et al. (2011) analysed how the Australian press represented a scientific report on the long-term consequences of 'Australia's expanding waistline' for cardiovascular disease. The press framed the report as showing that Australia was the fattest nation in the world, overtaking America. This frame was prompted by comments by the lead author when publicizing the report. However the coverage failed to note that the scientific report itself did not include any international comparisons and was only based on data from middle-aged Australians. As Holland et al. stress, there was a lack of critical commentary on the report and a failure to test the obesity claims of its lead author. As a result, preconceptions of the putative 'problem' were reinforced at the expense of findings about 'potential solutions' (or other crucial concerns, such as the ethics of obesity discourse and the unintended consequences of declaring a war on obesity) (see also Monaghan et al., 2019).

The relationship between lay and expert knowledge has also been explored more broadly by social theorists in the context of declining trust in expert authority in late modern society. Giddens (1990), for example, has suggested that the judgements of experts are now under increasing scrutiny and are either accepted or rejected by lay people who are making 'pragmatic calculations' about the risks involved. In these circumstances the most cherished beliefs underpinning expert systems are open to revision and alteration, thereby challenging a dominant source of authoritative interpretation. The degree to which people feel alienated from or at least ambivalent towards experts also relates to the German sociologist Beck's (1992, 2009) argument that we now live in a world 'risk society' that is increasingly interdependent and thus vulnerable to major socio-technical disruption. Social and economic developments have created global hazards, ranging from nuclear accidents to ecological disasters, for which there is no adequate aftercare. These structural features highlight the need for trust in expert authority at a time when greater reflexivity and awareness of the indeterminate status of knowledge about risk combine to undermine it. One of the main criticisms of this 'reflexive modernization' thesis is that it is based on broad generalizations of structural and organizational processes that lack grounding in actual processes and experiences of institutional and everyday life. Nonetheless, this approach has been enormously influential and has provided valuable insights on the structural and political aspects of risk.

While the risk society, like the other approaches outlined above, has adopted a weak constructionist position about risk, accepting that risk is an objective hazard that is mediated through social and cultural processes, there is one approach that takes a strong constructionist position – that concerned with risk and governmentality. From this standpoint there is no such thing as an objective risk; rather risks are solely a product of discourses, strategies, practices and institutions around phenomena that turn them into risks (Lupton, 1999). This Foucauldian inspired perspective is particularly interested in the way in which risk operates in relation to the political ethos of advanced liberalism. The latter conceptualizes individuals as rational agents who should take responsibility to protect themselves from risks rather than rely on the state to protect them. Rather than assume that individuals pre-exist as rational consumers, Foucauldians argue that they have to be configured as such through governmental practices. The approach can be illustrated by Harvey's (2010) study of commercially produced documents related to direct to consumer genetic testing services for diet-related disease. She focuses on how genetic susceptibility testing is positioned as a healthcare resource by these commercial providers. She argues that the documents configure individuals as being empowered to choose health by using the testing service and that this will facilitate their journey towards a healthy selfhood. Configured in this way users of the service become 'good citizens' of an advanced liberal democracy, increasing their own vital capital and contributing to the prosperity of all.

In sum, the social analysis of risk now incorporates a variety of approaches ranging from Douglas' cultural analysis through interpretivist and structural approaches to Foucauldian analyses of risk and governmentality. While there has been some debate about the continuing value of risk as a framework for analysis (Green, 2009), the approaches reviewed here suggest that each of them still has something to offer in helping us make sense of the meaning and nature of risk as a dominant feature of late modern society. Never has this been more apparent than during the COVID-19 pandemic where further investigation is urgently needed into how different national governments have adopted a variety of approaches to make sense of and minimize the risk of COVID and how the risks of mitigation strategies have been compared to those of viral infection. Likewise we need research into how cultural understandings of risk have shaped responses to COVID in everyday life and amongst those working 'on the front line' in the healthcare system in different countries.

See also: Citizenship and Health; Consumerism; Lay Knowledge; Pandemics and Epidemics; Pharmaceuticalization.

REFERENCES

Armstrong, N. and Murphy, E. (2008) 'Weaving meaning? An exploration of the interplay between lay and professional understandings of cervical cancer risk', *Social Science & Medicine*, 67 (7): 1074–1082.

Beck, U. (1992) *Risk Society*. London: SAGE.

Beck, U. (2009) *World at Risk*. Cambridge: Polity Press.

Brown, P. (2020) 'Studying COVID-19 in light of critical approaches to risk and uncertainty: research pathways, conceptual tools, and some magic from Mary Douglas', *Health, Risk & Society*, 22 (1): 1–14.

Douglas, M. and Wildavsky, A. (1982) *Risk and Culture: An Essay on the Selection of Technological and Environmental Dangers*. Berkeley: University of California Press.

Giddens, A. (1990) *The Consequences of Modernity*. Cambridge: Polity Press.

Green, J. (2009) 'Is it time for the sociology of health to abandon "risk"?' *Health, Risk & Society*, 11 (6): 493–508.

Harvey, A. (2010) 'Genetic risks and healthy choices: creating citizen-consumers of genetic services through empowerment and facilitation', *Sociology of Health & Illness*, 32 (3): 365–381.

Holland, K.E., Warwick Blood, R., Thomas, S.I. et al. (2011) '"Our girth is plain to see": an analysis of newspaper coverage of "Australia's Future Fat Bomb"', *Health, Risk & Society*, 13 (1): 31–46.

Lupton, D. (1999) *Risk*. London: Routledge.

Lyng, S. (1990) 'Edgework: a social psychological analysis of voluntary risk taking', *American Journal of Sociology*, 95 (4): 851–886.

Martin, G.P., Hanna, E., McCartney, M. and Dingwall, R. (2020) 'Science, society, and policy in the face of uncertainty: reflections on the debate around face coverings for the public during COVID-19', *Critical Public Health*, 30 (5): 501–508.

Monaghan, L.F., Rich, E. and Bombak, A.E. (2019) 'Media, "fat panic" and public pedagogy: mapping contested terrain', *Sociology Compass*, 13 (1): e12651.

Tulloch, J. and Zinn, J.O. (2011) 'Risk, health and the media', *Health, Risk & Society*, 13 (1): 1–16.

Webster, M. (2020) 'Childhood epilepsy in contemporary society: risk perceptions among children and their family members', *Health, Risk & Society*, 22 (1): 53–68.

Zinn, J.O. (2020) 'Health and illness as drivers of risk language in the news media – a case study of *The Times*', *Health, Risk & Society*, 22 (7-8): 437–455.

SUGGESTED FURTHER READING

- Alaszewski, A. (2015) 'Anthropology and risk: insights into uncertainty, danger and blame from other cultures', *Health, Risk & Society*, 17 (3–4): 205–225.

An illuminating review of the contribution of social anthropology to the study of risk, based on studies of non-Western cultures.

- Calnan, M. and Douglass, T. (2020) 'Hopes, hesitancy and the risky business of vaccine development', *Health, Risk & Society*, 22 (5-6): 291–304.

A valuable review of vaccine hesitancy and vaccine development. It considers among other issues how people personalize or individualize the perceived risk of vaccine uptake in the context of an atomized neoliberal society in which individual responsibility and choice are emphasized. The financial risks for pharmaceutical companies of developing a vaccine and the willingness of governments to share these risks in the face of COVID-19 are also discussed.

- Gabe, J. (1995) 'Health, medicine and risk: the need for a sociological approach', in J. Gabe (ed.), *Medicine, Health and Risk: Sociological Approaches*. Oxford: Blackwell Publishers.

An early but still useful discussion of different approaches to risk, from the risk industry and psychological risk analysis to a variety of cultural and social theories of risk.

- Rossiter, K. and Godderis, R. (2020) 'Essentially invisible: risk and personal support workers in the time of COVID-19', *Sociology of Health & Illness*, 42 (8): e25–e31.

An important commentary which draws attention to the gendered dynamics of risk that have emerged during COVID-19 for personal support workers such as nursing assistants – an often invisible but essential labour force in many healthcare systems.

25

The Sick Role

Lee F. Monaghan and Mike Bury

> *Intended as an ideal type, the sick role refers to the set of rights and obligations surrounding illness that could shape the actions of doctors and patients.*

American sociologist Talcott Parsons (1951) is generally credited for formulating the concept of 'the sick role'. Whilst Parsons recognized that health and illness have a biological basis, his account contributed to the early development of medical sociology by underscoring the social implications of illness and medical practice. For Parsons, 'the sick role' was central to this account, encapsulating in an 'ideal typical' or analytical sense those rights and obligations that surround illness when normal roles are relinquished or suspended. The concept emerged from the 'moral economy' (Varul, 2010) of mid-20th-century US society. He thus offered a socio-historical account of the normative expectations surrounding illness, sanctioned by physicians and defined as unmotivated deviance or the incapacity to perform valued social roles. For Parsons, the sick role had a nominal focus on the actions of a rational, income-generating masculine employee within a gendered division of labour, where paid work and doctors' judgements were privileged. Despite much social change, such values have not been entirely erased and, arguably, the sick role concept retains relevance.

Parsons first used the sick role concept in his description of 'The case of modern medical practice' in *The Social System* (1951). Adopting a functionalist approach that has antecedents in Durkheimian sociology, Parsons regarded the role of medical care as meeting certain 'prerequisites' that underpin the functioning of all social systems, especially modern ones. Within this theoretical framework, 'health' is crucial for the functioning of the social system, meaning that if the population's general health is 'too low' and 'the incidence of illness' 'too high' then this is 'dysfunctional' for society (p. 430). Accordingly, the key social function of medical practice is to help maintain an 'optimal' level of health in society.

Whilst there are two different models of illness in Parsons' work (Gerhardt, 1989), the more complex and interesting model treats illness as deviance, and the sick role as a mechanism of social control. Illness constitutes 'deviance' in a dynamic work-oriented society because it disrupts everyday role requirements and obligations; correspondingly, in order to regulate this, doctors act as gatekeepers to the sick role. The sick role is important because it allows individuals temporary exemption from their ordinary role obligations, and provides the mechanism for returning people to health and therefore to normal role performance. Of course, in providing such exemption, the sick role may become an attractive alternative to everyday pressures, providing a way of 'evading social responsibilities' (Parsons, 1951: 431) and offering 'secondary gain'. Hence, the sick role is 'contingent'. It is dependent on medical approval so that malingering, or motivated avoidance of role responsibilities, does not become too easy or 'dysfunctional' from a system viewpoint. In all modern societies absence from work due to ill health is heavily regulated, often requiring medical certification. In short, medical practice is part of society's social control apparatus.

Parsons identifies two sets of four, mutually reinforcing, dimensions to the sick role; four for the performance of the doctor's role and four for the performance of the patient's. Together they constitute the necessary elements for a functional 'sick role'. We will elaborate upon each of these ideal typical obligations and rights below, focusing first upon doctors and then patients.

First, Parsons (1951) argues that doctors have the obligation to be technically competent and meet 'selection criteria' separate from other elements of the person's social status (p. 434). In other words, the appointment of doctors and their practice should be based on technical expertise and not on their personal or social background. Second, the practitioner should be 'affectively neutral', tackling the medical problem in an 'objective way'. The doctor should thus have the welfare of the patient at heart and not personal or commercial considerations – 'the "profit motive" is supposed to be drastically excluded from the medical world' (p. 435). Parsons was keen, in this respect, to contrast medicine in the USA with the world of business. Doctors should be 'collectivity oriented' and serve the community.

In return for meeting these obligations, two rights flow. First, doctors are treated by society as professional practitioners, with a degree of independence and self-regulation. This treatment flows from the exercise of 'functional specificity' and 'universalism' so that doctors are expected to be expert in specific areas and utilize a body of knowledge that has universal application. The exercise of these skills allows doctors to claim a degree of freedom from the organizational and commercial constraints in which they work. Second, doctors are allowed access to tabooed areas such as the sick person's body. This access may involve physical examination or, more dramatically, surgery (see Parsons, 1951: 451–452).

The exercise of this set of obligations and rights on the part of the doctor provides the basis for the patient entering the sick role. If the patient felt, for example, that the doctor was technically incompetent, was acting because of personal feelings, or was crossing boundaries in tabooed areas such as access to the body, then the sick role would be likely to break down immediately. Indeed, many high profile controversies and scandals in countries such as the UK in recent decades have involved just such elements, indicating the degree to which the sick role concept is an analytical abstraction that may not describe actual conduct in the empirical world. For instance, official complaints about doctors being unfit to practice, culminating in hearings by the General Medical Council, have provided grist for media reporting that contradicts Parsons' idealized account. Such coverage, especially in the tabloid press, has tended to focus on and dramatize alleged sexual misconduct by male general practitioners (Bradby et al., 1997).

In the presence of effective and safe medical practice, however, it is anticipated patients can enter the sick role with some degree of confidence. For those entering this role, Parsons identifies two rights and two obligations. The first right, noted above, is exemption from normal role responsibilities. This has to be legitimated, often by a doctor in the last analysis, thereby protecting the patient against the charge of 'malingering' (Parsons, 1951: 437). Second, the individual has the right not to be held responsible for their sickness. These rights are conditional on two obligations. First, the person must demonstrate a motivation to get well. Second, they must seek technically competent medical help and also cooperate with the clinician, producing a 'complementary role structure'. In this way the 'secondary gain' of the sick role is limited and the return to health is maintained as a primary goal.

The sick role concept has been criticized. It raises many questions, especially concerning its relevance to the wide range of illness states and forms of medical practice that exist in modern societies. Among other things, Freidson (1970) discussed how stigmatized illnesses may be treated as illegitimate with implications for the person's ability to access the rights and privileges of the sick role – an issue that resurfaces in more recent writings that engage the politics of stigma in neoliberal modernity. Also, empirically, it has long been recognized that not all forms of illness lead to the adoption of the sick role (Bloor and Horobin, 1975). In many cases being 'legitimately ill' does not need the sanctioning of a doctor, and much self-treatment and self-help are employed in dealing with illness. Gallagher (1976) also identifies various problems. For example, in Parsons' scheme the sick role is essentially temporary; it is assumed the role will be occupied for a period leading to recovery and the resumption of normal roles. Yet, this is often contradicted by chronic illness, which, by definition, is long term and enduring. Gallagher also challenges what he takes to be Parsons' overly 'medico-centric' view of illness, the sick role and medical practice. In particular, Gallagher notes that whilst Parsons underscores the centrality of doctors (especially hospital doctors) in healthcare organizations, other healthcare workers (including family practitioners) as well as lay support and family structures are equally important. Moreover, Parsons' claims about the need for an optimal level of health in the social system were contradicted by the low priority given by the medical profession to prevention at that time, where 'training and orientation [were] attuned to illness rather than toward the maintenance of health' (Gallagher, 1976: 215).

When evaluating the sick role concept, it could be argued that not all criticisms can be taken at face value and the concept remains relevant for medical sociology. For example, despite Gallagher's (1976) telling points about the sick role's *temporary* character, the situation is often more complex than he allows. When defending his argument, Parsons (1978: 28) stated that even in the case of chronic disorders, such as diabetes, the physician has an obligation 'to reinforce the patient's motivation to minimize the curtailment of his [or her] capacities'. Parsons also recognized that a 'fulltime' occupancy of the sick role does not apply to all forms of illness, especially chronic illness. Furthermore, whilst Parsons may have been too prone to present the sick role as a means of providing an asymmetrical but complementary role structure (playing down its potential for conflict), when it is placed in his full discussion of health and medicine it does address issues of abiding concern. As Gerhardt (1979) notes, these range from the psychodynamic aspects of illness and treatment, to the structural issues of illness and incapacity, and thus to matters of social control and power. For Gerhardt, the sick role is part of a 'structural' view of illness, locating individual needs in the wider society. Young (2004) offers compatible reasoning when discussing 'illness behaviour', noting there is much outside of the doctor–patient relationship that matters, including government and world systems. Of course, such observations prompt questions concerning how we might conceptualize a changed and changing society and, relatedly, socially embedded responses to health matters. These are not trivial concerns, especially in the context of emerging infectious diseases and public health and state enforceable mandates that go way beyond the doctor–patient dyad – macrosocial power relations that also capitalize upon fear and moralizing action and which embody potential or actual conflict. Note, for example, the polarizing debate about lives versus livelihood early during the COVID-19 pandemic and responses to various mandates that were introduced thereafter (notably surrounding face coverings and then vaccine requirements).

Parsons' (1951) sick role concept, if read in line with a structural–functionalist emphasis on equilibrium and consensus rather than coercion and conflict, thus has its limitations. And, following Burnham (2014), who uses the language of 'abandonment', a case might be made for omitting discussion on the sick role from this third edition of *Key Concepts in Medical Sociology*. However, the sick role concept has not vanished from 21st-century sociology. Indeed, sociologists and scholars from other disciplines, such as psychology, still draw from, defend and/or extend it with reference to various contexts of illness and health.

Cheshire et al. (2021), in their study of chronic fatigue syndrome/myalgic encephalomyelitis in England, use Parsons' (1951) sick role as a theoretical lens with which to explore the varied meanings of recovery. They observe that for many research participants, recovery had more to do with freedom from the sick role than from symptoms. Researching high-stake sickness insurance meetings in Sweden, Flinkfeldt (2017) also draws from Parsons' (1951) concept and develops it with a focus on the obligation placed upon the sick person to want to get well. They assert 'analysing psychological matters as they are oriented to by participants renders sick role theory relevant for a wide range of settings' (Flinkfeldt, 2017: 1149). Hallowell et al. (2015), researching women undergoing elective risk-reducing breast surgery in Australia, seek to 'rehabilitate' Parson's work amidst 'renewed scrutiny'; for them, 'the concept of the sick role may provide useful insight into women's experiences of risk-management today' (p. 186). Also in Australia, Lohm et al. (2020) describe how a hybrid and relational mode of practice has emerged among the public amidst concerns about antibiotic risks and antimicrobial resistance. Those with chronic illness, for example, 'combined a Parsonian endorsement of' medical authority and expertise 'with reflexive risk management' (p. 237). These recent examples of empirical research are worth reading alongside more theoretically focused work on the sick role (Shilling, 2002; Varul, 2010; Williams, 2005), outlined in the second edition of *Key Concepts in Medical Sociology*. Attuned to the moral economy of capitalism and associated sociological concerns (for example, reciprocity, health seeking, productivity and body projects) such literature informed our conclusion that the sick role concept has continued salience.

Future studies might build upon this literature, including much needed research on the potential relevance of the sick role in the Global South and how 'sickness as potentially disruptive deviance' is institutionally managed in the (post) COVID world. The latter area of research would appear to be particularly salient given what we noted above on how a high level of sickness in the population is dysfunctional for society, with doctors serving as gatekeepers or agents of social control who have the power to grant or withhold access to the sick role. Important questions might be explored here not only in relation to consensual doctor–patient relations, as per Parsons' heuristic, but also negotiation and/or potential conflict amidst uncertainty about the possible long-term health consequences of the virus and the impact of extended public health restrictions on people's well-being. One would also need to add to this approach socio-historical, structural and discursive analyses of changes in the doctor–patient relationship and challenges to medicine – for instance, in terms of lay expertise and trust.

See also: Illness and Health Behaviours; Practitioner–Client Relationships; The Medical Model; Trust in Medicine.

REFERENCES

Bloor, M. and Horobin, G. (1975) 'Conflict and conflict resolution in doctor–patient relationships', in C. Cox and A. Mead (eds), *A Sociology of Medical Practice*. London: Collier-Macmillan.

Bradby, H., Gabe, J. and Bury, M. (1997) '"Sexy docs" and "busty blondes": press coverage of professional misconduct cases brought before the General Medical Council', *Sociology of Health & Illness*, 17 (4): 458–476.

Burnham, J.C. (2014) 'Why sociologists abandoned the sick role concept', *History of the Human Sciences*, 27 (1): 70–87.

Cheshire, A., Ridge, D., Clark, L.V. and White, P.D. (2021) 'Sick of the sick role: narratives of what "recovery" means to people with CFS/ME', *Qualitative Health Research*, 31 (2): 298–308.

Flinkfeldt, M. (2017) 'Wanting to work: managing the sick role in high-stake sickness insurance meetings', *Sociology of Health & Illness*, 39 (7): 1149–1165.

Freidson, E. (1970) *Profession of Medicine: A Study of the Sociology of Applied Knowledge*. New York: Harper & Row.

Gallagher, E. (1976) 'Lines of reconstruction and extension in the Parsonian sociology of illness', *Social Science & Medicine*, 10 (5): 207–218.

Gerhardt, U. (1979) 'The Parsonian paradigm and the identity of medical sociology', *The Sociological Review*, 27 (2): 229–251.

Gerhardt, U. (1989) *Ideas About Illness: An Intellectual and Political History of Medical Sociology*. Basingstoke: Macmillan.

Hallowell, N., Heiniger, L., Baylock, B. et al. (2015) 'Rehabilitating the sick role: the experiences of high-risk women who undergo risk reducing breast surgery', *Health Sociology Review*, 24 (2): 186–198.

Lohm, D., Davis, M., Whittaker, A. and Flowers, P. (2020) 'Role crisis, risk and trust in Australian general public narratives about antibiotic use and antimicrobial resistance', *Health, Risk & Society*, 22 (3–4): 231–248.

Parsons, T. (1951) *The Social System*. London: Routledge and Kegan Paul.

Parsons, T. (1978) *Action Theory and the Human Condition*. New York: The Free Press.

Shilling, C. (2002) 'Culture, the sick role and the consumption of health', *British Journal of Sociology*, 53 (4): 621–638.

Varul, M. (2010) 'Talcott Parsons, the sick role and chronic illness', *Body & Society*, 16 (2): 72–94.

Williams, S.J. (2005) 'Parsons revisited: from the sick role to … ?' *Health*, 9 (2): 123–144.

Young, J.T. (2004) 'Illness behaviour: a selective review and synthesis', *Sociology of Health & Illness*, 26 (1): 1–31.

SUGGESTED FURTHER READING

- Willis, E. (2015) 'Talcott Parsons: his legacy and the sociology of health and illness', in F. Collyer (ed.), *The Palgrave Handbook of Social Theory in Health, Illness and Medicine*. New York: Palgrave Macmillan.

This chapter revisits Parsons' broader theorizing and sick role concept and flags changed social conditions that often render his sociology of historical interest rather than direct relevance. However, viewing him as a 'pre-eminent founder' of health or medical sociology, Willis explains that Parsons first established illness and healthcare as profoundly social and asserts that his concerns are of perennial sociological interest.

- Mik-Meyer, N. and Obling, A.R. (2012) 'The negotiation of the sick role: general practitioners' classification of patients with medically unexplained symptoms', *Sociology of Health & Illness*, 34 (7): 1025–1038.

Inspired by Parsons' (1951) focus on the institutional requirements of the sick role, these researchers explore how general practitioners in Denmark classify patients with medically unexplained symptoms. Also utilizing a symbolic interactionist perspective, the authors consider the external or institutional validation of the sick role.

- Boersma, J.J. and Brown, P. (2020) 'The tired hero and her (il)legitimation: re-working Parsons to analyse experiences of burnout with the Dutch employment system and lifeworld', *Social Science & Medicine*, 265: 113471.

An informative article that draws upon Habermas' classic reworking of Parsons when analysing interview data generated with 'burnout sufferers and diagnosing professionals'. The authors offer a conceptually informed empirical study of a phenomenon that has particular cultural and economic salience in the Netherlands.

26

Practitioner–Client Relationships

Alison Pilnick

The practitioner–client relationship encompasses the ways in which healthcare workers and lay people interact during health-related consultations and activities. This relationship can be affected by the context of the consultation, the nature of the communication that takes place, and broader factors such as policies, protocols and the use of technologies.

Healthcare today is more diverse than ever, and this diversity encompasses not just the range of personnel who deliver care, but the settings in which they do so, the tools which they employ, the tasks they accomplish and the dilemmas they confront. There is a long history of addressing these relationships from a sociological perspective, focusing initially on the doctor–patient encounter in primary care.

The study of doctor–patient relationships has its beginnings in the 1930s, and Henderson's (1935) description of interactions between physicians and patients as processes of mutual feedback, where each is constantly affecting the behaviour of the other. These observations influenced the work of Parsons (1951), who understood medicine as a way of practising social control. Sickness was seen by Parsons as a form of deviance, albeit unmotivated, and as such it had to be managed at a societal level to prevent or minimize the social disruption it could cause. This meant that interactions between doctors and patients were mediated by normative role expectations shared by all members of a society: that being sick was an undesirable state; that patients would want to get well; and that they would both seek medical help when appropriate and comply with the resulting recommendations. For such an interaction to be successful, participants must adopt the appropriate role expectations of doctor and patient and bring these to the interaction. From this viewpoint, the relationship operates as a consensus model, in that the uncontested or paternalistic authority of the doctor is seen as unproblematic or legitimate on the basis that s/he will always act in the best interests of the patient. How these interests are in fact to be established falls outside of the scope of the model.

Subsequent work by Szasz and Hollender (1956) proposed three distinct types of doctor–patient relationship: activity-passivity (likened to a parent–infant relationship); guidance-co-operation (likened to a parent–adolescent relationship, where authority is still unequally distributed); and mutual participation (seen as adult to adult). They noted, however, that these relationships were fluid, and could change over time or were dependent upon the nature of a specific illness. Szasz and Hollender argued that doctors had traditionally limited their concern to bodily matters rather than relationships with patients, and this criticism was echoed in Balint's (1957) advocacy of a psychodynamically informed approach to medical consultations that would elicit and address the patient's problems as well as diagnose and treat the illness. These two works had a pervasive influence on the sociological study of doctor–patient relationships for much of the rest of the 20th century. The attainment of a mutual and collaborative approach has come to dominate recent policy, and since the 1960s doctor–patient relationships have often been found wanting by researchers, and have become the object of various reform efforts.

One consequence of this is that researchers have often treated doctor–patient interaction as a site where doctors exercise power over patients, as demonstrated by the lack of mutuality or collaboration in evidence in consultations analysed from a variety of perspectives (see, for example, Byrne and Long, 1976; Waitzkin, 1991). At the same time, other sociologists have attempted to explain this failure to achieve mutuality, with Freidson (1970) detailing the inherent differences doctors and patients bring to the relationship (such as the fact that for the doctor this may be a 'typical' case whereas for the patient it is specific and personal) as an inevitable source of conflict. Freidson argues that it is the function of the doctor to apply general knowledge to a particular patient, whereas patients seek to retain an acknowledgement of their particularity, and hence an element of control over their future. This mismatch of perspectives results in conflict which can only be overcome by the doctor obtaining the patient's trust.

Despite work suggesting that some conflict within the doctor–patient relationship is inevitable, the perceived inadequacy of prevailing practice has led to an emphasis on an alternative model of doctor–patient relationships. This negotiated model emphasises both doctor and patient as active, and what is commonly referred to as 'shared decision-making' is increasingly held up as best practice. However, what counts as shared decision making is often poorly defined and hence difficult to assess. On a more fundamental level, its desirability and achievability have also been questioned, on the basis that the competence gap between doctor and patient exists necessarily, and as a result some patients will prefer that this competence is used by the doctor to direct treatment choices.

At the same time, some sociologists have taken a rather different approach to what is generally identified as the problem of medical dominance. Researchers working from a conversation analytic viewpoint have demonstrated how an asymmetry of interaction is not automatically derivable from institutional processes, but is instead constituted by both doctor and patient (e.g. Maynard, 1991). In part, this is a way of handling the interactional difficulties the encounter presents, since part of what might be read as interactional dominance arises from the fact it is the patient's condition that is under review and the doctor who is expected to propose some solution (ten Have, 1991). As a result, patients actively choose to listen to doctors and to take advantage of the greater knowledge and expertise of doctors. From this point of view, apparent dominance may not always be problematic.

One final perspective on this is that Frank et al. (2010) suggest we will make little progress in researching how treatment decisions might best be shared between practitioners and patients until we recognize that this is a distributed process. In other words, we need to recognize that it moves beyond the doctor–patient dyad and can be affected by multiple other mediators beyond client participation, including: policies, protocols and the use of technologies. For example, it is often argued that in the last two decades, patients have become more autonomous, assisted by digital resources which make previously inaccessible medical information available to them or enable them to engage with practitioners in different ways. Empirical research in this field presents a more nuanced picture, dependent on both the technology and the context. For example, studies of remote monitoring technologies conclude that greater intimacy can be fostered between patients and providers as a result, but that this is a consequence of the overall increase in the quantity and quality of communication rather than anything inherent in the technology itself (Piras and Miele, 2019). We must also remember that it is not only patients who use or benefit from technology, and research on English general practitioners' use of online resources during medical consultations shows how these resources can actually be used to emphasize rather than diminish medical knowledge (Stevenson et al., 2019).

Bury (1997) situates changes to the doctor–patient relationship in a wider argument, suggesting there has been an erosion of hierarchical relationships more generally in late modern cultures, and a corresponding trend in the reduction of professionals' power. As an example, He's (2014) research on the problem of over-prescription in China concludes that it is driven by a desire not just to avoid litigation, but also to avoid conflict with patients. Another example is Brown et al.'s (2015) work with general practitioners in England, which suggests that younger doctors tend to more informal relationships with their patients but also to more limited engagement with the communities they serve. The shift, Bury (1997) suggests, is also reflected in the widespread introduction of the Expert Patients Programme in England, aimed at adults living with a chronic disease. People with experience of managing a chronic condition are trained as tutors who then deliver courses to others living with the same condition, where the emphasis is on user-led self-management. The advent of organizations such as the UK's National Institute for Health and Care Excellence (NICE), which places limits on the treatments that can be offered for particular conditions, alongside the introduction of clinical governance, also have an impact. Unless we widen our research lens to take this distribution of treatment decisions into account, we can only ever achieve a partial picture, and any recommendations for practice made as a result will not necessarily be realistic or desirable.

So far, and despite the title of this entry, we have only considered the doctor–patient relationship. Historically there has been some significant work, particularly in a US context, on other practitioner–client relationships, such as Coser (1963) on nurses. However, it is only in the past 15 or 20 years that we have seen a significant increase in the number of sociological studies that consider settings and activities beyond the doctor–patient consultation. As well as nursing, these include: health visiting, physiotherapy, pharmacy, the use of health-related helplines etc. As Pilnick et al. (2010) note, whereas doctor–patient consultations in primary care may be fundamentally concerned with issues of diagnosis and treatment, other sites of practitioner–client interaction have very different concerns. For instance, visits may be therapeutic in nature (for example, in physiotherapy), administrative (for example, admitting a patient to hospital) or related to teaching or training (for example, supervising a junior surgeon during an operation). This diversity of settings and activities raises a different set of issues, and we cannot assume models, principles or policies developed based on doctor–patient interaction in primary care can be transplanted wholesale. This problem is illustrated by a range of studies that demonstrate how 'blanket' recommendations for best practice can be problematic in the face of local contingencies. For example, Allwood et al. (2018) show how importing recommendations from another setting can create problems in dementia care. Other studies underline the importance of local culture in understanding practitioner–client relationships, for example Penn et al.'s (2011) work on adherence to antiretroviral drugs for HIV/AIDS in South Africa. Taken together, this research suggests that to better understand practitioner–client relationships in the 21st century we need to move beyond the restriction of traditional models, rooted in Western doctor–patient encounters, towards an analysis which recognizes the significant breadth and diversity the term encompasses.

See also: Consumerism; Digital Health; Professions Allied to Medicine; The Sick Role; Trust in Medicine.

REFERENCES

Allwood, R., Pilnick, A., O'Brien, R. et al. (2018) 'Should I stay or should I go? How healthcare professionals close encounters with people with dementia in the acute hospital setting', *Social Science & Medicine*, 191: 212–225.

Balint, M. (1957) *The Doctor, His Patient and the Illness*. London: Pitman.

Brown, P., Elston, M.A. and Gabe, J. (2015) 'From patient deference towards negotiated and precarious informality: an Eliasian analysis of English general practitioners' understandings of changing patient relations', *Social Science & Medicine*, 146: 164–172.

Bury, M. (1997) *Health and Illness in a Changing Society*. London: Routledge.

Byrne, P. and Long, B. (1976) *Doctors Talking to Patients: A Study of the Verbal Behaviours of Doctors in the Consultation*. London: Her Majesty's Stationery Office.

Coser, R.L. (1963) 'Alienation and the social structure: case analysis of a hospital', in E. Freidson (ed.), *The Hospital in Modern Society*. New York: Free Press.

Frank, A.W., Corman, M.K., Gish, J.A. and Lawton, P. (2010) 'Healer–patient interaction: new mediations in clinical relationships', in I. Bourgeault, R. Dingwall and R. de Vries (eds), *The SAGE Handbook of Qualitative Methods in Health Research*. London: SAGE.

Freidson, E. (1970) *Profession of Medicine: A Study of the Sociology of Applied Knowledge*. Chicago: University of Chicago Press.

ten Have, P. (1991) 'Talk and institution: a reconsideration of the "asymmetry" of doctor–patient interaction', in D. Boden and D. Zimmerman (eds), *Talk and Social Structure: Studies in Ethnomethodology and Conversation Analysis*. Cambridge: Polity Press.

He, A.J. (2014) 'The doctor–patient relationship, defensive medicine and overprescription in Chinese public hospitals: evidence from a cross-sectional survey in Shenzhen city', *Social Science & Medicine*, 123: 64–71.

Henderson, L.J. (1935) 'Physician and patient and a social system', *New England Journal of Medicine*, 212: 448–495.

Maynard, D. (1991) 'Interaction and asymmetry in clinical discourse', *American Journal of Sociology*, 97 (2): 448–495.

Parsons, T. (1951) *The Social System*. New York: Free Press.

Penn, C., Watermeyer, J. and Evans, M. (2011) 'Why don't patients take their drugs? The role of communication, context and culture in patient adherence and the work of the pharmacist in HIV/AIDS', *Patient Education and Counseling*, 83 (3): 310–318.

Pilnick, A., Hindmarsh, J. and Gill, V.T. (eds) (2010) *Communication in Healthcare Settings: Policy, Participation and New Technologies*. Oxford: Wiley-Blackwell.

Piras, E.M. and Miele, F. (2019) 'On digital intimacy: redefining provider–patient relationships in remote monitoring', *Sociology of Health & Illness*, 14 (S1): 116–131.

Stevenson, F., Hall, L., Seguin, M. et al. (2019) 'General Practitioners' use of online resources during medical visits: managing the boundary between inside and outside the clinic', *Sociology of Health & Illness*, 14 (S1): 65–81.

Szasz, T.S. and Hollender, M.H. (1956) 'A contribution to the philosophy of medicine: the basic models of the doctor–patient relationship', *Archives of Internal Medicine*, 97 (5): 589–592.

Waitzkin, H. (1991) *The Politics of Medical Encounters*. New Haven, CT: Yale University Press.

SUGGESTED FURTHER READING

- www.gov.uk/government/case-studies/the-expert-patients-programme

The above website gives an introduction to the Expert Patients Programme, which began in England as a Department of Health funded research project, and was devolved to become a Community Interest Company operating nationally.

- Armstrong, D. (2014) 'Actors, patients and agency: a recent history', *Sociology of Health & Illness*, 36 (2): 163–174.

This article describes a number of strategies that have served to encourage patients to exercise more autonomous behaviour in relation to their health. Drawing on the introduction of concepts such as 'risk factors' and 'self-management', it traces a shift from the 1950s 'passive patient' to the active patient of the 21st century.

- Pilnick, A. and Dingwall, R. (2011) 'On the remarkable persistence of asymmetry in doctor/patient interaction: a critical review', *Social Science & Medicine*, 72 (8): 1374–1382.

Whilst 'patient-centred medicine' has become accepted best practice in many healthcare fields, the evidence that this has a positive impact on health outcomes is scarce. This article suggests that rather than using training programmes to try and reduce or remove the asymmetry between doctors and patients, we should instead recognize that this asymmetry is embedded within the wider functionality of medicine in society.

27

Quality of Life

Mary Boulton

Quality of life refers to an individual's sense of social, emotional and physical well-being which influences the extent to which she or he can achieve personal satisfaction with their life circumstances.

The term 'quality of life' first came into common parlance in the USA at the end of the Second World War and referred to the possession of material goods – for example, a car, telephone, or washing machine – which made life 'better'. Since then, however, it has increasingly been recognized that material standard of living, as assessed by traditional economic measures such as gross domestic product (GDP), may be important to quality of life but is not the same as quality of life. Although difficult to define, quality of life refers to a broader range of aspects of personal well-being, happiness and life satisfaction. In recent years this has given rise to considerable efforts to develop measures of quality of life which are not reducible to material wealth (Maridal, 2017).

Despite its widespread use, quality of life has remained a vague and abstract concept. It has been viewed as the extent to which basic human needs have been satisfied; satisfaction or dissatisfaction with various aspects of life has been felt; and pleasure and satisfaction are considered to characterize human existence. From a phenomenological perspective, quality of life is seen as reflecting the gap between the hopes and expectations an individual holds and actual experience. Other definitions have variously emphasized the capacity of an individual to realize life plans; the ability of an individual to manage life as he or she evaluates it; or the ability to lead a 'normal' life. A particularly influential definition within social gerontology identifies two objective conditions – general health and functional status, and socio-economic status – and two subjective evaluations – life satisfaction and self-esteem – as at the core of quality of life (Bowling, 2017).

Within the health field, interest has focused on health-related quality of life (HRQL), a term which refers to a loosely related body of work on functional ability, health status and subjective well-being. The conceptual framework for this work derives largely from the World Health Organization's definition of health, which points to the need to take physical, mental and social well-being into account in assessing the health of individuals and populations. Debate continues over the specification of the domains which comprise HRQL. Some present it as characterized by resilience, health perception, physical function, symptoms and duration of life while others employ related concepts like health status, cognitive function, emotional state, social function, role performance and subjective well-being to define and assess HRQL.

Although HRQL has been investigated using qualitative methods, most effort has focused on the development of quantitative measurement instruments. While some early measures were designed to be used by clinicians to obtain 'objective' assessments of physical or mental functioning, more recent measures have been designed to obtain the patient's subjective assessments and to reflect lay perceptions of the impact of illness on their lives. Generic instruments – for example, the SF-36, the WHOQOL-BREF and the EQ-5D – are designed for use with any population group and provide a broadly based assessment. Disease specific instruments have also been developed to provide greater sensitivity in measuring aspects of symptoms and functioning relevant to particular conditions. A concern sometimes expressed about these instruments, which aim to obtain standard information from all patients with the same condition, is that they impose on individuals an external value system which may not reflect their own values. In an attempt to address this, individualized measures such as the Patient Generated Index have also been developed, which ask people to specify for themselves the domains of life that are most affected by their condition and the degree of disruption they experience. Such measures are more sensitive to differences between individuals or population groups with regard to the significance of illness and its effects on day-to-day life but are also more difficult to analyse and interpret. New technical developments make it possible to 'square the circle' by asking respondents to report their quality of life through standard questionnaire items, but where items are selected or chosen according to respondents' responses to initial items. Computerized adaptive testing, as it is known, also results in respondents being asked many fewer items.

A further complication is that many measures are not actually about quality of life per se but negative consequences of health problems such as pain, disability and social isolation. A range of measures are now available which attempt to focus on positive aspects of HRQL. For example, the ICCAP-O focuses attention on Amartya Sen's concept of capabilities – what the individual is capable of doing despite their health problems (Proud et al., 2019) – while the Long Term Conditions Questionnaire (LTCQ) assesses how good a quality of life individuals can enjoy despite having significant long-term conditions (Potter et al., 2017).

Measures of HRQL can be used in a variety of ways, from screening for and monitoring of psychosocial problems in individual patients, to assessing perceived health problems in population surveys. They are most commonly used, however, in clinical trials and evaluation research where they provide subjective, patient-based assessments for evaluating the effects of healthcare interventions. In this context, they have been invaluable in drawing attention to outcomes which may be missed by more traditional clinical measures, in highlighting differences in assessments between patients and clinicians and in demonstrating the limitations and deleterious side-effects of medical interventions. For example, in an early, highly influential study, Croog et al. (1986) carried out a randomized control trial among 625 men with moderate hypertension to determine the effects of three commonly used drugs which act in different ways to control blood pressure. After six months, patients in all three treatment groups had similar levels of blood pressure control. However, clear differences were found between the groups in a range of measures of quality of life, including general well-being, physical symptoms and sexual dysfunction, cognitive function, work performance and satisfaction with life.

Quality of life measures are now routinely used in evaluation research and clinical trials to assess the outcomes of healthcare interventions. An interesting development of this has been the use of HRQL instruments in clinical practice to follow up patients and assess the quality of service they receive. For example, in both England and Sweden, self-reported questionnaires about their health have been successfully introduced and integrated into routine care to assess the performance of providers of hip and knee replacements. This has transformed our understanding of the benefits of these procedures but it is still not clear how far the evidence produced has impacted on quality of services (Prodinger and Taylor, 2018).

Measures of quality of life have also been used by doctors as an adjunct to the clinical interview to improve their management of patients. For example, in a study designed to evaluate the impact of routine use of HRQL measures in a medical oncology clinic, Velikova and colleagues (2004) reported that physicians who received the feedback found it useful and explicitly referred to it in the majority of consultations. Patients in turn showed clinically meaningful improvements in their quality of life. However, the introduction of a questionnaire into a clinical consultation is still an unfamiliar experience for both patient and health professional and can change the interaction in unpredictable ways (Greenhalgh et al., 2018). It may, for example, improve communication and facilitate more shared decision-making between the two but this is a far-reaching cultural change in how care is delivered and further research is needed to understand its wider implications.

More controversially, quality of life measures are also used by health economists to provide a single index of the benefits of medical interventions, the quality adjusted life year (QALY). QALYs are a measure of life extension gained by a specific medical treatment adjusted by a 'utility' weight which reflects the relative value of the health status attained. For example, a year with side-effects of anti-hypertensive treatment has been judged to be equivalent to 0.98 of a year of full health. Calculations of costs per QALY gained can then be made for different healthcare interventions. There has been some scepticism about the meaningfulness of QALYs and unease about using them in making complex choices in resource allocation (Nord et al., 2009). Despite these criticisms, measures of quality of life are now a standard element in the decisions made by the UK's National Institute for Health and Clinical Excellence (NICE) about priorities for public funding of healthcare interventions. Another significant development is the commitment of major regulatory bodies such as the Food and Drugs Administration (FDA) in the USA and the European Medicines Agency to incorporating quality of life data into the regulatory process for development and approval of new drugs and medical devices.

In an effort to develop a theoretical foundation for HRQL research, Wilson and Cleary (1995) have outlined a model which links clinical measures, measures of HRQL and measures of quality of life at a more global level. The model proposes causal linkages between five types of outcome of healthcare, which move from the cell to the individual to the interaction of the individual as a member of society. At each subsequent level, concepts are increasingly integrated and increasingly difficult to define and measure and the factors influencing them increasingly complex and outside the control of the healthcare system.

According to Wilson and Cleary's model, *biological and physiological measures* assess the function of cells and organs and are usually made by clinicians. *Symptom reports* shift the focus to the individual and depend on subjective assessments. *Measures of functional status* assess the ability of the individual to perform particular tasks and are influenced by symptom experience and other factors in the individual (e.g. personality, motivation) and the social environment (e.g. income, housing, social support). *General health perceptions* are the global perceptions that individuals hold about their health and take account of the values which they attach to different symptoms or functional impairments. Finally, *overall quality of life* is a measure of life satisfaction that represents a synthesis of a wide range of experiences and feelings that people have, including HRQL but also other salient life circumstances such as economic, political and spiritual factors.

This model highlights the complex factors which influence quality of life and which may at times produce what appear to be counter-intuitive or paradoxical assessments. For example, in a study of individuals with moderate to severe disabilities, Albrecht and Devlieger (1999) found that the majority reported a good to excellent quality of life despite experiencing severe difficulties performing daily tasks, being socially isolated and having limited incomes. Such findings point to the way the range of social and psychological processes involved in accommodating to illness or disability can produce changes in the internal standards for appraising current health status, or a redefinition of notions of what constitutes a good quality of life, which may in turn influence perceptions of quality of life independently of 'objective' health status or functional ability.

The use of HRQL measures in longitudinal research has increased interest in the cognitive mechanisms underlying this process, known as 'response shift'. For example, in a study of patients with advanced cancer Aburub et al. (2018) looked at the extent to which changes over time in what constitutes quality of life were the result of cancer progression (true change) or adaptation to the experience (reconceptualization response shift). Two different reconceptualizations were identified: a shift away from the negative aspects of life when areas initially identified as negative were no longer regarded as significant and a shift towards the negative when newly problematic areas were encountered.

In summary, HRQL represents an attempt to treat health as multi-dimensional, social and subjective in ways that sociologists have long advocated. Because much of its development has been in the context of applied policy considerations, theoretical and conceptual developments have been neglected. The emphasis has also been on quantitative assessment which misses out the rich descriptions of patients' experiences provided by more qualitative approaches. Nevertheless, attention to quality of life in assessing the outcomes of medical care has served to draw attention to the broader impact of illness and healthcare on patients' daily lives and to provide a framework for incorporating a wider range of social and psychological factors in considerations of health and healthcare.

See also: Chronic Illness; Disability; Evaluation.

REFERENCES

Aburub, A.S., Gagnon, B., Ahmed, S. et al. (2018) 'Impact of reconceptualization response shift on rating of quality of life over time among people with advanced cancer', *Supportive Care in Cancer*, 26: 3063–3071.

Albrecht, G.L. and Devlieger, P.J. (1999) 'The disability paradox: high quality of life against all odds', *Social Science & Medicine*, 48 (8): 977–988.

Bowling, A. (2017) *Measuring Health: A Review of Quality of Life Measurement Scales*. Buckingham: Open University Press.

Croog, S.H., Levine, S., Testa, M.A. et al. (1986) 'The effects of antihypertensive therapy on the quality of life', *The New England Journal of Medicine*, 314: 1657–1664.

Greenhalgh, J., Gooding, K., Gibbons, E. et al. (2018) 'How do patient reported overcome measures (PROMS) support clinician–patient communication and patient care? A realist synthesis', *Journal of Patient-Reported Outcomes*, 2: 42.

Maridal, J.H. (2017) 'A worldwide measure of societal quality of life', *Social Indicators Research*, 134 (1): 1–38.

Nord, E., Daniels, N. and Kamlet, M. (2009) 'QALYs: some challenges', *Value in Health*, 12 (supplement 1): S10–S15.

Potter, C.M., Batchelder, L., A'Court, C. et al. (2017) 'Long-Term Conditions Questionnaire (LTCQ): initial validation survey among primary care patients and social care recipients in England', *BMJ Open*, 7: e019235.

Prodinger, B. and Taylor, P. (2018) 'Improving quality of care through patient-reported outcome measures (PROMs): expert interviews using the NHS PROMs Programme and the Swedish quality registers for knee and hip arthroplasty as examples', *BMC Health Services Research*, 18: 87. https://doi.org/10.1186/s12913-018-2898-z

Proud, L., McLoughlin, C. and Kinghorn, P. (2019) 'ICECAP-O, the current state of play: a systematic review of studies reporting the psychometric properties and use of the instrument over the decade since its publication', *Quality of Life Research*, 28: 1429–1439.

Velikova, G., Booth, L., Smith, A.B. et al. (2004) 'Measuring quality of life in routine oncology practice improves communication and patient well-being: a randomised controlled trial', *Journal of Clinical Oncology*, 22 (4): 714–724.

Wilson, I.B. and Cleary, P.D. (1995) 'Linking clinical variables with health-related quality of life: a conceptual model of patient outcomes', *Journal of the American Medical Association*, 273: 59–65.

SUGGESTED FURTHER READING

- Verkerk, M.A., Busschbach, J.J.V. and Karssing, E.D. (2001) 'Health related quality of life research and the capability approach of Amartya Sen', *Quality of Life Research*, 10 (1): 49–55.

In the context of his work on low-income countries, the economist Amartya Sen developed the Capability Approach to quality of life which focuses on the quality of life that individuals are able to achieve. This paper outlines the core concepts of his approach, which include 'functionings', 'capability' and, in this account, 'resources'. While Sen's work does not relate directly to HRQL research, the authors suggest that his theoretical framework could facilitate its development beyond current limitations.

- Armstrong, D., Lilford, R., Ogden, J. and Wessely, S. (2007) 'Health-related quality of life and the transformation of symptoms', *Sociology of Health & Illness*, 29 (4): 570–583.

Measures of HRQL now play an important role in healthcare but where did they come from? This paper outlines the origins and development of HRQL instruments over the last century in the context of increasing interest in 'distal' symptoms, their location in the social rather than the biological realm and the growth in questionnaire technology. Quality of life is now established as a fundamental goal of healthcare and the patient's self-report is at its core.

- Karimi, M. and Brazier, J. (2016) 'Health, health-related quality of life, and quality of life: what is the difference?' *PharmacoEconomics*, 34 (7): 645–649.

Much confusion has arisen in relation to the terms quality of life, health-related quality of life and health. This short paper reviews the history and definitions of these terms and argues that definitions are problematic because some fail to distinguish between HRQL and health or between HRQL and quality of life and that some HRQL questionnaires measure self-perceived health status rather than HRQL. Given this underlying confusion, the authors raise the question of whether returning to only two, distinct types of measures – health status and of quality of life – might be a way forward.

- MacKillop, E. and Sheard, S. (2018) 'Quantifying life: understanding the history of Quality Adjusted Life Years (QALYs)', *Social Science & Medicine*, 211: 359–366.

QALYs is a generic measure of disease burden, which takes account of both the quality and the quantity of life lived. While it is now widely used internationally in economic evaluations to assess the value of medical interventions, it was many years before the use of QALYs was fully accepted. This article draws on extensive qualitative data and Multiple Streams Analysis to examine the roles of health economists, 'policy entrepreneurs' and the wider social environment in eventually enabling QALYs to be adopted within UK health policy.

28

Sleep

Simon J. Williams

> *Sleep involves a loss of waking consciousness and the temporary relinquishing of our social roles and responsibilities, whilst also being a social role itself. As a socially, culturally and historically variable matter, which is vital for our health and well-being, sleep links to many topics in medical sociology from health inequalities to medicalization and new digital technologies.*

Sleep is not perhaps the first thing that springs to mind when you think of sociology. In fact it has traditionally been a neglected matter, even amongst those more corporeally minded sociologists. Early sociological insights on the social dimensions of sleep however – including the rights and responsibilities of the 'sleep role' (Schwartz, 1970) – have now been supplemented by a variety of other engagements with sleep matters in sociology, both theoretical and empirical in kind. Not just sociology either, but many other branches of the social sciences and humanities are also contributing to this field in an interdisciplinary fashion.

What these engagements clearly show us is that sleep, far from being simply a biological matter, or the sole province of sleep science and sleep medicine, is socially and culturally variable, including the very ways we sleep, the methods of managing it and the multiple meanings we accord it. Sleep is historically variable too, as Ekirch's (2001) research on the 'segmented slumber' of pre-industrial times clearly illustrates. Important questions therefore arise, in this historical light, regarding our contemporary norms and ideals of consolidated nocturnal slumber in the Western world today. These issues too are political through and through, including the governance of sleep in contemporary times within and beyond the clinic (Williams, 2011).

Sleep, as this suggests, is not simply a rich and fascinating topic in its own right. It also links or intersects with many if not all other topics in the social sciences and humanities, from intimacy to interrogation, embodiment to enhancement, science and technology to health, medicine to the media, and social inequalities to time or lack of it in contemporary society.

As for the intersections between these engagements with sleep and the sociology of health and illness, several strands of research are identifiable. One key strand of sociological research has explored the social patterning of sleep across the lifecourse with particular reference to age and gender. Findings here, based on qualitative research, include the *negotiated* nature of sleep amongst couples, how women tend to be more disadvantaged sleepers than men given their caring roles and responsibilities (Hislop and Arber, 2003) and how men tend to view sleep in more functional ways related to work roles (Meadows et al., 2008). Research in this vein too, using survey data, has revealed how sleep problems increase with age and associated events such as bereavement (Arber et al., 2007) and how sleep varies according to socio-economic status, with sleep seen as a potential 'mediator' between social position and health (Arber et al., 2009). As for the coronavirus crisis, well that too has impacted sleep in complex ways, including the potential to widen these existing sleep inequalities both during and post-pandemic (Williams and Meadows, 2020).

Another important strand of sociological research has explored the degree to which sleep has become *medicalized* – i.e. 'made medical' – and/or *pharmaceuticalized* – i.e. rendered amenable to pharmaceutical intervention of some kind. Moloney (2017), for example, in a North American study, notes how physicians and patients alike consistently expressed reluctance toward the use of sedative hypnotics, thereby using the term 'reluctant medicalisation' to capture these concerns. Coveney and colleagues (2019a) too, in their interviews with general practitioners, sleep scientists, patients and a wide range of other stakeholder groups in England, note how the medicalization of sleeplessness is at most a *partial* and *problematic* process and how recourse to the sociological notion of pharmaceuticalization provides further important insights on the dynamics of these processes over time *within* and *beyond* medicalization. These studies in turn have been augmented by research which points to a variety of *moral repertoires* drawn on in relation to hypnotic use. Associated typifications include the '*deserving*' *patient*, the '*responsible*' *user*, the '*compliant*' *patient*, the '*addict*', the '*sinful*' *user* and the '*noble*' *non-user*, incorporating other cross-cutting themes such as *addiction* and *control*, *ambivalence* and *reflexivity* (Gabe et al., 2016).

It is not just a question of prescription sleep medicines, however. Research has also focused on the experiences of sleep amongst recovering heroin users and the challenges involved in their attempts to restore normative sleeping patterns during recovery (Nettleton et al., 2011). This work in turn has been augmented in two ways. First, by exploring how sleep is 'assembled' in these rehabilitation settings through a variety of social, normative, material, affective processes and practices, thereby extending the notion and ontology of sleep in a fulsome fashion through what these authors refer to as 'sleepfulness' (Nettleton et al., 2017). Second, through research using the concept of '*sleep waves*' to explore the biological, experiential, temporal and social rhythms in play within residential settings (Meadows et al., 2017). In doing so Meadows and colleagues show how these sleep waves may in time become relatively stabilized within these settings, yet disrupted once more through the anxieties which anticipation of moving on engender.

Another important strand of work pertains to relations between sleep and health as such. Clearly, as we have seen, the medicalization and pharmaceuticalization of sleep is partial and problematic. At one and the same time, the importance of sleep for health is increasingly emphasized by sleep experts and more widely within popular culture and self-help genres. The *healthicization* of *sleep* therefore is a relevant concept here too given: (1) the ways in which sleep or lack of it is now regarded as an at-risk state in terms of health and safety; (2) the multiple links now drawn between sleep, health and lifestyles; and (3) the numerous exhortations to improve our sleep in the name of health and well-being. Yet, despite such matters, we return to the point raised above that sleep is not necessarily considered a health matter in people's minds, particularly among men where more 'functional' notions of sleep seem to prevail (Meadows et al., 2008).

As for public health initiatives with the sleep of the nation in mind, Meadows and colleagues (2021) identify three key issues. First, sleep is 'liminal' and therefore beyond the limits of our conscious agency and voluntary control. Second, sleep is linked to structural inequalities. Third, sleep is never just one thing, but many or multiple insofar as it is not simply *embodied* but *embedded* and *enacted* in a variety of different settings and contexts across culture, time and place. Public health therefore, Meadows and colleagues argue, would be better served by pursuing a 'ground-up' rather than a 'top-down' approach to these sleep matters, which explores 'good' and 'poor' sleep in these three key ways.

Three further *interrelated* issues are also important to mention here in closing, albeit briefly.

The first concerns the advent of new digital technologies to track and improve or optimize our sleep in various ways far beyond the lab or clinic: a case of what Williams and colleagues (2015) term the '*m-apping*' of sleep through these mobile technologies and apps. Concerns on this count are now being raised, by sleep experts themselves, as to whether or not these technologies cause more harm than good, particularly if they fuel our sleep anxieties. Other more general concerns regarding these new digital technologies – from the big data they generate to the issues of privacy and surveillance they raise – apply equally well here too.

The second closely related issue concerns the use of other biomedical technologies, such as pharmaceuticals, for non-medical purposes in order to enhance, hack or optimize our sleep in various ways. Coveney and colleagues (2019b), for example, have recently explored public understandings of cognitive enhancing and wakefulness promoting drugs for non-medical purposes. In doing so they reveal a range of public views on their possible or prospective uses, including: becoming the best version of oneself; gaining a competitive edge; personal achievement or well-being; and to promote personal or public safety.

These developments in turn raise a third critical issue concerning the *future* of sleep. Whilst the era of biomedical enhancement may suggest that *sleepless* futures are not too far away, if not already with us, most of us are likely to continue to sleep in one form or another, not least because we like, if not love, it as a welcome release from the waking world. Even so, the future of sleep looks set to become ever more entangled with these new digital ways of tracking, treating, managing, monitoring, improving and optimizing it beyond the clinic. Existing sleep inequalities may consequently widen or new ones may emerge, depending on who does and does not avail themselves of these new technologies. As for the future of sleep medicine, well this too looks set to become increasingly bound up with big data, artificial intelligence (AI) and machine learning, as the latest *American Academy of Sleep Medicine* (Goldstein et al., 2020) position statement suggests, including more personalized and predictive forms of sleep medicine in future in the service of better patient care and outcomes.

Sleep then to conclude, as these examples amply demonstrate, adds important new dimensions to many existing topics within medical sociology, from gender and ageing across the lifecourse to the complexities and contradictions of health, and from the medicalization and pharmaceuticalization of life to contemporary health inequalities and new digital technologies. Whilst more research is needed on all these counts, within and beyond medical sociology, four areas of future study are particularly important to note in closing. First, the reciprocal relationship between sleep and mental health is a topic ripe for further sociological investigation. Second, the effects of the coronavirus crisis on our sleep, both during and post-pandemic, will be important to study (Williams and Meadows, 2020), including the impacts for health and social care workers on the frontline, the intersectional dimensions of these issues, and their relationship to health inequalities. Third, the implications of smart digital technologies and associated AI developments for our sleep, within and beyond the lab and the clinic, will be another critical issue to study as part and parcel of the future of sleep itself. Finally, in a reflexive vein, future research may profitably build on what Gilliat-Ray (2021) usefully terms the 'sleepwork' involved in our own research, particularly qualitative fieldwork, including the ways we may (or may not) 'sleep on' our writing and data analysis for insights and inspiration. Something to ponder perhaps with your own sleep and research in mind…

See also: Ageing and the Lifecourse; Digital Health; Gender; Medicalization; Pharmaceuticalization; Social Class.

REFERENCES

Arber, S., Bote, M. and Meadows, S. (2009) 'Gender and socio-economic patterning of self-reported sleep problems in Britain', *Social Science & Medicine*, 68 (2): 281–289.

Arber, S., Hislop, J. and Williams, S.J. (2007) 'Editors' introduction: gender, sleep and the lifecourse', *Sociological Research Online*, 12 (5): 19. Online: www.socresonline.org.uk/12/5/19.html

Coveney, C., Williams, S.J. and Gabe, J. (2019a) 'Medicalisation, pharmaceuticalisation or both? Exploring the medical management of sleeplessness as insomnia', *Sociology of Health & Illness*, 41 (2): 266–284.

Coveney, C., Williams, S.J. and Gabe, J. (2019b) 'Enhancement imaginaries: exploring public understandings of pharmaceutical cognitive enhancing drugs', *Drugs: Education, Prevention and Policy*, 26 (4): 319–328.

Ekirch, A.R. (2001) 'The sleep we have lost: pre-industrial slumber in the British Isles', *The American Historical Review*, 106 (2): 343–386.

Gabe, J., Coveney, C. and Williams, S.J. (2016) 'Prescriptions and proscriptions: moralising sleep medicines', *Sociology of Health & Illness*, 38 (4): 627–644.

Gilliat-Ray, S. (2021) 'Sleeping on the job: where qualitative fieldwork meets the sociology of sleep', *Qualitative Research*, 21 (2): 145–160.

Goldstein, C., Berry, R.B., Kent, D.T. et al. (2020) 'Artificial Intelligence in sleep medicine: an American Academy of Sleep Medicine position statement', *Journal of Clinical Sleep Medicine*, 16 (4): 606–607.

Hislop, J. and Arber, S. (2003) 'Sleepers wake! The gendered nature of sleep-disruption among mid-life women', *Sociology*, 37 (4): 695–711.

Meadows, R., Arber, S., Venn, S. and Hislop, J. (2008) 'Engaging with sleep: male definitions, understandings and attitudes', *Sociology of Health & Illness*, 30 (5): 696–710.

Meadows, R., Nettleton, S., Hine, C. and Ellis, J. (2021) 'Counting sleep? Critical reflections on a UK national strategy', *Critical Public Health,* 31 (4): 494–499.

Meadows, R., Nettleton, S. and Neale, J. (2017) 'Sleep waves and recovery from drug and alcohol dependence: toward a rhythm analysis of sleep in residential settings', *Social Science & Medicine*, 184: 124–133.

Moloney, M.E. (2017) '"Sometimes, it's easier to write the prescription": physician and patient accounts of the reluctant medicalisation of sleeplessness', *Sociology of Health & Illness*, 39 (3): 333–348.

Nettleton, S., Meadows, R. and Neale, J. (2017) 'Disturbing sleep and sleepfulness during recovery from substance dependence in residential rehabilitation settings', *Sociology of Health & Illness*. 39 (5): 784–798.

Nettleton, S., Neale, J. and Pickering, L. (2011) 'Techniques and transitions: a sociological analysis of sleep practices amongst recovering heroin users', *Social Science & Medicine*, 72 (8): 1367–1373.

Schwartz, B. (1970) 'Notes on the sociology of sleep', *The Sociological Quarterly*, 11 (4): 485–499.

Williams, S.J. (2011) *The Politics of Sleep: Governing (Un)Consciousness in the Late Modern Age*. Basingstoke: Palgrave.

Williams, S.J., Coveney, C. and Meadows, R. (2015) 'Mapping sleep: trends and transformations in the digital age', *Sociology of Health & Illness*, 37 (7): 1039–1054.

Williams, S.J. and Meadows, R. (2020) 'Coronavirus: why sleep gaps may widen during and after the crisis', *Discover Society*, 12 April. Online. https://discoversociety.org/2020/04/12/coronavirus-why-sleep-gaps-may-widen-during-and-after-the-crisis/

SUGGESTED FURTHER READING

- Coveney, C. (2013) 'Managing sleep and wakefulness in a 24-hour world', *Sociology of Health & Illness*, 36 (1): 123–136.

An illuminating and insightful exploration of sleep-wakefulness promoting practices and subjective sleep experiences, based on semi-structured interviews with 25 shift workers and students.

- Hale, B. and Hale, L. (2009) 'Is justice good for your sleep? (And therefore good for your health?)', *Social Theory & Health*, 7 (4): 354–370.

A thought-provoking study of the relationship between social justice and sleep, and the implications of these relations for health.

- Moriera, T. (2006) 'Sleep, health and the dynamics of biomedicine', *Social Science & Medicine*, 63 (1): 54–63.

A science and technology studies (STS) informed look at the *dynamic* biomedical processes of contestation and divergence involved in the emergence of the category of 'obstructive sleep apnoea' as a disorder and the associated health technologies deployed for treating it.

- Kroll-Smith, S. (2003) 'Popular culture and "excessive daytime sleepiness": a study of "rhetorical authority" in medical sociology', *Sociology of Health & Illness*, 25 (6): 625–643.

A great study of the increasing significance of popular culture in the creation of 'medical troubles', taking excessive daytime sleepiness as its problematic and revisiting the medicalization thesis in the process.

29

Death and Dying

Gitte H. Koksvik and David Clark

Death and dying are social processes that encompass a variety of dimensions ranging from what constitutes a 'good death' to the influence of place, culture, social
structures and policies on how, where and when we die.

Sociologists have used the subject of death and dying as a lens through which to
understand wider structures and cultures, linking human mortality to the underlying question of what makes and shapes human society itself. The study of 'death
and dying', seen as a specific subgenre of the wider sociological discipline, has now
itself gathered momentum and we are seeing considerable interest in such areas as
end of life care and decision-making, assisted dying and bereavement.

The first classical sociological studies in this field emerged in works such
as *Awareness of Dying* (Glaser and Strauss, 1965) and *Passing On* (Sudnow,
1967), which examined the experience and management of dying in American
hospital settings. These ethnographies detailed highly bureaucratized institutions where the lives of dying patients were characterized by experiences of
meaninglessness and isolation and where the dying person's autonomy was
overridden by hospital staff and hospital routines. Since then, sociologists have
also turned their attention to end of life 'trajectories' in specific high intensity,
technological medical environments like intensive care or emergency resuscita-
tion wherein death is often preceded by clinical decision-making to forego life-
prolonging interventions, in ways that are sometimes seen as the antithesis to a
'natural death' (Stanton-Chapple, 2010).

Death and dying, as key concepts in medical sociology, relate in large part
to the phenomenon of medicalization, which intensified in the last half of the
20th century. Indeed, medicalization emerges simultaneously as the key framework for research but also as its major foe. In many parts of the world, where
death has increasingly followed a protracted period of illness and decline,

most deaths occur in an institutional setting, subsequent to medical treatment. Modern medicine and healthcare systems are therefore instrumental in shaping people's understanding and experiences of the end of life and dying and in achieving what is considered a *good* or acceptable death (Kaufman, 2005). Much sociological research on death and dying has used ethnographic fieldwork as its methodological orientation, creating significant overlap with cultural or social anthropologists who have also taken a keen interest in meaning-making and experiences surrounding illness and death. Sociologists in this field have garnered understanding both of the experiences of carers, next of kin and people facing end of life and of the institutional management of death and dying. This work has contributed to a persistent concern with the 'good death'.

Indeed, sociological interest in death and dying in a medical context largely coincides with wider critiques articulated by a variety of new social movements, such as Hospice, Patient's Rights, Death Awareness, and the supporters of Assisted Dying. The hospice and palliative care movement developed as a reaction to the shortcomings of modern medicine at the end of life and championed a philosophy centred on accompaniment and holistic care of dying individuals to counter the perceived medical neglect of the dying. The concept of 'total pain', capturing the multifaceted experiences of suffering that a person might experience at the end of life and to which care-givers should attend, has generated a significant amount of subsequent sociological commentary. In North America, the hospice movement grew as a response to excessive medical intervention and futile aggressive treatments near the end of life. Hospice and palliative care furthered an ideal of a good death as one centred on accompaniment, symptom management, open awareness and acceptance (see *Awareness Contexts* in the second edition of this text). Yet as the movement has transitioned to become an integrated and medicalized part of the healthcare system, concerns have been raised about its increasing routinization and institutionalization. Sociologists have also highlighted the constraining elements of this particular philosophy of a good, accompanied, death in which the guiding principles might become prescriptive benchmarks for patient behaviour, thereby furthering issues of control and creating categories not only of good and bad deaths, but also of good and bad *patients* (McNamara et al., 1994). Recently, it has been argued that this ideal of dying, which emphasizes awareness and acceptance as a possibility for personal (spiritual) growth, is losing influence. A discrete period of decline associated with dying is increasingly considered negative or even unnecessary (Cottrell and Duggleby, 2016).

The contemporary 'Right to Die' movement and the associated practice of *assisted dying*, whereby individuals can legally obtain medically administered or self-administered medication to end their own lives upon their own competent request, evidence this turn. Advocates focus on autonomy and choice, applied to issues like the right to select the place, timing and manner of one's own death. Assisted dying may create new forms of caring relationships through planning death and the potential to choreograph experiences of dying.

Likewise, ethnographic research has illustrated how 'euthanasia talk' in the clinical encounter may help patients maintain a sense of autonomy and agency while facing the end of life (Norwood, 2009).

Although only legal in a small number of jurisdictions worldwide, assisted dying is currently gaining traction and has become an integral part of the way death and dying are considered in many parts of the world. Advocates of the 'Right to Die' sometimes position this as an explicit corrective to medical-ization, and as a way for individuals to reclaim from the medical complex a measure of power and ownership over their own lives – including hospice and palliative care. Nevertheless, 'right to die' discourse increasingly draws on the language and imagery of suffering and pain, and legalized assisted dying is in almost all cases advocated for and framed within a state's healthcare provision. Some sociological commentators argue that assisted dying does not oppose medicalization but rather constitutes a demand for it of a dif-ferent kind, wherein notions of individual control and choice remain crucial (Karsoho et al., 2016).

Another important element of the contemporary landscape of dying and death is 'talking', and there is growing interest in and advocacy for 'conversations' about future wants and preferences – with family, friends or professionals. This is often linked to the policy drive, seen in many countries, towards advance care planning, statements of preferences, and do-not-resuscitate orders. Barriers to the uptake of these 'technologies' are often framed as the negative disposition in modern culture to talking about death and dying. Death Cafés, where people gather to talk about death and dying, death salons, popular non-fiction, films and series can all be seen as taking a stance against the death 'taboo' in the interest of a valorized 'open-ness' or 'conversation' about mortality and its dis-contents. Such trends can be seen as democratizing and liberating, or as further manifestations of inscription on modern subjectivity.

Death is sometimes referred to as the great equalizer. Nevertheless, as explained in other entries in this book, notably in Part 1, socio-economic, geographic and cultural/behavioural factors play an important role in deter-mining a person's health, their access to and experience of healthcare delivery, their life expectancy and ultimately the manner of their dying. People from lower socio-economic backgrounds experience less access to certain types of care. Moreover, most societies today have diverse populations that hail from different cultural, ethnic and religious backgrounds. Sociologists have taken an interest in exploring conceptions of end of life care among minority groups, identifying different interpretations of illness, pain and conceptions of good death. Gunaratnam's (2013) work on the end of life of migrants in the UK illustrates some of the issues that may arise when people become ill and face death away from their country of origin, as well as the logistical and emo-tional navigation involved in disposition and potential repatriation before or after death.

Conceptions of good and bad dying vary significantly across cultures and populations. The greatest burden of dying today is found in low- and middle-income countries, where 80 per cent of global death takes place. Here too, dying is increasingly the result of non-communicable diseases and is thus preceded by protracted periods of illness and decline. However, there is a dearth of sociological research on death in these settings. Existing studies often describe situations of resource scarcity prompting inventiveness among caregivers whilst also exposing deep frustrations, suffering, premature and avoidable deaths. End of life care in many low and middle-income countries is further rendered difficult due to limited access to and restrictive legislation on pain medication (Knaul et al., 2018). Researchers also note the impoverishing effects of healthcare where treatment provided by privatized medical systems may have devastating economic consequences for individuals and households, even at the end of life (Wagstaff et al., 2017).

Drawing on subaltern theory, Zaman et al. (2017) employ the concept of 'the waiting-room of history' to question the standard Global North view of end of life care in the Global South. This notion rests on a world-view according to which history is linear and so-called 'developing countries' are expected to go through the same process as the 'developed' in order to reach their supposedly 'ideal' level and way of organization. As such, differences in the organization and delivery of healthcare in these countries are taken to be shortcomings or stepping stones on the path of 'development'. This assumption, however, is a cultural construct and there has been some sociological interest in so-called 'reverse' learning, whereby it is posited that 'developed' countries might have something to learn from the organization of end of life care in 'developing' ones. Examples of this include efforts to develop compassionate communities and community-based approaches that counter medicalization and bureaucratization, fostering greater community involvement and ownership in end of life – such as those that have been widely described for Kerala (Kumar, 2012).

Medical sociologists, and their colleagues in cognate disciplines, can be seen addressing contemporary challenges in the delivery of end of life care in a world characterized by population growth and ageing. Some are engaged in studies that illuminate and critique contemporary orthodoxies – such as the work of palliative care or ideologies of the good death. Others are tracing the practical, moral and clinical contours of a world which is slowly adopting the practice of legalized assisted dying. Most recently the pandemic associated with COVID-19 has created a surge of new interest in death from infectious disease, where some of the established principles of modern dying (advance care planning, communication with the dying person and close ones, shared decision-making, the option of assisted dying, personalized funerals and memorialization) are being challenged in multiple ways. Death and dying therefore remain important areas for theoretical and methodological innovation, as well as new empirical enquiry.

See also: Ageing and the Lifecourse; Medical Technologies; Medicalization; Practitioner–Client Relationships.

REFERENCES

Cottrell, L. and Duggleby, W. (2016) 'The "good death": an integrative literature review', *Palliative & Supportive Care*, 14 (6): 686–712.

Glaser, B.G. and Strauss, A.L. (1965) *Awareness of Dying*. New Brunswick and London: Aldine/Transaction.

Gunaratnam, Y. (2013) *Death and the Migrant: Bodies, Borders and Care*. London: Bloomsbury Academic Press.

Karsoho, H., Fishman, J.R., Wright, D.K. and Macdonald, M.E. (2016) 'Suffering and medicalization at the end of life: the case of physician-assisted dying', *Social Science & Medicine*, 170: 188–196.

Kaufman, S.R. (2005) *And a Time to Die: How American Hospitals Shape the End of Life*. Chicago: University of Chicago Press.

Knaul, F.M., Bhadelia, A., Rodriguez, N.M. et al. (2018) 'The Lancet Commission on Palliative Care and Pain Relief: findings, recommendations, and future directions', *Lancet*, 6, Special Issue, S5–S6.

Kumar, S. (2012) 'Public health approaches to palliative care: the Neighbourhood Network in Kerela', in L. Sallnow, S. Kumar and A. Kellehear (eds), *International Perspectives on Public Health and Palliative Care*. London: Routledge.

McNamara, B., Waddell, C. and Colvin, M. (1994) 'The institutionalization of the good death', *Social Science & Medicine*, 39 (11): 1501–1508.

Norwood, F. (2009) *The Maintenance of Life: Preventing Social Death Through Euthanasia Talk and End-of-Life Care – Lessons from the Netherlands*. Durham: Carolina Academic Press.

Stanton-Chapple, H. (2010) *No Place for Dying. Hospitals and the Ideology of Rescue*. Walnut Creek, CA: West Coast Press.

Sudnow, D. (1967) *Passing On: the Social Organization of Dying*. Englewood Cliffs, NJ: Prentice-Hall.

Wagstaff, A., Flores, G., Smitz, M.-F. et al. (2017) 'Progress on impoverishing health spending in 122 countries: a retrospective observational study', *Lancet Global Health*, 6: e180–e192.

Zaman, S., Inbadas, H., Whitelaw, A. and Clark, D. (2017) 'Common or multiple futures for end of life care around the world? Ideas from the "waiting room of history"', *Social Science & Medicine*, 172: 72–79.

SUGGESTED FURTHER READING

- Clark, D. (2002) 'Between hope and acceptance: the medicalisation of dying', *British Medical Journal*, 324: 904–907.

Clark writes about the origins and development of palliative care and the attendant notions of good death in relation to modern critiques of medicalization.

- Seymour, J.E. (1999) 'Revisiting medicalisation and "natural" death', *Social Science & Medicine*, 49: 691–704.

Seymour writes about intensive care, questioning some of the criticisms levied against end of life and dying in this high-tech unit as being inherently unnatural and, as such, a bad death.

- Buchbinder, M. (2018) 'Choreographing death: a social phenomenology of medical aid-in-dying in the United States', *Medical Anthropology Quarterly*, 32 (4): 481–497.

Buchbinder uses ethnographic methods and illustrates in an accessible manner how new ways of dying, caring relationships and dependencies emerge with the practice of assisted dying.

- Seale, C. (ed.) (2008) 'Death, dying and bereavement Virtual Special Issue' (VSI), *Sociology of Health & Illness*. Online: https://onlinelibrary.wiley.com/page/journal/14679566/homepage/death__dying_and_bereavement_virtual_special_issue.htm

Edited by Seale, this VSI compiles articles written by a range of authors on various topics all relating to end of life care and decision-making, dying, death and bereavement.

PART 3

HEALTH, KNOWLEDGE AND PRACTICE

30

The Medical Model

Lee F. Monaghan and Mike Bury

> *The idea of a singular medical model is contested but it is often used within sociology to refer to the conception of disease established in the late 19th and early 20th centuries, based on an anatomo-pathological view of the individual body.*

Modern medicine is heterogeneous and undertaken in various contexts (clinics, specialties, research and science); hence, the idea that there is one practically adequate medical model is contested. Whilst Kontos (2011) makes this point in the field of academic medicine and philosophy, Strong (1979), a medical sociologist, indicated as much when writing 'the medical model' as a sociological descriptor is a source of 'irritation' for 'some doctors' given the 'fractional nature' of their enterprise and how medical knowledge has changed since the 19th century (p. 211). Despite such observations, the medical model (or what is also termed the biomedical model) is often used by sociologists and others as a shorthand way of describing the dominant approach to disease in Western medicine. Besides locating this model and core elements of it in its historical context, this entry outlines critical responses (within and outside of medicine) before noting certain complexities that necessitate a nuanced appraisal. We finish by identifying some possible issues to consider following the outbreak of COVID-19.

In the 19th century, the medical model, based on a pathological anatomy of the body, broke away from earlier conceptions to establish the idea of specific diseases with specific causes. Earlier, disease in Western societies had been largely based on humoral theories and on exhaustive descriptions of symptoms. Scepticism about scientific and laboratory-based medicine was common in the early modern period and in some contexts persists to this day. However, by the mid-19th century various alternative models of disease, including those based on 'bedside medicine' (Jewson, 1976), were made to give way to a view that located disease in specific organs. Indeed, in 1800, Bichat had argued that the pathological processes giving rise to disease might not even be located in an organ, but in a specific tissue. By the 1880s bacteriology had begun to show that particular micro-organisms were responsible for specific diseases; for example, the tubercle bacillus for tuberculosis and the vibrio cholerae for cholera. Predictably, many physicians, who were wedded to the idea that disease involved the whole person and must be systemic in origin and character, resisted these findings.

By contrast, the new model of disease contained three main dimensions: (1) that a specific aetiology could be found underlying specific diseases; (2) that diseases caused lesions in the body which altered its anatomy and physiology; and (3) that these two processes, in turn, gave rise to symptoms. Though successes in applying this new approach were not immediate, by the end of the 19th century the antitoxin for diphtheria was showing dramatic results and the adoption of antisepsis was beginning to make hospital care and especially surgery safer. The development of antibiotics, especially following the identification by Fleming of penicillin in 1928, and its final introduction in 1941 (Porter, 1997), showed that the medical model of disease could produce lasting and beneficial results.

The impact of the new medical model on the doctor–patient relationship was equally profound. As the conception of disease focused on processes inside the body, the task of the doctor was to elicit information about the signs and symptoms of the disease – respectively, that which is objectively observable (for example, infected secretions) and subjectively experienced (for example, tiredness) – and then locate these in the new nosology. Thus, the ability to diagnose became highly prized and was based on test results and judgements about deviations from 'the normal', rather than on observations of departures from the patient's 'natural state' (Lawrence, 1994: 45). From the patient's viewpoint, the task now was to pay attention to signs and symptoms and present them to the doctor at the appropriate time. As disease was seen to reside in the individual body, it could best be diagnosed and treated in a one-to-one situation by the clinician. Doctors were increasingly oriented towards individual 'presentation', rather than tackling the complexities and heterogeneity of the patient's familial, social or moral worlds. The medical model can be seen, therefore, as reinforcing individualism as a dimension of modern experience – an 'obviously' culturally bound or circumscribed view, as explained by those drawing from Indigenous perspectives when critiquing the Western biomedical model (see Suggested Further Reading).

During the late 19th and especially early 20th centuries, the association of the new approach to disease with social and sometimes political reform in the West partly explained doctors' growing allegiance to the medical model. Gender, intersecting with class, ethnicity and national identity, also exerted their effects. Even in the early 19th century, as novels such as Eliot's *Middlemarch* made clear, the reforming medical man, increasingly under the influence of the medical model, was part of the changing fabric of (in this case) English society.

The medical model did not simply develop in a particular historical context: it was an important constitutive part of society's changing character. 'Medical progress' was but one element linked to modernity and the transformation of cultural and social structures.

Focusing on the making of modern Britain, Lawrence (1994) argues that, by 1920, the idea of disease as individual pathology had become almost entirely dominant, pushing other theories and approaches aside. This model underpinned and legitimated the development of a 'bounded' medical profession, which increasingly exercised jurisdiction over designated medical matters (p. 77). State regulation of medicine and a ceding of quasi-judicial powers to the profession, for example its ability to register or de-register ('strike off') practitioners, gave it enormous powers of autonomy and control. Senior hospital doctors, in particular, and those organized in the various Royal Colleges had, and arguably still have, particular access to these levers of power. Not surprisingly, therefore, even those doctors sympathetic to a scientific medicine have not always met the development of the medical model with unqualified acceptance. Some within the profession, especially those in specialties such as public health and psychiatry, and in general practice, have argued against the complete subsuming of medicine under the aegis of the medical model.

Various critiques emerged from within medicine in the 1960s and 1970s. Szasz, a medically trained psychoanalyst, and Laing, an ex-army psychiatrist, among many others, issued broad critiques of the application of the medical model to mental illness. Also working within psychiatry, Engel (1977) proposed the now well known 'biopsychosocial model', given the perceived neglect of psychological and social factors (typically understood in behavioural terms) (for a critique, see Kontos, 2011). Furthermore, the 1970s saw strong reactions by leading epidemiologists in public health to what they perceived as the public's overreliance on (unevaluated) curative medicine, and too great an influence on the part of the medical establishment. McKeown (1976), for example, examined the historical role of medicine and showed that for many if not all infections, mortality had fallen substantially before the medical model had uncovered their causes or, indeed, fashioned any preventative or curative responses. McKeown demonstrated that public health measures and better living standards were responsible for improvements in health in the 19th and 20th centuries. Part of the problem with the 'mechanistic' medical model's focus on 'engineering' interventions at the individual level was that the broader determinants of health were overlooked.

In medical sociology, early theorizing regarded medicine as socially functional. Parsons (1951) held medicine and the medical model of disease to be rational, counteracting the 'needs dispositions' of the ill. By addressing the individual's problems in medical terms, the tendency towards deviance, represented by illness states, could be safely channelled, pending the return of the individual to their former roles. However, by the 1970s, medical sociologists were also becoming highly critical of the medical model and its application by the medical profession. Freidson (1970), in particular, set out a full-blown critique of the profession and, quite unlike Parsons, challenged the apparent objectivity of the medical model. The belief in illness as an objective entity, Freidson argued, stemmed from the perception of 'viruses and molecules ... [as a] physical reality independent of time, space and changing moral evaluation' (p. 208). However, Freidson insisted, 'biological deviance or disease is defined socially and is surrounded by social acts that condition it' (p. 209). Hence, far from acting as a socially functional institution, medicine left the patient in a passive position, with lay constructions given little or no credence. The 'clash of perspectives' between the patient's world and that of the doctor led to an underlying conflict: 'Given the viewpoints of the two worlds, lay and professional, in interaction, they can never be wholly synonymous' (p. 321). Freidson's argument rested on a distinction between illness (the experience of the patient) and disease (the conception of the doctor). Whilst the application of the medical model of biological disease could vary depending on the cultural context, Freidson was more concerned to contrast the different perspectives of patients and doctors than present a detailed critique of the 'social construction' of disease.

It has perhaps been Foucault's critique of the medical model that has proven most influential. His writings on 'bio-power' set out what he took to be the social significance of the pathological anatomy view of disease. In his book, *The Birth of the Clinic*, Foucault (1976) centres his argument on Bichat and his dictum to 'open up a few corpses'. The significance of this move was, as noted earlier, to locate disease in what Foucault terms the 'volumes and spaces' of the body. This individuating and internalizing of disease, for Foucault, was the hallmark of the 'new' medical model. The increasing dominance of this model, together with the associated growth in power and influence of the medical profession, demonstrated for him the intimate relationship between knowledge and power.

Like Freidson, medicine's monopoly over disease and illness for Foucault stemmed from the power to name and locate disease in the individual. Bringing the individual under 'the gaze' of medical perception was part of a growing tendency in modernity to rely on the 'discursive practices' of experts in effecting social order. These practices divided populations according to their 'disciplinary' codes. For Foucault the term 'discipline' had a double meaning: the 'discipline' of medicine at one and the same time located the individual in a scientific schema, and, on the other, added to the tendency to create 'docile bodies' by regulating them in specific ways. The expansion of medicine, psychology and the human sciences in general, no less than the growth of the clinic and hospital (like the school and the prison), was the institutional expression of 'disciplinary power' shaping and reshaping modern life.

The point of Foucault's critique was that the enormous expansion in the power of medicine and the medical conception of disease was neither inevitable nor irreversible. He stated: 'this order of the solid, visible body is only one way – in all likelihood neither the first, nor the most fundamental – in which one spacialises disease' (p. 3). The message is clear: things could have been otherwise, and therefore can be otherwise in the future. The apparent objectivity of the body and the permanence of the medical model are open to question and change. These critical views have done much to contest the medical profession's power and to fuel some of the challenges to 'medical dominance' now found in public and academic circles. However, despite the persuasiveness of these critiques, there are limitations which suggest that the medical model is more complex than envisaged. Two must suffice here.

First, the idea that the medical model is neither the first nor likely the last way of conceptualizing disease may be literally true, but, paradoxically, it understates the transformations that the medical model and other features of modernity have created. Whilst alternative ways of conceptualizing disease and illness have emerged (health promotion, public health and the myriad of 'alternative practices' that have all grown in recent decades), the medical model shows little sign of disappearing. Developments in pharmacology, genetics and the neurosciences suggest that the power of medical knowledge and of the profession has grown in scope and reach, however problematic this sometimes appears. When highlighting the continuing development of scientific and medical thought, as well as their ongoing cultural significance, the entry on 'the medical model' in the second edition of *Key Concepts in Medical Sociology* referred to 'recent' work on 'the new genetics' (Atkinson et al., 2009), and normality and pathology in modern biomedicine (Rose, 2009). A decade later, as reported in the UK, biomedical research and development (R&D) has expanded. Jones and Wilsdon (2018) critically refer to a 'doubling down on biomedical science', resulting in a 'biomedical bubble'. Rather than a speculative mania, the term 'bubble' denotes other meanings here. For instance, it refers to how certain groups are ignored (epistemic bubble) and how advocates' interactions reinforce 'networks, feedback loops and commitments beyond anything that can be rationalised through cost–benefit analysis' (social bubble) (p. 26).

Second, despite the attention given to infectious diseases in pandemic times, further inflating 'the biomedical bubble', countervailing tendencies persist. The ongoing challenges associated with chronic illness, especially among ageing populations, has meant that numerous areas of medical practice have moved away from a complete reliance on a narrow, 'mechanistic' view of the body or of illness, if indeed they ever accepted it fully. Many of those working with the chronically ill are as concerned with the physical, social and psychological functioning of the individual and with the pattern of informal care as they are with diagnosis or medical treatments. Whilst dementia, for example, has attracted large-scale investments in laboratory research, medical practitioners have remained concerned with its observable effects on individuals and their families. Such concerns have also buttressed significant investment in social research over the past decade. From this viewpoint, the medical model may never have been quite as fundamental to everyday medical practice as Foucault and others believed. Such caveats concerning the medical model suggest that its role is at one and the same time more powerful and more limited than critics have recognized.

Given the above complexities and co-existing trends, sociologists interested in the medical model should have plenty to consider when undertaking further work. In so doing, there is scope to contribute to debates concerning the authority and investments in the medical model and alternative approaches in unequal societies (notably, approaches emphasizing the fundamental socio-economic causes of health inequalities). Related topics for investigation, connecting with other concepts in this volume, include 'pharmaceuticalization' or socio-technical processes that incorporate promised drug-based biomedical 'fixes'. For instance, what might medical sociologists have to say in regard to the epistemic and political authority granted to recurrent biomedical responses to COVID-19 (including mandating mass inoculation and booster vaccines), especially given this disease's emergence and patterning within broader environmental/material conditions of existence? Following the entry on 'pandemics and epidemics', also in this volume, to what extent have societal responses to COVID-19 reflected medical imperialism and thus the biomedical focus on the body's interiority to the relative neglect of society? Such questions deserve sociological attention. In so doing, we would return to Strong (1979) who also cautions against an alternative 'fully social model of health' (p. 212). Although much depends on how society is viewed and who controls the model (see also the Suggested Further Reading on the dynamic modelling of obesity), a social model could have 'disturbing political implications' (Strong, 1979: 212) where wide-scale interventions target individual behaviours rather than inequitable structures. Consider, for example, how a restrictive view of society (as an aggregate of individuals or groups of individuals rather than as a network of unequal power relations) has arguably downplayed social inequalities in government responses to the COVID-19 crisis. A key challenge, going forward, will be to critically engage such matters, analysing how different and cross-cutting models frame 'problems' and proposed 'solutions' in health, medicine and society.

See also: Complimentary and Alternative Medicine; Geneticization; Illness and Health Behaviours; Medical Autonomy, Dominance and Decline; Medicalization; Pandemics and Epidemics; Pharmaceuticalization; Practitioner–Client Relationships; Social Constructionism; The Sick Role.

REFERENCES

Atkinson, P., Glasner, P. and Lock, M. (eds) (2009) *The Handbook of Genetics and Society*. London: Routledge.

Engel, G.L. (1977) 'The need for a new medical model: a challenge for biomedicine', *Science*, 196 (4286): 129–136.

Foucault, M. (1976) *The Birth of the Clinic*. London: Tavistock.

Freidson, E. (1970) *The Profession of Medicine: A Study of the Sociology of Applied Knowledge*. Chicago: University of Chicago Press.

Jewson, N. (1976) 'The disappearance of the sick man from medical cosmology 1770–1870', *Sociology*, 10 (2): 225–244.

Jones, R. and Wilsdon, J. (2018) *The Biomedical Bubble: Why UK Research and Innovation Needs a Greater Diversity of Priorities, Politics, Places and People.* Nesta. Online: https://media.nesta.org.uk/documents/The_Biomedical_Bubble_v6.pdf

Kontos, N. (2011) 'Biomedicine – menace or straw man? Reexamining the biopsychosocial argument', *Academic Medicine*, 86 (4): 509–515.

Lawrence, C. (1994) *Medicine in the Making of Modern Britain 1700–1920.* London: Routledge.

McKeown, T. (1976) *The Role of Medicine: Dream, Mirage or Nemesis?* Oxford: Blackwell.

Parsons, T. (1951) *The Social System.* New York: The Free Press.

Porter, R. (1997) *The Greatest Benefit to Mankind: A Medical History of Humanity from Antiquity to the Present.* London: HarperCollins.

Rose, N. (2009) 'Normality and pathology in a biomedical age', *Sociological Review*, 57 (s2): 66–83.

Strong, P.M. (1979) 'Sociological imperialism and the profession of medicine: a critical examination of the thesis of medical imperialism', *Social Science & Medicine*, 13A: 199–215.

SUGGESTED FURTHER READING

- West-McGruer, K. (2020) 'There's "consent" and then there's consent: mobilising Māori and Indigenous research ethics to problematise the western biomedical model', *Journal of Sociology*, 56 (2): 184–196.

West-McGruer draws from a Māori perspective on research ethics when critiquing the biomedical model, including assumptions about individual informed consent, universality and the prioritization of scientific discovery. Mindful of colonialism and the historical pathologization and mistreatment of Indigenous peoples, the issues raised in the article are also of contemporary concern amidst extractive, technologically enabled practices.

- Harrison, S. (2010) 'Co-optation, commodification and the medical model: governing UK medicine since 1991', *Public Administration*, 87 (2): 184–197.

Harrison argues that, at least in the UK, the medical model has been co-opted for managerial purposes to support commodified care and, in the process, weaken rather than strengthen medical dominance. In discussing such matters, the article adds another perspective to those debates, discussed elsewhere in this volume, on 'managerialism' as well as 'medical autonomy, dominance and decline'.

- Chang, V.W. and Christakis, N.A. (2002) 'Medical modelling of obesity: a transition from action to experience in a 20th century American medical textbook', *Sociology of Health & Illness*, 24 (2): 151–177.

Exploring transitions in the conceptualizing of obesity in a leading medical textbook between 1927 and 2000, this article shows how medicine may incorporate broader contextual (environmental) concerns as well as those at the individual (including genetic) level. The authors also connect with debates engaged in by Strong (cited above), and others, on the possible consequences of a social model relative to a medical model (revolving around the question of what the social denotes) and thus the potential to facilitate or constrain medicalization.

- Manago, B., Davis, J.L. and Goar, C. (2017) 'Discourse in action: parents' use of medical and social models to resist disability stigma', *Social Science & Medicine*, 184: 169–177.

Drawing from interviews with parents of disabled children, Manago et al. explore how participants' responses to stigma variously drew from the medical model (emphasizing diagnostic labels, treatment and individual deficit) and the social model (emphasizing disabling social structures). Invocation of these models served diverse ends and sometimes in counterintuitive ways as parents challenged and/or deflected disability stigma.

31

Social Constructionism

Orla McDonnell

> The basic premise of social constructionism is that reality is a product of definitional practices and the task of sociology is to explain the social processes involved in the production of knowledge pertaining to, or which constitutes, this reality.

In their influential book *The Social Construction of Reality*, Berger and Luckmann (1967) bring together the key theoretical strands of classical sociology: the first, which emphasizes the objective structures of society and their influence in shaping human action (constraining individual action), and the second, which emphasizes the role of human agency in constructing the social world through (inter)subjective meanings. Berger and Luckmann are concerned with everyday knowledge, that is, the social stock of knowledge that constitutes the background cultural assumptions orientating our everyday social actions. This knowledge becomes coextensive with, although not reducible to, what is knowable, in the sense of how social actors come to perceive a fit between their subjective realities and what they know to be the objective world. This alignment is why the world appears to societal members as an objective reality. Berger and Luckmann 'define "reality" as a quality appertaining to phenomena that we recognize as having a being independent of our own volition (we cannot "wish them away")' (p. 1). This classic 'treatise in the sociology of knowledge' underscores the importance of understanding social processes and people's definitional practices when seeking to make sense of their beliefs about reality. This premise is a staple across interpretivist and symbolic interactionist theories that emphasize how the meanings and experiences of illness are shaped by socio-cultural contexts (Atkinson and Housley, 2003). The original idea of the social construction of illness was not whether illness has an independent reality as a disease entity existing in nature. Instead, the concept referred to the social conventions established in particular spheres of relevance in which illness acquires meaning (Freidson, 1970).

In the context of the so-called science wars, which arose when social constructionism was applied to scientific as opposed to everyday knowledge, the concept became more troubling and subsequently became mired in a theoretical division between relativism and realism. Social constructionism became a controversial concept largely because of 'post-structuralist' theoretical trends that conflate questions concerning ontology (what exist as external realities in the social and natural worlds) and epistemology (what we can know about these realities). This stance is known as radical constructionism: it rejects the notion that the foundation of knowledge is based on an external reality and denies that there is any rational basis for deciding between alternative conceptualizations of reality. However, just as there are a variety of constructionist approaches to knowledge, there are a variety of realist positions. As we will see below, different versions of social constructionism are compatible with different realist epistemologies. The following focuses on one current of constructionist thought as applied to medical knowledge, namely: the sociology of scientific knowledge (SSK).

Sociology seeks explanations for scientific knowledge by exploring science as a social institution. In paying attention to the social organization of knowledge, sociologists focus on the social forces and processes that shape knowledge production. Such accounts can be both structuralist and constructionist. The former analyse the broader structures of power that influence scientific knowledge and its applications. This approach also addresses the social reproduction and transformations that knowledge brings about. For example, 'new' knowledge such as genetics can reproduce or alter cultural norms, institutional structures and discourses in terms of how diseases are understood and social issues, such as risk, are problematized. The focus of the constructionist approach is on the 'doing' of science. Constructionism emphasizes the culturally constructed character of scientific knowledge and how this is influenced by local contingencies such as professional turf wars, dominant cognitive frameworks, professional credibility strategies and the alignment of different vested interests (scientific elites, practitioners, healthcare policy-makers and funders, and patient groups and advocates who politicize medico-scientific research).

While both approaches can overlap, there are tensions. The starting point for SSK lies in its fundamental challenge to the classical view of scientific knowledge, based on positivism, which claims that scientific knowledge is determined by the distinct properties of its objects of study in the natural world. In structuralist accounts, this classical view of scientific knowledge is sometimes assumed or left unquestioned. The analytical focus is to show how representations of reality are distorted in line with ideological interests reflecting the way power is played out according to pervasive social structures. Conversely, SSK takes a relativist approach, highlighting the cultural character of scientific knowledge. This approach also traces the social processes and forces that are involved in the production of knowledge. However, it engages with the *content* of scientific knowledge as an empirical object of sociological investigation rather than taking social structures based on established interests and power as its analytical starting point. Whereas structuralists take a stance on the validity of knowledge claims, largely in relation to the predetermined structures that shape knowledge and its social implications, constructionists are agnostic on this point. This agnosticism stems from the principle of 'methodological relativism', which is adopted as a strategy of objectivity in SSK. The basic theoretical precept guiding this approach is that since scientific knowledge is socially produced then it should be studied empirically like all other forms of knowledge. In short, it should be studied as sets of beliefs and conventions that are bound up with the context of knowledge production itself (Bloor, 1970). However, for those who see common ground between structuralist and constructionist positions, the agnostic stance taken by SSK towards the truth or falsity of knowledge claims limits constructionism as a form of sociological critique.

Empirical studies in SSK focus on scientific controversies and the social processes at play. In their case study of a medico-scientific dispute between vascular and immunological theories of the pathogenesis of multiple sclerosis (MS), Nicolson and McLaughlin (1988), following the principle of methodological relativism, give equal explanatory weight to the rival theories. They show how experts put their own competing constructions on the reality of MS depending on their different professional traditions and demonstrate how new knowledge is filtered through existing beliefs and theories, affording rival experts a considerable degree of flexibility in interpreting the same body of evidence. They argue that the immunological account of MS continues to hold sway over its rival because there is a stronger cognitive fit between this model and the clinical expertise involved in the management of the disease. Furthermore, the mode of treatment suggested by this model is in keeping with conventional drug treatment, which can more readily be accommodated within existing clinical practice than the alternative therapy developed on the basis on vascular theory. They argue that enrolling support for an unorthodox therapeutic approach depends on the relative power of its supporters, irrespective of the evidence. Here we see common ground with a structuralist approach when local contingencies associated with knowledge production are further contextualized in relation to broader political, cultural and economic structures in society.

Other areas of research and debate are also noteworthy. While the complex and contested nature of mental illness raises concerns about the weak construct validity of diagnostic categories, sociologists who follow a social constructionist approach are not, per se, concerned with the ontological status of mental disorders. Instead, sociological studies emphasize the social processes that constitute and legitimate particular knowledge claims in clinical practice and mental health policy discourse. Mayes and Horwitz (2005; see also Horwitz, 2012) offer an exemplary study, which combines a structuralist and constructionist approach. They explore the shift from the minority and controversial position that mental illness is akin to physical illness to the whole-scale biologization of mental illness. In their analysis of the history of the third edition of the *Diagnostic and Statistical Manual* (DSM-III), Mayes and Horwitz demonstrate how this paradigm shift within psychiatry arose from a confluence of social factors and forces rather than any new knowledge. The social processes involved in the making of the DSM included a crisis of legitimacy in psychiatry, professional turf wars, competing economic and political interests, political controversy and expediency. While this study emphasizes macro political and social processes, we see another variant of the social constructionist approach drawn from micro-sociological perspectives in Whooley's (2010) study of how psychiatrists negotiate biologically reductive understandings of the complexity of mental illness, which nonetheless underpin their professional standing as experts. Other disciplines also contribute to related debates about clinical diagnosis, in accord with social constructionist principles. For instance, on autism assessment, Hayes et al. (2021) take a discursive psychology approach to explore how uncertainty and contradiction undermine the 'straightforward notion of diagnosis as a way to identify underlying biological problems that cause disease' (p. 1).

The main controversy about constructionism centres on relativist claims about knowledge. The implication of a constructionist approach for medical knowledge is that it has no objective basis in the properties of the 'things' that medical practitioners claim to know about. Logically, this argument also applies to sociological knowledge. Hence, for medical sociologists, the same propositions that constructionists apply to scientific knowledge may be used to undermine the very basis on which sociology engages with medical knowledge (Bury, 1986; Williams, 2001). A naïve constructivist epistemology is absurd to medical sociologists who wish, for example, to engage medicine in the context of social structures as independent realities that impact on health and that can be changed by human actions. A weaker version of constructionism, which is core to much sociological thinking, accepts epistemological relativism (rejecting the naïve realism of positivism), while accepting ontological realism (rejecting naïve constructionism). Nicolson and McLaughlin (1987) insist that constructionist theory is realist in the ontological sense that it neither denies the physical reality of disease nor treats the objects of medico-scientific knowledge as mere artefacts. In characterizing the SSK version of constructionism as 'constructionist realism', they state that 'knowledge may be regarded not as a unique representation or mirror of external reality, but as an instrument by which we may operate with that reality' (1988: 251). Thus, the explanatory power of constructionism demonstrates that the contrasting perspectives and evaluations of medical knowledge are underdetermined by the properties of an external physical reality, while overdetermined by social processes. Their version of constructionist realism shares similar premises to Pilgrim's (2014) application of 'critical realism' to the contested field of mental health research.

For some medical sociologists, constructionism has gone too far in countering biological reductionism (Williams, 2001). In the field of mental illness, Busfield (2000) even suggests abandoning the term 'social construct' because of its anti-realist connotations, which itself is revealing of the politics of knowledge. Most sociologists recognize that ontological relativism is an unfeasible proposition for the discipline. Since constructionism has many meanings and theoretical antecedents, the concept continues to be debated. On the one hand, constructionism is accused of undermining sociological realism by placing too strong an emphasis on interpretative practices or local social contingencies, while underplaying the role that pervasive social structures play in the formation of knowledge and the accomplishment of reality. On the other hand, it is accused of challenging natural realism by embracing a relativist epistemology that cuts the ground from under science itself. Moreover, a relativist epistemology, when applied to constructionism itself, undermines it as a form of sociological critique. In practice, most sociologists seek common ground between constructionist and structuralist approaches. Their theoretical choices are more likely to be determined by the focus of analysis and the degree of contextualization demanded of any explanatory approach.

In sum, social constructionism remains an important concept that aligns with different theoretical approaches concerned with the production of knowledge. For medical sociologists, public controversies about science and its uses are fertile ground for investigating the socio-political priorities enacted in health policies, public health interventions and clinical work. Today, this research is of urgent relevance not only in the context of escalating concerns about mental health but also of the COVID-19 pandemic, including the political task of managing controversy and risks amidst uncertain evidence and policy ambiguities (see Suggested Further Reading). There may also be more sustained controversies, not only of a manufactured kind – for example in relation to 'vaccine hesitancy' – but also with respect to the contested medical realities of what has been called 'long COVID' plus the psychosocial effects of prolonged lockdowns, unemployment, domestic abuse, etc. Indeed, one may expect sustained controversy about the structural inequalities highlighted and, in some contexts, accentuated by the pandemic and associated societal responses (including controversy about the narrow technocratic discourse of 'pandemic preparedness' to which sociologists are lending their voices). The pandemic (response) also harbours latent controversies about the production of knowledge, for example with respect to the role of a powerful but weakly regulated technology industry in creating and managing big data for pandemic surveillance. Going forward, medical sociologists will find useful applications of social constructionism in case studies on scientific disputes and public health controversies in the cognate scholarship of science and technology studies, and critical public health, respectively.

See also: Geneticization; Medicalization; Surveillance and Health Promotion; The Medical Model.

REFERENCES

Atkinson, P. and Housley, W. (2003) *Interactionism: An Essay in Sociological Amnesia*. London: SAGE.

Berger, P.L. and Luckmann, T. (1967) *The Social Construction of Reality: A Treatise in the Sociology of Knowledge*. New York: Anchor Books.

Bloor, D. (1970) *Knowledge and Social Imagery*. London: Routledge and Kegan Paul.

Bury, M.R. (1986) 'Social constructionism and the development of medical sociology', *Sociology of Health & Illness*, 8 (2): 137–169.

Busfield, J. (2000) 'Rethinking the sociology of mental health', *Sociology of Health & Illness*, 22 (5): 543–558.

Freidson, E. (1970) *The Profession of Medicine: A Study of the Applied Sociology of Knowledge*. New York: Dodd Mead.

Hayes, J., McCabe, R., Ford, T. et al. (2021) '"Not at the diagnosis point": dealing with contradiction in autism assessment teams', *Social Science & Medicine*, 268: 113462.

Horwitz, A.V. (2012) *All We Have to Fear: Psychiatry's Transformation of Normal Anxieties into Mental Disorders*. New York: Oxford University Press.

Mayes, R. and Horwitz, A.V. (2005) 'DSM-III and the revolution in the classification of mental illness', *Journal of the History of Behavioural Sciences*, 41 (3): 249–267.

Nicolson, M. and McLaughlin, C. (1987) 'Social constructionism and medical sociology: a reply to M.R. Bury', *Sociology of Health & Illness*, 9 (2): 107–126.

Nicolson, M. and McLaughlin, C. (1988) 'Social constructionism and medical sociology: a study of the vascular theory of multiple sclerosis', *Sociology of Health & Illness*, 10 (3): 234–261.

Pilgrim, D. (2014) 'Some implications of critical realism for mental health research', *Social Theory & Health*, 12 (1): 1–21.

Whooley, O. (2010) 'Diagnostic ambivalence: psychiatric workarounds and the Diagnostic and Statistical Manual of Mental Disorders, *Sociology of Health & Illness*, 32 (3): 452–469.

Williams, S.J. (2001) 'Sociological imperialism and the profession of medicine revisited: where are we now?' *Sociology of Health & Illness*, 23 (2): 135–158.

SUGGESTED FURTHER READING

- Decoteau, C.L. and Sweet, P.L. (2016) 'Psychiatry's little other: DSM-5 and debates over psychiatric science, *Social Theory & Health*, 14 (4): 414–435.

Psychiatry and the field of mental illness constitute fertile ground for social constructionist approaches to scientific controversies, including recent debates about the DSM-5. This article traces the different ways that the 'social' has been banished from psychiatric science, its existence in practice ignored and its influence in the profession's history denied.

- Dixon, J. and Richter, D. (2018) 'Contemporary public perceptions of psychiatry: some problems for mental health professions', *Social Theory & Health*, 16 (4): 326–341.

This article foregrounds the practice implications of a social constructionist approach for mental health work. It explores how different constructions of mental disorder, which manifest in tensions between patients and carers, between different healthcare policies and between mental health professions, can be negotiated in practice.

- Mykhalovskiy, E. and French, M. (2020) 'COVID-19, public health, and the politics of prevention', *Sociology of Health & Illness*, 42 (8): 4–15.

What gets counted as evidence in the production of epidemiological knowledge and modelling is key to revealing the assumptions that guide how we come to know the reality of pandemics and interventions that are deemed actionable and legitimate as preventative strategies. This article is a call to arms for critical engagement with scientific knowledge and technical expertise that mask and may exacerbate structural and systemic inequalities.

- Rhodes, T. and Lancaster, K. (2020) 'Mathematical models as public troubles in COVID-19 infection control: following the numbers', *Health Sociology Review*, 29 (2): 177–194.

These authors argue that public controversies surrounding epidemiological modelling provide sociologists with a lens for understanding how the technical products of science produce social effects (read 'realities'). A particular version of social constructionism is found in this study – one associated with the 'doing' of science. The authors focus on the 'work' that predictive modelling does in rendering uncertain futures knowable as 'anticipated potentials' and in translating theoretical (mathematical) abstractions into 'material practices' (p. 179).

32

Lay Knowledge

Gareth H. Williams, Eva Elliott and Jennie Popay

Lay knowledge refers to the ideas and perspectives employed by people to interpret their experiences of health and illness in everyday life.

The concept of lay knowledge within medical sociology was developed as a critical response to the literature on lay beliefs (Popay et al., 1998; Williams and Popay, 2006). The study of people's beliefs about illness, health and medical care initially provided a way of understanding different forms of 'illness behaviour' and 'lay referral', particularly where 'non-compliant' behaviour suggested differences between the perspectives of patients and their physicians. Research on these themes provided an empirical foundation for the argument that patients' behaviours were influenced by their personal beliefs, and that these beliefs were reasoned attempts to deal with the sometimes intensely contradictory demands of illness and its treatment in everyday life. However, a second line of thought was emerging.

Drawing on the Durkheimian tradition of sociological theorizing about the conscience collective, Herzlich (1973), casting a respectful but sociologically critical eye on her respondents' accounts, moved away from the methodological individualism characteristic of much work on lay beliefs at the time. She argued that individual beliefs about health and illness are representations of the culture and society in which people live. While these representations may include medical ideas about pathology and aetiology, lay perspectives express a certain cultural autonomy and embody a wider theorization of health and illness in relation to society. Herzlich's work provided an important bridge between the highly focused empirical studies of individual patients within medical sociology and the panorama of social theorizing about the relationships between self and society. In so doing it marked out a set of themes that would remind future social scientists that lay beliefs represented far too fecund a field to be left to the withering attention of health services researchers or government civil servants.

As awareness of lay knowledge grew, so too did interest in how it could be harnessed to the service of healthcare delivery and research. However, evaluations of early policy initiatives that aimed to do this, such as the UK Expert Patients Programme, suggested that these responses to lay knowledge and expertise remained top-down, normative and individualistic, drawing on psychological rather than sociological concepts (Taylor and Bury, 2007). More recent attempts to harness the experiential knowledge of patients and publics in healthcare and research decision-making processes have also been criticized by Maguire and Britten (2018) as forms of 'colonization'. They argued that in an ideal scenario different forms of knowledge would be treated as equal, albeit different. However they observed that research networks that aim to involve patients and publics continue to privilege scientific and professional discourses and requirements.

Herzlich (1973) provided the intellectual foundation for two key arguments about lay knowledge to develop. First, that lay ideas are not 'primitive' residuals stuck in the otherwise smoothly functioning bowels of modern 'scientific' societies. Rather they are complex bodies of knowledge and forms of rationality that are central to our understanding of culture and society. Second, 'lay knowledge' has two key dimensions. On the one hand, it contains a robust empirical approach to making sense of the contingencies of everyday life: notably of the occurrences of health and illness in ourselves, our families and the wider communities in which we live. On the other hand, especially in situations in which the illness is particularly serious or frightening, the construction of lay knowledge represents a search for meaning that goes beyond the straightforwardly empirical, situating personal experiences of health crisis in relation to broader frameworks of morality, politics and cosmology.

Comaroff and Maguire's (1981) classic study of 'the search for meaning' in childhood leukaemia illustrates this complexity. Modern medicine, they argue, supplies an empirical basis for explaining to parents what is happening to their children. However, it provides no overarching framework through which parents can 'make sense' of what is happening. The parents in their study were asking not only what causes childhood leukaemia, but why has my child developed this disease, and why now? Perhaps it is not the business of good doctoring to answer these questions, but they point to the tension between 'evidence-based' and 'narrative-based' approaches to health knowledge. Lay people need the evidence, but that will not be enough to support the wider framework of interpretation required to make sense of a particular illness. The tension between evidence (how things work) and meaning (what gives life its purpose) reflects different ways of understanding the world. The point is not that one 'way of knowing' is better than another but that their separation impoverishes knowledge itself (Elliott et al., 2016).

Since the 1990s sociologists have been increasingly interested in lay knowledge about health risks as well about health and illness. For Herzlich's (1973) middle-class Parisians the 'way of life' in modern societies, defined in terms of social and environmental circumstances rather than individual behaviours, produced ill health. Later work revealed a tendency for personal responsibility explanations for ill-health to be prevalent in both 'rich' and 'poor' populations. This possibly reflects the enduring values of a Protestant ethic in some of the communities studied, and the effects of the ideology of 'possessive individualism' that were ripping through Western societies at the time (Blaxter, 1983).

However, the key characteristic of lay knowledge is that it is integrative and holistic. It draws on multiple sources: scientific, professional and experiential. While the resulting syncretic lay knowledge reflects the cultural values and ideological interests of the times, it can also provide an incisive moral and political critique of them. A good example of this is to be found in Davison et al.'s (1991) qualitative study in naturalistic settings examining the relationships between lay perspectives on coronary heart disease and the orthodox doctrine promulgated in a nationwide health promotion campaign – Heartbeat Wales. This study uncovered a strong strand of lay thinking that emphasized personal responsibility for health and a close correspondence between lay views and the simple, linear causal models of health educators linking diet, exercise, blood pressure, serum cholesterol and heart disease.

Davison et al. also argued that in situations when explanation is needed – for example, when a person becomes ill or a relative dies prematurely – these lay views become more complex. They coined the term 'lay epidemiology' to describe the way in which people may use a combination of personal, familial and social sources of knowledge, alongside professionally delivered information, to try and make sense of these situations. People develop a notion of who is a 'candidate' for a coronary that corresponds quite closely with risk factor epidemiology. However, the reality of lay experience is that we come across many individuals who smoke, eat fatty foods, consume a lot of alcohol, have a stressful life, take no exercise and live to a ripe old age and conversely there are those who live an Aristotelian 'good life' of balance, frugality, virtue and restraint but collapse and die in their 40s. Like the parents of children with leukaemia in Comaroff and Maguire's (1981) study, abstract descriptions of 'risk factors' are not enough to explain why a much-loved mother or brother has died too young. And as science has evolved so too has lay epidemiology, with molecular and genetic models becoming part of the cultural representations through which lay people 'make sense' of their experience of health in general and specific diseases (Jenkins et al., 2013).

The articulation of meanings through 'lay knowledge' provides a lens through which we can better understand the dynamic relations between the micro features of everyday human action and agency and the wider social structures that generate inequalities in health (Elliott et. al., 2016; Popay et al., 1998). Much health policy and research assumes a freedom to make healthy choices that is out of line with the reality of many people's everyday lives: a reality revealed in

lay knowledge. For people living in conditions of poverty, behavioural risks –
smoking, poor diet, drinking alcohol, lack of exercise – are better understood as
coping mechanisms, embedded in the material and environmental conditions,
in which they live. Mirroring Herzlich's (1973) middle-class Parisians, the 'way
of life' for disadvantaged groups – unemployment, poor housing, low income
and chronic stress – provides a context for making sense of 'risky' behaviours.

This more political expression of lay knowledge finds its most radical form
in the 'popular epidemiology' examined by Brown (1995), and others, where it
becomes a form of 'civic intelligence' deployed in the contestation of scientific
expertise. Studies of popular epidemiology take situations in which lay people
have become concerned about a public health problem in their locality – the
numbers of children with cancer, the high prevalence of asthma, an increase in
road traffic accidents – and seek some explanation for it. In these circumstances
popular epidemiology begins with lay people linking the observed increase in
the health problem to a social or environmental hazard: traffic density/speed,
factory emissions, toxic waste, nuclear power, etc. Having made the connection,
lay people then try to do something about it, and find themselves in conflict
with local politicians, business corporations and/or professional experts who
disagree with the connection being made. In these situations, local people may
be forced to move beyond stating a point of view to a process in which a social
movement develops. Evidence is systematically collected and analysed, scientific arguments are developed and sometimes tested in court. In the process
boundaries between 'lay people' and 'experts' and between scientific rationality,
personal beliefs and political interests are blurred.

The devaluing of lay knowledge about health, particularly its more political
expression, is evident in the myriad examples of articulated lay observations
and experience rendered invisible, silenced or weaponized into accusations
of individual or collective misdemeanour. For example, blaming high rates of
parental smoking for the prevalence of respiratory problems in children, rather
than damp housing. A recent study of the resurgence of coal workers' pneumo-
coniosis, or 'black lung' disease in Appalachia in the USA, outlined how pol-
luting industries succeed in undermining screening programmes through fear
of unemployment and claims for compensation through exploiting uncertainty
over diagnosis and its status as a contested illness (Shriver and Bodenhamer,
2018). In the UK, the detailed lay knowledge of hazards from the external
cladding added to Grenfell Tower in London – which, if acted on, could have
prevented the fire that killed 72 council residents in 2017 – was dismissed by
the Local Council who judged it to be defamatory, political, 'oppositional' and
therefore irrelevant (Popay, 2018).

The sociological study of lay knowledge about health and illness provides a
lens through which the generation of, and interaction between, different forms
of knowledge and expertise, through conflict and consensus, can be seen and
the implications better understood. These dynamic processes reveal themselves
most dramatically at times of personal, community or societal crisis, when the
taken-for-grantedness of everyday life is disturbed. As we were writing this

entry, the COVID-19 pandemic was generating research into how ordinary people were responding to, and making sense of, the risks posed by the virus itself and by the unequal impacts of policy and technical responses to these risks. Together with the Black Lives Matter movement, COVID-19 has forced us to attend to the knowledge of the most marginalized and how it is shaped by the intersections of class, race, gender and disability. To paraphrase the historian E.P. Thompson (1963), to value lay knowledge is to rescue the wisdom of experience, and what we can learn from it, from the enormous condescension of professional experts.

It has been argued that the concept of lay knowledge oversimplifies the sociology of the 'lay expert' and understates the importance of professional and/or 'scientific' expert knowledge (Prior, 2003). Whatever one's position on these issues, it is undeniable that the exploration of lay knowledge throws into sharp relief major enduring social concerns about the relationship between authority and expertise, the problem of meaning in a pluralistic society, the incommensurability of different frameworks of interpretation, and the challenges of developing a society that is both democratic and knowledge-based.

See also: Illness Narratives; Risk; Social Movements and Health.

REFERENCES

Blaxter, M. (1983) 'The causes of disease: women talking', *Social Science & Medicine*, 17 (2): 59–69.

Brown, P. (1995) 'Popular epidemiology, toxic waste, and social movements', in J. Gabe (ed.), *Medicine, Health and Risk*. Oxford: Blackwell.

Comaroff, J. and Maguire, P. (1981) 'Ambiguity and the search for meaning: childhood leukaemia in the modern clinical context', *Social Science & Medicine*, 15 (2): 115–123.

Davison, C., Davey Smith, G. and Frankel, S. (1991) 'Lay epidemiology and the prevention paradox: the implications of coronary candidacy for health promotion', *Sociology of Health & Illness*, 13 (1): 1–19.

Elliott, E., Popay, J. and Williams, G. (2016) 'Knowledge of the everyday: confronting the causes of health inequalities', in K.E. Smith, C. Bambra and S.E. Hill (eds), *Health Inequalities: Critical Perspectives*. Oxford: Oxford University Press.

Herzlich, C. (1973) *Health and Illness: A Socio-Psychological Approach*. London: Academic Press.

Jenkins N., Lawton, J. and Hallowell N. (2013) 'Inter-embodiment and the experience of genetic testing for familial hypercholesterolaemia', *Sociology of Health & Illness*, 35 (4): 529–543.

Maguire, K. and Britten, N. (2018) '"You're there because you are unprofessional": patient and public involvement as liminal knowledge spaces', *Sociology of Health & Illness*, 40 (3): 463–477.

Popay, J. (2018) 'What will it take to get the evidential value of lay knowledge recognised?' *International Journal of Public Health*, 63: 1013–1014.

Popay, J., Williams, G., Thomas, C. and Gatrell, A. (1998) 'Theorising inequalities in health: the place of lay knowledge', *Sociology of Health & Illness*, 20 (5) 619–644.

Prior, L. (2003) 'Belief, knowledge and expertise: the emergence of the lay expert in medical sociology', *Sociology of Health & Illness*, 25 (3): 41–57.

Shriver, T.E. and Bodenhamer, A. (2018) 'The enduring legacy of black lung: environmental health and contested illness in Appalachia', *Sociology of Health & Illness*, 40 (8): 1361–1375.

Taylor, D. and Bury, M. (2007) 'Chronic illness, expert patients and care transition', *Sociology of Health & Illness*, 29 (1): 27–45.

Thompson, E.P. (1963) *The Making of the English Working Class*. London: Penguin.

Williams, G. and Popay, J. (2006) 'Lay knowledge and the privilege of experience', in D. Kelleher, J. Gabe and G. Williams (eds), *Challenging Medicine*, 2nd edn. London: Routledge.

SUGGESTED FURTHER READING

- Elliott, E., Harrop, E. and Williams, G.H. (2010) 'Contesting the science: public health knowledge and action in controversial land-use developments', in P. Bennett, K. Calman, S. Curtis and D. Fischbacher-Smith (eds), *Risk Communication and Public Health*, 2nd edn. Oxford: Oxford University Press.

This chapter uses two case studies (regarding landfill waste sites and opencast mines) to elaborate the process whereby ordinary people contest and challenge the work and judgement of scientific experts in relation to the 'toxic' impact of environmental interventions. Both case studies emphasize the importance of seeing knowledge about public health issues in the round, recognizing that 'science' is often flawed and inadequate. Case study research of these kinds of environmental dispute illustrate how experiences of flawed or discredited science act as an important source of contention in conflicts over environmental health issues.

- Popay, J., Bennett, S., Thomas, C. et al. (2003) 'Beyond "beer, fags, egg and chips"? Exploring lay understandings of social inequalities in health', *Sociology of Health & Illness*, 25 (1): 1–23.

This paper explores lay understandings of the causes of health inequalities. Using both quantitative and qualitative methodology, the views of people living in contrasting socio-economic neighbourhoods are compared. It highlights ways in which different methodologies provide different and not necessarily complementary understandings of lay perspectives on the causes of health inequalities.

33

Medical Tourism

Neil Lunt

Medical tourism occurs when patients travel across borders or to overseas destinations for planned treatments including fertility, cosmetic, dental and elective surgery.

Medical tourism is a subset of the wider notion of patient mobility that also includes temporary visits abroad, long-term residency, residence within common border areas, and outsourcing. There is a diversity of terms that capture patient travel for healthcare and there is little prospect of agreement in the near future (Connell, 2015). Although controversial, the strength of the term 'medical tourism' lies in signalling the commodified nature of activities associated with patient travel and the role of business and ancillary interests that promote such services.

Medical tourism has historical antecedents. In 19th-century Europe, a growing middle-class travelled to spa towns for the health-enhancing qualities of mineral springs. Alongside changes in transportation technology, scientific and surgical developments (internal medicine, surgical techniques and biochemistry) encouraged patient travel for more medicalized experiences. During the 20th century, wealthy people from low- and middle-income nations travelled to high-income nations to access better facilities and highly trained clinicians. Patient movement was also evident within developed health systems, to obtain treatments that were not available or legal within their home country. By the late 20th century, flows of wealthy patients were strongly shaped by the experience of history, including migration patterns and elites from the Global South now receiving treatment in the capital cities of their former colonial rulers. The explosion of oil wealth also saw increased patient travel from Gulf states to British, German, French and American health systems.

A broad range of drivers have facilitated the emergence of contemporary patient travel, including: transformations of economic production and trade, regional political and trade cooperation, technological shifts, migratory flows, and socio-cultural trends and developments. Many domestic health systems continue to experience significant challenges and strain – tightened eligibility criteria, waiting lists and shifting priorities for healthcare impact on consumer decision-making. There is also the emergence of patient choice and forms of consumer identity in healthcare, including within countries that traditionally have had publicly funded services. As well as growing consumer citizenship, the European Union (EU) enables citizens, under specific circumstances, to access medical care in other EU Member States and their national purchaser reimburses these treatment costs.

Much medical travel scholarship has focused on patient travel primarily from the Middle East, North America and Western Europe, including patients funded by insurance and public health systems as well as those making out-of-pocket payments. There is growing awareness of more diverse travel, from higher- to lower- and middle-income nations, and involving regional, diasporic and South–South exchanges (Connell, 2016; Lunt et al., 2014a). For example, the past colonial connection between the UK and India appears to have encouraged a medical market between these countries. Diasporas may return to India for family visits, festivals and holidays but also combine such trips with healthcare treatments. Travel to places of cultural affinity engenders familiarity and trust. Frequently, transnational lenses are invoked to explain health mobility and travel for treatment situated within a broad range of health-seeking behaviours (Phillimore et al., 2019).

As discussed below, four distinct traveller conceptualizations – tourist, pilgrim, exile and nomad – emphasize elements of motivation, treatment type, domestic context and travellers' connections to treatment destinations. Such concepts owe much to medical anthropologists working within the emerging field and their emphasis on travel, culture and fieldwork conducted overseas.

Medical tourism is a concept used to describe travel outside of a person's home country jurisdiction and it has been widespread in the marketing, health and social science literature. The term is controversial for both its accuracy and implications for understanding travelling experience, linking medical travel and leisure to foreground tourist-like activities (accommodation, flights and recreation). Whilst the term captures the commodified nature of activities, including business and ancillary roles, criticism is levelled at its overemphasis on choice, connotations of pleasure and promotion of a marketplace model (Whittaker, 2015). Medical tourist narratives of patients travelling from the Global North to poorer countries in the Global South also risk reinforcing stereotyped assumptions about race, nation and class.

Second, some view cross-border travel for healthcare as a *medical pilgrimage* (Song, 2010), exploring interconnections of faith, technology, travel and healthcare research and treatment. Salvation, optimism and breakthrough are associated with stem cell science and biogenetics, with medical journeys entailing both sacrifice and tribulation (Kangas, 2010). Pilgrimage has some parallels to diasporic tourism, including return visits of members of migrant communities to their homeland or places where there are strong ties. Trips serve numerous functions – visiting friends and relatives, searching for roots and attending celebrations – and may include healthcare utilization where travel for medical treatment is secondary.

Research on travel for assisted reproductive technology talks of *medical exile*. This denotes travellers who experience rejection and structural disadvantage in domestic health systems. This patient-centred term highlights social, cultural, financial and legal constraints among populations that are seemingly given little option but to travel abroad for treatment (Inhorn, 2015). Associated ideas emerge in Whittaker's (2015) examination of outsourced patients: those sponsored by governments, or healthcare insurers, and subsequently treated in another country due to domestic health system weaknesses or cost (also Ormond, 2013). Use of the term 'exile' among medical sociologists and anthropologists is also controversial because treatments in hospitals of the Global North may be associated with choice and volition and perceived by patients as having many advantages.

Medical nomadism emphasizes movement and freedom of groups that were never fully territorialized, i.e. resisting integration within a single place or nation-state. Foregrounding a high degree of mobility and strong social networks, nomadism signals a de-territorialized healthcare experience. Travel to countries for treatment may include homelands and third country settings. Such mobility is shaped by various factors. On the one hand, travel overseas may increase choice options and empower individuals. On the other hand, nomadic health mobility is shaped by a context where services may be formally available but there are systemic barriers to their consumption.

Such terms have value in clarifying previously overlooked aspects of mobility. The terms may work in tandem and denote overlapping characteristics, routes and destinations. For example, commercial considerations so fundamental to medical tourism are also relevant when researching medical exile and medical pilgrimage. A number of overseas clinics target returning diasporas who have greater resources than do domestic patients, or travellers for whom treatments are not legally available at home.

Medical travellers paying out-of-pocket expenses continue to attract attention, with web-based resources providing consumers with information about treatments and destinations. Such sites may convey information unevenly regarding benefits and risks of medical procedures and in framing provider credibility. Information from lay referral (including online) networks of friends and peers also help shape decision-making. Medical tourism facilitators, intermediaries and brokers have emerged to help travellers locate appropriate destination hospitals and clinics and manage arrangements, including translation and treatment.

Insofar as medical travel is underpinned by private treatment, it is difficult to obtain clear information on patient numbers, provider activities and patient outcomes. When making decisions, medical travellers often pay more attention to 'soft' information (i.e. from peers, direct from websites and internet marketing) than 'hard' clinical information (i.e. data on outcomes and treatment risk) (Lunt et al., 2014b). There is little evidence about the clinical outcomes for particular treatments, institutions, clinicians and localities. Commercial providers' results may not undergo robust verification. Furthermore, the cross-national comparison of surgeons offering similar treatments is difficult because of differences in caseload composition. Overemphasis on patient satisfaction measures, as an index of success, could lead to overtreatment, overprescribing of antibiotics and over-diagnosis. Some treatments militate against objective outcomes (for example, cosmetic treatments), and some measures, such as those pertaining to fertility, may become skewed by more immediate outcomes that fail to acknowledge longer-term risks and complications.

The wider shores of medical travel harbour treatments for which there are no clinical trials to support efficacy. Under a regime of commercialization and commodification, relationships are increasingly governed by commercial regulation (tort and contract) rather than professional ethics. There is no internationally agreed framework to regulate medical tourism and prospective patients are rarely fully aware of the lack of clear avenues for redress should treatment abroad lead to unexpected complications. Legal uncertainty and complexity bedevil all phases of treatment abroad: access to information, treatment itself, aftercare and follow-up. There are also questions about appropriate jurisdiction and the time-period to seek legal redress (Lunt et al., 2014b).

System-level implications exist for countries of origin and destination. Delivering care to patients from abroad contributes to a receiving nation's direct foreign exchange earnings. Also, sectors other than medical care – hospitality and travel – benefit financially. However, if provision is by transnational and global corporations, resulting profits may leak overseas. This is noteworthy given several major private providers in international patient markets are subsidiaries of overseas parent companies.

Medical travel could provide incentives for clinical and ancillary staff from lower-income countries to return, thereby helping to reverse the 'brain drain' of qualified clinicians and health professionals. There are, however, concerns over international patient flows that induce an internal brain drain within lower-income countries, with professionals moving to private providers and abandoning the public health system to pursue better salaries and work opportunities irrespective of national clinical needs. From an economic perspective, medical travel could, potentially, exert competitive pressure within a country and help drive down the costs and prices offered in domestic systems. 'Demonstration effects' of healthcare workers observing best practice in treatment, clinical care and technological diffusion may benefit countries providing care for medical tourists, irrespective of whether treatment is via public or private providers.

The costs of rectifying the problems caused by poor treatment overseas, or treatments that require extensive follow-up, may fall on local facilities when travellers return. There are equity concerns and dangers of a two-tier health system emerging or being compounded. Large numbers of medical tourists travelling overseas (for dental care or cosmetic treatments) will have implications for the domestic health system, potentially accentuating trends that are encouraged by current domestic private provision. These trends include being able to avoid (perceived) long waiting lists, to access treatments not routinely provided within the public health system and to seek a high level of 'customer service' (private rooms, higher staffing ratios and on-site facilities).

In situations where eligibility has been tightened (for example, for fertility and dental services), or procedures are illegal, people with private resources 'choosing' to access these overseas may normalize such treatments and prompt discussions at home about the importance of providing them locally. However, that numbers of people willingly pay out-of-pocket for treatment overseas may only ease political pressures within publicly funded healthcare. The exodus of largely middle-class patients as medical tourists may have the effect of undermining the solidarity of healthcare provision and of reproducing or amplifying divisions pertaining not only to social class but also place, as discussed in Part 1 of this book.

In short, explanations for medical travel include motivations that relate both to domestic and destination health systems: reputation, perceived quality, cost, availability, as well as cultural and familial reasons. The healthcare citizenship rights offered by somebody's country of residence (coverage, eligibility) and other factors, including discrimination, are all crucial considerations in this field of research. When exploring health treatment abroad it is necessary to keep in mind that there is diversity in treatments and destinations, industry imagery and normalization, and various mechanisms (including virtual and social networks) are used to build trust and convert a latent willingness to travel into a patient journey overseas.

Alongside health policy, medical anthropology and health economics, medical sociology can make a distinctive contribution to the study of medical tourism. It has the potential to address gaps in our knowledge of doctor–patient relationships surrounding medical treatments abroad, and our understanding of decision-making and treatment experience, particularly the intersection with health status and social stratification. It promises greater insight around how commercialization and commodification (by clinics, hospital and aftercare settings) shape patients' experiences. Finally, medical sociology understands the social context of decisions and treatment, highlighting lay referral and support networks, travel companions and wider family and community contributions that are practical, financial and emotional.

See also: Citizenship and Health; Consumerism; Privatization; Reproduction; Risk.

REFERENCES

Connell, J. (2015) 'Medical tourism – concepts and definitions', in N. Lunt, D. Horsfall and J. Hanefeld (eds), *Elgar Handbook on Medical Tourism and Patient Mobility*. Cheltenham: Edward Elgar.

Connell, J. (2016) 'Reducing the scale? From global images to border crossings in medical tourism', *Global Networks*, 16 (4): 531–550.

Inhorn, M.C. (2015) *Cosmopolitan Conceptions: IVF Sojourns in Global Dubai*. Durham, NC: Duke University Press.

Kangas, B. (2010) 'Traveling for medical care in a global world', *Medical Anthropology*, 29 (4): 344–362.

Lunt, N., Horsfall, D., Smith, R. et al. (2014a) 'Market size, market share and market strategy: three myths of medical tourism', *Policy & Politics*, 42 (4): 597–614.

Lunt, N., Smith, R.D., Mannion, R. et al. (2014b) 'Implications for the NHS of inward and outward medical tourism: a policy and economic analysis using literature review and mixed-methods approaches', *Health Services and Delivery Research*, 2 (2). https://doi.org/10.3310/hsdr02020

Ormond, M. (2013) *Neoliberal Governance and International Medical Travel in Malaysia*. London: Routledge.

Phillimore, J., Bradby, H., Knecht, M. et al. (2019) 'Bricolage as conceptual tool for understanding access to healthcare in superdiverse populations', *Social Theory & Health*, 17 (2): 231–252.

Song, P. (2010) 'Biotech pilgrims and the transnational quest for stem cell cures', *Medical Anthropology: Cross-Cultural Studies in Health and Illness*, 29 (4): 384–402.

Whittaker, A. (2015) 'Outsourced' patients and their companions: stories from forced medical travellers', *Global Public Health: An International Journal for Research, Policy and Practice*, 10 (4): 485–500.

SUGGESTED FURTHER READING

- Connell, J. (2011) *Medical Tourism*. London: CABI.

Connell's book explores the background and rise of health tourism. It also examines how medical tourism benefits local healthcare providers, economies and tourism.

- Holliday, R., Jones, M. and Bell, D. (2019) *Beautyscapes: Mapping Cosmetic Surgery Tourism*. Manchester: Manchester University Press.

Holliday et al. offer a social and cultural analysis of travel for cosmetic surgery, drawing on an Economic and Social Research Council project. This qualitative cross-national study of cosmetic tourists and the cosmetic travel industry offers valuable insights on patient decision-making, travel and treatment experience.

- Lunt, N., Horsfall, D. and Hanefeld, J. (eds) (2015) *The Handbook of Medical Tourism and Patient Mobility*. Cheltenham: Edward Elgar.

This multidisciplinary handbook contains 46 chapters, examining medical travel from global, regional and country perspectives.

34

Reproduction

Jane Sandall, Lee F. Monaghan and Jonathan Gabe

> *Incorporating complex social, cultural and biological processes, reproduction refers to pregnancy, birth and the use of various technologies.*

The shared ideas, values and practices of any society are central to how women, men and children orient themselves towards the major events of birth, illness and death. By extension, reproduction is an area that reveals the relations between healthcare as a social practice, dominant cultural values and gendered ideas or expectations. There is considerable cultural variation in how pregnancy and childbearing are defined and managed in everyday life. Crucial to the sociological view of reproduction is that it happens to, and within, society, as well as to individuals, who may, or may not, be subject to medical control. Thus, the way reproduction is 'managed' has important implications for society as a whole: for how people as social agents view reproduction, how they relate to one another in various institutional contexts and how they perform roles such as parent, worker and patient.

An examination of literature in this field shows that an early, narrow definition of the sociology of human reproduction – relating to conception, pregnancy, birth and motherhood – has been broadened. The literature now encompasses, inter alia, the study of sexualities, masculinities, New Reproductive Technologies (NRTs) and selective NRTs (for example, genetic screening of egg and sperm donors, preimplantation genetic diagnosis), and the social relations involved in the provision of reproductive health services. This expansion has resulted in writings examining the sexual politics of reproduction, the construction of biomedical knowledge and intersections with other fields, such as science and technology studies and research on parenting cultures. Such writings have aimed to move away from definitions of reproductive processes as biological events, isolated from shifting social realities and intersecting identities in local and global contexts. At the same time, writers stressing social aspects, including embodiment, have been cautious not to mask biological matters.

There has been much recent work in medical sociology on reproduction. We introduce some of that literature below (see also Suggested Further Reading) after first revisiting certain classic texts, themes and debates. Although published several decades ago Macintyre's (1977) review still endures in its identification of four types of sociological approach to the management of childbirth and sets out a sociological research agenda more generally. These approaches are: (1) historical, drawing on the sociology of professions and science perspectives; (2) anthropological, focusing on the management of birth in different cultures; (3) 'patient'-oriented, focusing on user views and experiences; and (4) 'patient'–services interaction. Macintyre's review highlights two key themes that are directly related to areas of debate within the sociology of reproduction. The first has been the concept of *medicalization*, and the second has been a dualistic notion of *competing ideologies of reproduction*. We address these two themes in turn before noting subsequent criticisms and debates, some recent insights from the sociology of NRTs and, finally, possible areas for future research.

Medicalization, a key concept in medical sociology, draws attention to medicine as a powerful institution of social control. Women have been seen as particularly vulnerable to medicalization, and it is in relation to reproduction that the concept has been much debated. Sociologists have drawn attention to the medicalization of various aspects of the reproductive process. An early development of the medicalization concept was the work of feminists who identified patriarchal society and its extension – patriarchal medicine – as a key force behind the medicalization of women's health issues. These scholars analysed how previous religious justifications for patriarchy were transformed into scientific ones, and described how women's traditional skills for managing birth were expropriated by medical experts at the end of the 19th century. Such work examined the way services were organized, reproductive technologies controlled and sexuality constrained as particular manifestations of the patriarchal domination that shaped women's reproductive experiences. This early feminist literature identified the sexual politics of women's health and provided a theoretical basis for reclaiming knowledge about, and control over, women's bodies. It was polemical, intentionally political, and critical of the medical model imposed on pregnancy and birth.

Oakley's (1980) influential studies of pregnancy and childbirth in Britain provoked a wider public and professional debate (for recent autobiographical reflections on four decades of childbirth research, see Oakley, 2016). In her early work, Oakley demonstrated the ways in which the discourse of the medical world differs from the everyday language of women and their relatives, and how various understandings are associated with unequal authority and power. In a critical analysis of the profession of obstetrics, she theorized a dualistic notion of *competing ideologies of reproduction*. Here women see pregnancy as a social process over which they should exert active control, while medicine posits it as a potentially pathological event that must be controlled and managed. This theory assumed that women of all classes and ethnicities share the same view. This assumption was later challenged by writers who argued that discourses pertaining to reproduction cannot be reduced to dichotomies; rather, they are multiple and complex. For example, Riessman (1983) examined childbirth and reproduction, premenstrual syndrome and mental health. She claimed that what women have gained and lost with the medicalization of 'life problems' has not been documented. Nor has it been noted how women have actively participated in the construction of new medical definitions, or the reasons that led to such involvement. Riessman argued that both physicians and women have contributed to the redefining of women's experiences in terms of medical categories. Furthermore, physicians have sought to medicalize experience because of beliefs and economic interests, depending on specific professional developments and market conditions.

The work on childbearing in the 1970s and the 1980s provided the background for the subsequent focus on NRTs. By the mid-1980s attention was moving away from the experiences of the majority of women during pregnancy and birth towards a critique of NRTs. This move was spurred on by the birth of Louise Brown, the first test tube baby, in the UK in 1978. NRTs include surrogacy, assisted fertility techniques, prenatal screening and diagnosis, preimplantation diagnosis and foetal surgery. These technologies emerged from a scientific approach to reproduction, just like older techniques such as contraception that were developed to 'manage' pregnancy and childbirth. Questions asked about NRTs have comprised three dimensions. The first describes their nature and function; the second is the triad of women, gender and science; the third expands the above debates to encompass health system access issues and cross-cultural perspectives.

Drawing on feminist criticisms of scientific knowledge and the medicalization of women's lives, studies of reproduction have highlighted the power relations such practices mediate. Criticisms include: women being used as experimental material; women's bodies being commodified; and the construction of the conflicting status of women and foetuses. Writers have critiqued state control over access to services, and have also asked in whose interests have various technologies – such as prenatal screening and testing, infertility treatments, test tube babies, foetal imaging and surrogacy – been developed. The debate has focused on the extent to which these new technologies have been beneficial, or a form of oppression to women, setting up a binary divide of 'salvation or damnation'. Yet in reality the picture is more complex. In the USA, in an influential piece, Rothman (1986) reported that prenatal testing changed the way people thought about childbirth and parenthood. An open mind about the outcome of pregnancy had been replaced with a new norm of '*tentative pregnancy*', even though perfection could not be offered. She concluded that although prenatal testing had increased women's choices, it had also constructed women as genetic gatekeepers, with a new moral responsibility for the consequences of their decisions which had societal implications.

In the 1990s, contributors considered how biomedicine constructs the procreative body, the role of associated regulatory practices and how technology allows medical professionals greater jurisdiction over larger areas of reproduction. Stacey (1992) argued that NRTs, such as IVF, GIFT and the 'new genetics' that are based on the discovery of DNA, opened up new possibilities and created a 'scientific revolution in human reproduction', i.e. the teaming of real science with obstetrics, with implications for the way such technologies are managed and controlled. There has been a concern that women are not just seen as the passive recipients of reproductive technology, and that efforts should be made to explore how they contest and contribute to the construction of new medical definitions and the use of NRTs. Such work has disavowed technological and biological determinism and emphasized human agency. This has involved the delineation of the role of experts and the identification of resistance. Lock and Kaufert (1998) have pointed out how women make pragmatic use of reproductive technologies and have challenged the representation of women as the passive victims of surveillance. A subsequent review of the experience of infertility informed by social scientific studies of illness experience, gender, the body and stigma highlighted an increasing focus on the socio-cultural and health systems context (Greil et al., 2010). The infertility literature can also serve to remind us that it is not only women who reproduce, who undergo medicalization and who experience stigma; men should also be included in such research (e.g. Hannah and Gough, 2020).

The sociology of reproduction raises many other issues. Notably, there are questions about the underlying perspectives of writers in this field, ranging from those who seek to contribute and develop sociological theory, to writers explicitly aiming to improve women's experiences. This range of perspectives parallels debates within the study of illness narratives as well as public sociology, which is reflective of a broader division of labour where different types of knowledge are formulated for academic and/or extra-academic audiences. In the debate about *competing ideologies of reproduction*, Annandale and Clark (1996) have critically reviewed many of the underlying assumptions of writings in the domain of the sociology of childbirth. In so doing these authors have sought to further conceptual knowledge, though such thinking has also been drawn upon by others to inform public and policy debates. On the basis of a range of broad critiques of writings on the sociology of health and gender, Annandale and Clark have suggested that much of the literature has been sociologically naïve around the use of reproductive technology and the rhetoric of midwifery. Specifically, they have argued that much writing has been preoccupied with abnormalities in women's health; has universalized women's experiences regardless of ethnicity and class; has equated reproductive technology with the medicalization of reproduction; has assumed that an increased use of technology in childbirth is a 'bad' thing for women; and has implied that women are powerless victims or dupes in this process. Furthermore, in juxtaposing midwifery and obstetrics, much writing has given uncritical support to the notion that midwifery is 'better' for women than male-dominated obstetrics;

it assumes that midwifery has an underlying feminist viewpoint and implies that midwives are 'with women', ignoring issues of power between women and their female caregivers. Of course, and to refer to Annandale's entry in Part 1 of this volume, we might add to the above a need to engage with 'all forms of gender identity' within the realm of human reproduction, thereby affording more nuanced insights.

The entry on reproduction in the second edition of *Key Concepts in Medical Sociology*, referring to feminist perspectives and new directions for research in the sociology of reproduction, emphasized the need to deconstruct notions about what is 'natural' and explore the transformative possibilities of technology. There is much in leading journals, such as *Sociology of Health & Illness*, which attests to the vibrancy of such techno-social matters. One example is Baldwin's (2018) UK study of the use of social egg freezing to enable reproductive delay. Drawing on interviews with women who have used this technology, she demonstrates how their decisions are shaped by neoliberal discourses which position women as responsible for their fertility and heteronormative lifecourse expectations which valorize the nuclear family. Their decisions are also influenced by discourses of 'appropriate parenting' which prioritize the accumulation of suitable resources and the lack of a particular type of partner who might embrace new fatherhood. Doctors also have an important role to play in determining access to NRTs. This is illustrated in Shaw's (2019) study of medical professionals working in private fertility centres in Columbia. Through ethnographic observation and interviews with clinic staff and women patients, she shows how the praxis of assisted conception is impacted on three interrelated levels. The first level concerns the nature of the medical system, with limited regulation enabling treatment variation and competition between doctors. The second involves doctor–patient interaction, with lack of regulation encouraging doctors to negotiate treatments based on their own moral judgements and social understandings. The third level refers to the relationship between society and doctors' treatment decisions, with doctors effectively choosing who should be parents and how families should be formed.

Three last issues or potential lines of enquiry are worth highlighting, especially following the outbreak of COVID-19 in local and global contexts. First, how have COVID-19 related restrictions, such as barring partners from prenatal healthcare and constraints on home health visitors postpartum, impacted parents' mental and emotional life? Attentiveness to restrictions could also extend to the impact of international travel bans on what has been described as 'an increasingly globalized parenting culture' that includes 'border crossings' and 'appetites' for NRTs (Faircloth and Gurtin, 2017). Second, insofar as health authorities have advised pregnant women to get vaccinated, what might that mean in terms of pharmaceuticalization, relational understandings of risk and responsibility? Third, amidst reports that COVID-related disruptions could result in millions of women in the Global South losing access to contraception and facing other threats (for example, increases in maternal mortality, especially in 'fragile settings') (United Nations, 2020), how might a global sociology advance policy relevant insights amidst arguably blinkered efforts to protect lives? Through such work, medical sociologists will have much to focus on and contribute to in these challenging times. In so doing, the study of reproduction could also advance insights on matters such as social change, disaster responses and intersecting inequalities that pattern health and illness.

See also: Gender; Geneticization; Medical Technologies; Medical Tourism; Medicalization; Nursing and Midwifery as Occupations; Risk; Sexuality.

REFERENCES

Annandale, E.C. and Clark, J. (1996) 'What is gender? Feminist theory and the sociology of human reproduction', *Sociology of Health & Illness*, 18 (1): 17–44.

Baldwin, K. (2018) 'Conceptualising women's motivations for social egg freezing and experience of reproductive delay', *Sociology of Health & Illness*, 40 (5): 859–873.

Faircloth, C. and Gurtin, Z. (2017) 'Introduction – making parents: reproductive technologies and parenting cultures across borders', *Sociological Research Online*, 22 (2): 1–5.

Greil, A.L., Slauson-Blevins, K. and McQuillan, J. (2010) 'The experience of infertility: a review of recent literature', *Sociology of Health & Illness*, 32 (1): 140–162.

Hannah, E. and Gough, B. (2020) 'The social construction of male infertility: a qualitative questionnaire study of men with a male factor infertility diagnosis', *Sociology of Health & Illness*, 42 (3): 465–480.

Lock, M. and Kaufert, P.A. (1998) *Pragmatic Women and Body Politics*. Cambridge: Cambridge University Press.

Macintyre, S. (1977) 'The management of childbirth: a review of sociological research issues', *Social Science & Medicine*, 11 (8–9): 447–484.

Oakley, A. (1980) *Women Confined: Towards a Sociology of Childbirth*. Oxford: Martin Robertson.

Oakley, A. (2016) 'The sociology of childbirth: an autobiographical journey through four decades of research', *Sociology of Health & Illness*, 38 (5): 689–705.

Riessman, C.K. (1983) 'Women and medicalization: a new perspective', *Social Policy*, 14 (1): 3–18.

Rothman, B.K. (1986) *The Tentative Pregnancy: Amniocentesis and the Sexual Politics of Motherhood*. New York: Viking Penguin.

Shaw, M.K. (2019) 'Doctors as moral pioneers: negotiated boundaries of assisted conception in Colombia', *Sociology of Health & Illness*, 41 (7): 1323–1337.

Stacey, M. (ed.) (1992) *Changing Human Reproduction: Social Science Perspectives*. London: SAGE.

United Nations (2020) *Policy Brief: The Impact of COVID-19 on Women*, 9 April. Online: www.un.org/sexualviolenceinconflict/wp-content/uploads/2020/06/report/policy-brief-the-impact-of-covid-19-on-women/policy-brief-the-impact-of-covid-19-on-women-en-1.pdf

SUGGESTED FURTHER READING

- Almeling, R. (2015) 'Reproduction', *Annual Review of Sociology*, 41 (1): 423–442.

A useful review article that conceptualizes and seeks to develop an understanding of human reproduction as a social and biological process. Areas for further investigation are discussed, notably reproductive ageing, men and the need for both qualitative and quantitative research.

- Williams, G. and Jones, I.R. (2016) 'Editorial: childbirth and reproduction', *Sociology of Health & Illness*, Special Themed Section on Childbirth and Reproduction, 38 (5): 687–688.

This editorial introduces five articles on childbirth and reproduction. As well as Oakley's autobiographical reflections, cited above, articles explore: masculinity and the medicalization of infertility, biographical disruption in the context of couples living with endometriosis, emerging foetal monitoring technologies and professional practice, and uncertainty within families following a genetic diagnosis.

- Latimer, J. and Thomas, G.M. (2017) 'Editorial: the politics of reproduction and parenting cultures – procreation, pregnancy, childbirth and childrearing', *Sociology of Health & Illness*, 39 (6): 811–815.

Latimer and Thomas introduce several pertinent articles, emphasizing how medical sociology and science and technology studies interface. Articles address topics such as early-age mothers' birth stories, abortion, sister-to-sister egg donation, men's experiences of infertility, and ultrasound and reassurance in healthcare.

- Fairclough, C. and Gurtin, Z.B. (2018) 'Fertile connections: thinking across Assisted Reproductive Technologies and parenting culture studies', *Sociology*, 52 (5): 983–1000.

This article outlines a processual approach to studying reproduction and develops links between the assisted reproduction literature and parenting culture studies. Themes include stratified reproduction or how different social hierarchies intersect with reproduction, resulting in some reproductive futures being encouraged while others are despised.

35

Medical Technologies

Alex Faulkner

Medical technologies are social and industrial artefacts that may be diagnostic, monitoring, screening, preventive, therapeutic, prosthetic, palliative, regenerative, rehabilitative or assistive, with contemporary attention being greatly focused on innovations in genetics, data media, mobile and tele-health, and nano and human cell technologies.

It is impossible to think of contemporary medicine without considering the multitude of technologies that are now integral to medical practice and to healthcare worldwide. Such technologies are to be found inside healthcare systems, in domestic and personal spaces and in workplaces and public places. Increasingly, medical technology is provided, accessed and consumed outside of traditional medical and healthcare settings in various forms of self-administered or remotely connected care regimes. Medical technology can lead to the re-shaping and re-defining of the boundaries of healthcare and 'medicine' itself, and the subjective identities of ourselves as its users, be it as patients, consumers, citizens or health activists.

Technological trends including miniaturization, molecularization, geneticization, 'smart' connectivity, artificial intelligence (AI) and 'big data' are transforming healthcare, to some extent. However, it is easy to overestimate the extent of these innovative developments, because all societies globally, including the most industrially advanced, continue to rely on thousands of less eye-catching, long-established technologies such as defibrillators and wheelchairs. Nevertheless, information technology (IT) innovations are enabling important trends, especially in the re-location of care in 'near-patient', 'point-of-care' and some self-care technologies. These developments encompass primarily diagnostic and monitoring functions, though more therapeutic treatment innovations will undoubtedly appear. The advance of portable technologies offers particular opportunities in less developed economies and hard-to-reach populations in the Global South. In this context, the complexities of local healthcare systems and community relations play an important part in shaping the uptake of devices such as point-of-care diagnostics, where, for example, local laboratory practices may not match built-in standards of portable devices (Engel et al., 2017).

Medical technologies enter into the everyday 'lifeworld' experiences of user-ship and citizenship (Lauritzen and Hyden, 2006). Users of technologies may be construed as patients or citizens with subjective and social capacities and identities. Patients may organize themselves around technologies, for example cardiac pacemaker groups. The importance of this aspect of medical technologies is greatly increased by the escalation of mobile 'mHealth' online, portable and smartphone-based applications (apps). The uptake or incursion of mHealth into personal lives brings with it issues of the corporate use of 'big data', and questions are raised by such developments for personal self-efficacy, regulation and medical authority – is an app, which claims to enable self-measurement of blood pressure, recreational or medical? Where does liability for outcomes of such devices lie (Lynch and Farrington, 2018)? More radically still, does the lifeworld and even bodily incorporation of biomedical technologies lead citizens toward 'cyborg' identities? 'Cyborg bodies' become enmeshed in complex ways with gendered power relations, including masculinities and disability (Robertson et al., 2020).

Of particular interest and concern is the increasing incorporation of software and AI in many technologies, for example though 'biosensors' which can communicate data from *in vivo* to medical professionals. This greatly complicates the regulatory challenge, not least because software can be classified as a medical device if it has a 'medical function'. The classification of medical technologies is itself a matter deserving of sociological understanding, because different classifications are used by different social actors with different 'stakeholder' agendas. Processes of classification are at the heart of how societies make the world intelligible and meaningful and are central to the regulation of the safety of devices. Medical device regulation and healthcare systems use a range of risk classifications in attempting to balance industrial innovation and marketization against consumer safety, public health value and cost effectiveness. Judgements are made via clinical trials and other forms of evidential evaluation and 'Health Technology Assessment' (HTA) (Faulkner, 2009). In the European Union, new medical device regulations are being introduced at the time of writing following several scandals concerning failing devices.

HTA, developed since the late 1980s, attempts to rationalize healthcare by tying technology to robustly evaluated standards of research evidence. These movements have evolved large infrastructures across industrial countries, deploying complex methodologies for assessing technologies in terms of efficacy, effectiveness, safety and cost-effectiveness. In the UK, the movement is epitomized by the internationally-recognized National Institute for Health and Care Excellence (NICE), which commissions assessments and medical specialist opinion, and makes recommendations about the adoption and clinical use of medical devices and pharmaceuticals, acting as a gatekeeper. By having its decisions debated in the public realm, NICE effectively enables 'the politics' of conflicting stakeholders' views about technologies to be ventilated, thus providing some social legitimacy to often contentious healthcare technology policy decisions.

But where do these technologies come from? Many devices are invented and marketed by companies in the large medical device industrial sector. There are hundreds of small companies and a relatively small number of multinational companies. They tend to specialize in a few types of devices, for example joint replacements. Sociologists have conceptualized this medical device economy in terms such as a 'medico-industrial complex' or 'corporate health', pointing critically to the potential bias, for example, of technologies leading to supply-induced demand rather than meeting real perceived health needs. In the contemporary era, the relationship between academia and industry, often promoted by the state (the 'triple helix'), is especially important for innovation. Hence the processes of development of this innovating force have come under scrutiny, including, for example, the role of universities' technology transfer offices and policies about intellectual property. Hence, 'spin-off' companies in the medical devices sector have been studied as a site where conflicting expectations of clinical end-users, investors and entrepreneurial researchers meet. Unsurprisingly perhaps, a range of redirections, goal adjustments and radical adaptations of original 'value propositions' are likely to occur. In one study (Lehoux et al., 2014), a company developing a heart ablation (tissue surgery) monitor most successfully negotiated such tensions, including pressure from investors.

As mentioned above, medical devices sometimes fail at the point of application, as has been the case over the last two decades with various breast and hip implants (Wienroth et al., 2014), and recently transvaginal mesh for pelvic organ prolapse and urinary incontinence, giving rise to court cases and action by patient organizations. Issues of device failure, and indeed corrupt practices, are under-researched in medical sociology, though, as seen in McKelvey et al. (2018), there have been some notable recent cases (an Italian doctor-researcher imprisoned in 2019 for falsifying evidence about an allegedly regenerative tracheal (windpipe) implant). Aside from negligent and unethical practices such as counterfeiting, the quality of medical devices is a broad 'global health' issue. In 2010, the World Health Organization (WHO) reported that 8 per cent of the medical devices in circulation globally were potentially counterfeit.

The diffusion and quality of medical devices in low- and middle-income countries (LMICs) has begun to be addressed by the WHO in a series of reports and 'Global Forums' that debate issues with NGOs and others. The WHO collects examples of local communities' adoption of devices, including examples of 'frugal innovation', where devices are designed respecting local resource-poor circumstances. Many challenges face these endeavours, such as defining standards and regulatory oversight (Mori et al., 2011). Access to medical devices is important in LMICs, as is access to medicines. For example, the first advanced MRI scanners were introduced into public hospitals in Botswana and Ghana only in the early 2010s. Ethical issues for doctors are also exacerbated by sudden global crises such as the COVID-19 pandemic, highlighting potential shortages and global supply chains for respiratory devices, exacerbating clinical pressures (Truog et al., 2020) – problems which, of course, go beyond LMICs.

Social science's theoretical literature on health technologies is massive, comprising many approaches, and were outlined in some detail in the second edition of this *Key Concepts* handbook (2013). As in the 2013 overview, it remains useful to consider the question of the 'neutrality' of technology. Are medical technologies in themselves value-free, independent of their social, economic and healthcare contexts? It is obvious that the answer to this is negative, but the *relative* influence of 'social' or 'technological' forces is likely to differ from case to case (Faulkner, 2009). News headlines tend to deploy simplified messages and images ('new device set to revolutionize heart surgery'), which imply that medical technology has straightforward 'impacts', often framed in terms of stark benefits or risks. However, the above cases and discussion show that it is impossible to maintain a wholly technological, 'determinist' theory. The pathways from innovation to consumption, technologies' social, economic and personal significance, and stakeholders' alternative perceptions of value and evidence, all illustrate the entanglement of social and technological dynamics. Technological determinism ignores the socially based variability of both the design of technologies and what can be called their usership (Faulkner, 2009). Hence, the now more popular conceptual approaches which have developed from what has been called 'technology-in-practice' (Timmermans and Berg, 2003). This can be illustrated with examples.

One example is the social consequences of the practice of the prostate-specific antigen (PSA) blood test, which can indicate latent prostate cancer in men. Although PSA is widely used its benefits have proved equivocal, leading to dilemmas for men offered the test (Faulkner, 2009). It is also apparent that some technologies are quite closely aligned with an existing profession's practices (for example, stents in cardiovascular surgery), while others are much more 'configurational' in the sense that there are different ways of organizing their use and adapting the technology itself. Complex telemedicine systems are a good example. This 'technology-in-practice' or 'mutual constitution' approach has also been developed in 'actor-network theory' (ANT). A good example of applying ANT comes from the management of childhood asthma, where the commonly used metered-dose inhaler was shown to be a significant actor in a complex network including also parents, clinicians, scientists, children's lungs, aerosol gases and mechanical valves (Prout, 1996). Out of this ensemble, to simplify greatly, grew novel skills, novel biomedical organization and novel social identities, as well as care regimes. Hence, from this complex ensemble, a particular 'technology identity' (Ulucanlar et al., 2013) emerged.

Technologies and devices have become ever more important in medical sociology – and Science & Technology Studies (STS) – approaches to healthcare.

Sociological analysis can show the many ways in which they are not 'neutral' tools. Innovative devices and products disrupt existing social subjectivities, care organization and skills, and may be associated with classical sociological concerns of inequalities, medicalization, privatization, political economy, industrial power and collective identity. Scientific trends such as molecularization, nanotechnology and data science, produced through international innovation networks, are of undoubted importance for medicine's future. Nevertheless, an even-minded sociological approach should not be too distracted by high-tech visions. For a sociological understanding, it is important to consider also 'mundane', under-the-radar, taken-for-granted technologies, and a wide variety of geographical sites including deprived populations in global healthcare. In such a view, the surgical face mask or the wheelchair may be as sociologically interesting, and have just as important social significance, as the gene-edited cell therapy or the latest bio-electronic device.

See also: Bioethics; Digital Health; Geneticization; Medicines Regulation; Reproduction.

REFERENCES

Engel, N., Yellappa, V., Pant Pai, N. and Pai, M. (2017) 'Diagnosing at point of care in South India: coordination work and frictions', *Science & Technology Studies*, 30 (3): 54–72.

Faulkner, A. (2009) *Medical Technology into Healthcare and Society: A Sociology of Devices, Innovation and Governance*. Basingstoke: Palgrave Macmillan.

Lauritzen, S.O. and Hyden, L.-C. (eds) (2006) *Medical Technologies and the Life World: The Social Construction of Normality*. Abingdon: Routledge.

Lehoux, P., Daudelin, G., Williams-Jones, B. et al. (2014) 'How do business model and health technology design influence each other? Insights from a longitudinal case study of three academic spin-offs', *Research Policy*, 43 (6): 1025–1038.

Lynch, R. and Farrington, C. (2018) *Quantified Lives and Vital Data: Exploring Health and Technology through Medical Devices*. London: Palgrave Macmillan.

McKelvey, M., Saemundsson, R.J. and Zaring, O. (2018) 'A recent crisis in regenerative medicine: analyzing governance in order to identify public policy issues', *Science and Public Policy*, 45 (5): 608–620.

Mori, M., Ravinetto, R. and Jacobs, J. (2011) 'Quality of medical devices and *in vitro* diagnostics in resource-limited settings', *Tropical Medicine and International Health*, 16 (11): 1439–1449.

Prout, A. (1996) 'Actor-network theory, technology and medical sociology: an illustrative analysis of the metered dose inhaler', *Sociology of Health & Illness,* 18 (2): 198–221.

Robertson, S., Monaghan, L.F. and Southby, K. (2020) 'Disability, embodiment and masculinities', in L. Gottzén, U. Mellström and T. Shefer (eds), *Routledge International Handbook of Masculinity Studies*. Oxon: Routledge.

Timmermans, S. and Berg, M. (2003) 'The practice of medical technology', *Sociology of Health & Illness*, 25 (3): 97–114.

Truog, R.D., Mitchell, C. and Daley, G.Q. (2020) 'The toughest triage – allocating ventilators in a pandemic', *The New England Journal of Medicine*, 382: 1973–1975.

Ulucanlar, S., Peirce, S., Elwyn, G. and Faulkner, A. (2013) 'Technology identity: the role of sociotechnical representations in the adoption of medical devices', *Social Science & Medicine*, 98: 95–105.

Wienroth, M., McCormack, P. and Joyce, T.J. (2014) 'Precaution, governance and the failure of medical implants: the ASR(TM) hip in the UK', *Life Sciences, Society & Policy*, 10: 19. https://doi.org/10.1186/s40504-014-0019-2

SUGGESTED FURTHER READING

- Oudshoorn, N. (2011) *Telecare Technologies and the Transformation of Healthcare*. London: Palgrave Macmillan.

An important, well-theorized discussion using a 'technology-in-practice', 'material-semiotic' approach to analyse the redistribution of care organization, practices and identities both professional and patient, when remote care systems are introduced. An increased role for patients themselves is a key focus.

- Lehoux, P. (2006) *The Problem of Health Technology: Policy Implications for Modern Health Care Systems*. Abingdon: Taylor & Francis.

Lehoux's book is notable for addressing the pathways of medical technologies from design to usership, through evaluation and HTA procedures, and set within a framework that incorporates a focus on social values about what are desirable technologies for societies.

- *WHO Compendium of Assistive, Ehealth and Medical Devices 2014*. Geneva: WHO. Online: https://apps.who.int/iris/bitstream/handle/10665/108781/9789241564731_eng.pdf

A massive collection of examples of medical technology projects from all over the world. A good starting point for investigating local, real-world socio-economic and health system contexts, problems and achievements, especially in LMICs.

- MacKenzie, D. and Wajcman, J. (1999) 'Introduction', in *The Social Shaping of Technology*, 2nd edn. Buckingham: Open University Press.

An excellent, basic and still relevant introduction to the variety of theories of technology–society relations in general, showing how neither social nor technological determinism is likely to explain innovation and usership processes. 'Social construction of technology' and political economy perspectives are included.

36

Digital Health

Deborah Lupton

The term 'digital health' describes a diverse array of digital devices and software that are used for managing and promoting health and well-being, generating and archiving health and medical details, supporting medical education and training or offering medical services.

Across many countries, and particularly in the Global North, digital technologies are widely used for health and medical purposes (Lupton, 2017; World Health Organization [WHO], 2019). Digital health technologies have been in operation since the early years of mass personal computing. With the emergence of the internet and World Wide Web in the 1980s, information websites, online discussion forums, email lists and newsletters sprang up to provide health and medical information and support and to share lay knowledge. Lay people used search engines such as Google Search to find these resources and basic electronic health records and telemedicine services were established. During these early years, such services were accessed on desktop and laptop computers.

Even more digital technologies relevant to health emerged after the turn of the 21st century. The online encyclopaedia Wikipedia was invented, offering numerous entries on health and medicine. Mobile devices such as smartphones, tablet computers and wearable health and fitness trackers, together with Wi Fi technologies, expanded the opportunities for people both to seek and share health information and experiences, as well as generate information about their own bodies. Tens of thousands of mobile applications ('apps') are now offered to lay people to learn about health and medical topics, engage in self-diagnosis, participate in remote consultations with medical professionals, monitor their bodies and participate in self-care routines for chronic illness. Healthcare professionals can access apps to support their medical training and healthcare delivery. Social media and content-sharing services such as Facebook, YouTube, Tumblr, Twitter, Instagram, Pinterest, Reddit and TikTok generate and share a huge amount of health and fitness content by lay people and healthcare professionals alike. Robotic surgery is used in some procedures. Medical and health details are generated, archived and processed as 'big data' for medical and public health research.

From a sociological perspective, digital health raises a number of important questions. These include the following: How is the medical profession's authority and expertise supported, challenged or undermined when lay people use these technologies? How are public health services and healthcare delivery changed? What are the implications for the doctor–patient relationship and for how people understand their bodies and health status? Key theoretical perspectives in sociology can be used to examine these issues. In what follows, I will outline three perspectives – the political economy approach, Foucauldian theory and more-than-human theory – before applying these perspectives to a discussion of digital health in response to the COVID-19 pandemic.

The political economy approach is founded on the work of Karl Marx, whose critical scholarship published in the 19th century drew attention to the social structures and social class-related inequalities that emerged from the Industrial Revolution and the capitalist economic system. Applied to contemporary digital health, a political economy perspective demonstrates the continuing disparities in the benefits offered by these technologies. Social researchers have pointed out other social determinants of digital health use beyond social class, including factors such as geographical location, gender, age, ethnicity/race and level of health or disability and digital infrastructure access (Rice and Sara, 2019). They have emphasised that due to major differences between social groups and geographical regions in access to digital devices and software, some people simply lack the opportunity to go online or use apps for health-related purposes. For example, people living in low-income countries and in remote rural regions in mid- and high-income countries, are forced to deal with inadequate Wi Fi and mobile telephony services. Groups such as these are likely to miss out on the opportunities and benefits that digital health services can offer them (WHO, 2019).

The scholarship of the late philosopher Michel Foucault has been influential in medical sociology since the 1980s. His concepts of biopolitics and biopower have been taken up to address health and medical topics. The Foucauldian perspective highlights both the repressive and the productive nature of power: how it brings knowledge and practices into being and action. Biopolitics and biopower refer to the complex power relations involved when state agencies such as government health departments, non-government and commercial enterprises and lay people and healthcare professionals work together to manage the health and bodies of populations. Applied to digital health, the Foucauldian perspective highlights how certain ideals and practices are promoted as beneficial for people to take up in their own interests to improve their health and fitness (Guta et al., 2018). Technologies such as apps and wearable fitness trackers are positioned as helping people learn about their bodies and engage in self-care regimens as part of conforming to dominant ideals concerning how to be a 'responsible citizen' (Lupton, 2016).

In many areas of the humanities and social sciences, more-than-human theory (also referred to as 'new materialisms') has begun to make a major impact. As the term suggests, more-than-human theory devotes attention to the ways that humans come together with nonhumans to form collections ('assemblages') of things that generate forces and capacities for action. These nonhumans include living and non-living things such as other animals and plants, as well as elements of place and space such as mountains, bodies of water and urban landscapes and human-made objects such as houses, furniture, food and clothing. Health-related assemblages might include humans coming together with things such as hospitals, medical clinics, pharmaceuticals, vitamins and fitness apparel (Andrews and Duff, 2019). Digital technologies are viewed from this perspective as assemblages of these diverse agents of humans and nonhumans. A more-than-human analysis of people's use of digital health technologies, for example, can identify the ways in which assemblages of humans, digital devices, software, digital data and places are configured and experienced. This perspective can offer an analysis of affective forces and agencies such as pleasure, confidence, greater knowledge and the capacity to act to improve or manage one's health. More-than-human theory emphasizes too the anxiety, frustration and disappointment that are sometimes generated with and through the assemblages created when people go online or use apps for health-related purposes (Lupton, 2020).

The advent of the novel coronavirus (COVID-19) pandemic in early 2020 generated massive social and economic changes in people's everyday lives, including their use of digital health services. As part of physical distancing measures, many countries moved quickly to institute and dramatically expand telemedicine services so that people could contact healthcare providers online rather than attend surgeries or hospital waiting rooms. Online symptom or self-diagnosis platforms and apps appeared to help people determine whether they were at risk from contracting the virus or needed testing or healthcare. Digital technologies played an important role in population monitoring, containment and control measures. In some countries, a range of smartphone and social media apps were developed for use in surveillance and mapping of symptoms and viral spread, contact tracing and enforcement of quarantine or self-isolation measures.

A *political economy perspective* on the COVID-19 crisis emphasizes that not all citizens were able to engage with the digital health technologies that were on offer or to take up the practices of prevention that websites, apps and government advertising advocated, due to social determinants such as social disadvantage, area of residence or lack of education. Neoliberal and free market capitalist political systems were called to account and disrupted by the COVID crisis but also operated to protect the privileged and profit from what was termed 'disaster capitalism' or 'coronavirus capitalism' by Canadian activist, author and film-maker Naomi Klein (see Adams, 2020). These developments included the rapid growth and expansion of digitized surveillance technologies that have often been employed to discipline people for not being 'responsible citizens', even when their ability to conform to state imperatives was limited due to poverty, lack of digital access, overcrowding at home, fear of starvation or homelessness: particularly in low- or middle-income countries.

Foucauldian-inspired critiques taking up the concepts of biopolitics and bio-power discussed the political dimensions of how social groups and populations (the 'body politic'), as well as individual bodies, were managed, disciplined and governed in the COVID crisis. For some commentators, governance responses to the pandemic – such as using software to collect, quantify and model the spread of the virus and apps and drones to monitor people's health and behaviour – were evidence of a 'radical biopolitics' (Ecks, 2020). Emphasizing Foucault's key principle that the exertion of power can be both productive and repressive, it can be argued that some of the digital technologies adopted by various governments to intervene in and regulate the pandemic were restrictive of people's freedoms (such as the apps used to make decisions about whether people could leave their homes). However, this was part of a delicate balance sought by state agencies in an attempt to ensure that the pandemic did not become out of control, so as to limit its effects on the health of their citizens as well as the economy. In short, these measures, were designed (if not always sensibly implemented) to control and minimize viral transmission in the population rather than simply or only a quest for political control.

A more-than-human perspective identifies that in the case of COVID-19, constantly changing 'pandemic assemblages' (Fox, 2020) emerged as the pandemic ran its course. The virus itself (SARS-CoV-2) became a powerful agent of change, as it came into contact with humans and nonhumans (surfaces that were touched by humans) and rapidly moved from infecting the bodies of animals in Chinese wet markets to those of humans. Strategies of containment focused on limiting people's movements in space and place, as well as using a new testing regime to discover who was infected and to encourage people to engage in hygiene practices. Together, these human and nonhuman agents generated affective forces and agencies that enhanced or diminished humans' capacities for action. The capacity to protect oneself from the virus but also from effects of hopelessness or feelings of loss of control were important elements of the ways that humans engaged with digital health technologies such as telemedicine and symptom-checker and contract tracing apps. More broadly, social media, digital messaging services and video streaming platforms were important ways of supporting social connections, exercise regimens and mental well-being.

A multitude of novel digital health technologies will likely emerge in the future, responding to new outbreaks of infectious disease as well as longstanding health problems. As the world deals with and moves into a post-COVID future, many issues related to digital health technologies will require continuing sociological investigation. The impact on the healthcare system and healthcare delivery systems will need to be examined. Detailed investigation into what digital health technologies were most useful and helpful to both lay people and healthcare providers, and which failed to live up to their promise, are required. The (ab)uses of surveillance technologies for monitoring the health and movement of citizens and populations should come under scrutiny if they are continued beyond the immediate crisis and need for containment. How social media and other online resources contributed to – or perhaps undermined – mental health and well-being during the pandemic and beyond is another important area for sociological research.

See also: Medical Technologies; Risk; Surveillance and Health Promotion.

REFERENCES

Adams, V. (2020) 'Disasters and capitalism … and COVID-19', *Somatosphere,* 26 March. Online: http://somatosphere.net/2020/disaster-capitalism-covid19.html/

Andrews, G.J. and Duff, C. (2019) 'Matter beginning to matter: on posthumanist understandings of the vital emergence of health', *Social Science & Medicine*, 226: 123–134.

Ecks, S. (2020) 'Coronashock capitalism: the unintended consequences of radical biopolitics', *Medical Anthropology Quarterly blog*, 6 April. Online: http://medanthro quarterly.org/2020/04/06/coronashock-capitalism-the-unintended-consequences-of-radical-biopolitics/

Fox, N.J. (2020) 'Capitalism is the elephant in the COVID19 isolation room', *Discover Society*, 26 March. Online: https://discoversociety.org/2020/03/26/capitalism-is-the-elephant-in-the-covid19-isolation-room/

Guta, A., Voronka, J. and Gagnon, M. (2018) 'Resisting the digital medicine Panopticon: toward a bioethics of the oppressed', *The American Journal of Bioethics*, 18 (9): 62–64.

Lupton, D. (2016) *The Quantified Self: A Sociology of Self-Tracking*. Cambridge: Polity Press.

Lupton, D. (2017) *Digital Health: Critical and Cross-Disciplinary Perspectives*. London: Routledge.

Lupton, D. (2020) '"Better understanding about what's going on": young Australians' use of digital technologies for health and fitness', *Sport, Education and Society*, 25 (1): 1–13.

Rice, L. and Sara, R. (2019) 'Updating the determinants of health model in the Information Age', *Health Promotion International*, 34 (6): 1241–1249.

WHO (2019) *WHO Guideline: Recommendations on Digital Interventions for Health System Strengthening*. World Health Organization. Online: www.who.int/reproductivehealth/publications/digital-interventions-health-system-strengthening/en/

SUGGESTED FURTHER READING

- Henwood, F. and Marent, B. (2019) 'Understanding digital health: productive tensions at the intersection of sociology of health and science and technology studies', *Sociology of Health & Illness* special issue on 'Digital Health: Sociological Perspectives', 41 (S1): 1–15.

Henwood and Marent provide an editorial introduction to this special issue, containing 13 articles in which authors have adopted various sociological perspectives on digital health. Theoretical approaches include more-than-human and political economy perspectives as well as discussions of the concepts of trust, medicalization, temporalities and datafication.

- Lupton, D. (ed.) (2017) *Digitised Health, Medicine and Risk*. London: Routledge. (Also published as a special issue of *Health, Risk & Society*, 2015, 17 (7–8).)

This edited collection begins with an introductory chapter, followed by eight articles covering diverse social and cultural aspects of how digital health intersects with health, medicine and risk. The chapters refer to such topics as apps designed for health, pregnancy, asthma monitoring and health coaching, online forums for mothers discussing infant feeding, an online alcohol and drug screening intervention, digital media campaigning by health activists and citizens' views on technologies that use sensors to monitor body functions.

- Lupton, D. (ed.) (2018) *Self-Tracking, Health and Medicine: Sociological Perspectives*. London: Routledge. (Also published as a special issue of *Health Sociology Review*, 2017, 26 (1).)

This edited collection features seven chapters with an introduction that provides an overview of sociological approaches to self-tracking in the context of health and medicine. The book provides details from empirical studies on a range of self-tracking practices using digital devices, including heart rate, diabetes and drug use monitoring, health and fitness apps, and wearable devices.

- Roberts, C., Mackenzie, A. and Mort, M. (2019) *Living Data: Making Sense of Health Biosensing*. Bristol: Bristol University Press.

This book reports on empirical research conducted in the UK on a range of digital technologies using sensors for tracking health and body functions and how they are used by people in everyday life. There are discussions of fertility sensing and monitoring devices and remote monitoring technologies for older people as well as those used for stress and genotyping.

37

Geneticization

Rebecca Dimond, Heather Strange and
Jacqueline Hughes

> *Geneticization refers to the way in which diseases, conditions and behaviours may come to be regarded as being determined, wholly or in part, by genetic factors.*

Geneticization describes the extension and significance of genetic explanations within medical and social discourse (Lippman, 1991) and is associated with the 'new genetics': the development of recombinant DNA techniques and subsequent increased accessibility of genetic information about individuals, families and populations. Geneticization refers to the process by which disorders and behaviours typically deemed 'problematic' are increasingly described as genetically-determined, whereby research and policy become dominated by a genetic agenda. Medical science and research have focused on 'mapping' human genetic make-up in order to realize a new kind of 'truth' about individual bodies and humankind. Alcoholism, homosexuality and obesity have been described as 'genetic', and the identification of 'a gene for...' attracts intense media speculation, without subsequent confirmation or clear clinical application. From a critical sociological perspective such discourses are problematic: alternative contexts, models of health, and sources of treatment become discarded, and existing debates about medicalization are reproduced in a genetic context. Varying success in translation from research to clinical application has led to questions about the value of prioritizing genetic information over alternative frameworks or solutions. The concept of geneticization has most recently been critiqued within the social sciences for being overly simplistic and context specific (Arribas-Ayllon, 2016; Weiner et al., 2017).

Critics such as Weiner et al. (2017: 989) nonetheless argue that 'a genetic imaginary persists, which plays a performative role in driving investments in new gene-based developments'. Research promising significant, widespread health improvements via continued exploration of genetic information continues to attract large-scale investment. High-profile initiatives to collect, exploit and share genetic information are facilitated by rapid advances in 'big data' science – our increased ability to produce and store vast datasets. One of the first big data projects, the 2003 Human Genome Project (HGP), was an international collaboration designed to produce a 'map' of the human genome. The HGP was expected to identify a genetic basis for many diseases, and lead to enhanced treatments and cures. Genomics England's 100,000 Genomes Project completed the sequencing of 100,000 NHS patient genomes in 2018, with the intention of supporting scientific and clinical advances, and helping to develop 'personalized' medical care. Such large-scale, collaborative collections of DNA samples (genetic 'biobanks', sometimes matched with clinical data), provide opportunities to increase knowledge, develop diagnostic/predictive tests and identify treatments. Yet biobanks raise concerns about consent, anonymity, use and ownership of genetic data. They also raise questions about the nature of collaboration: about patient involvement in decision-making (Courbier et al., 2019) and who benefits from cross-border collaboration (Feld and Kreimer, 2019). Low- and middle-income countries have specific challenges in terms of researcher retention, access to funding and application of local context to knowledge (Reidpath and Allotey, 2019). Utilizing genetic medicine to enhance global health will require a greater emphasis on the recognition and funding priorities in the Global South (Gibbon et al., 2018).

Despite some success in the development of therapeutic applications, the 'promissory futures' of many genetic research projects remain, for the most part, unfulfilled. Clinical treatment is limited for most disorders thought to have a genetic component. Complex multifactorial diseases (such as cancer and major mood disorders) have been linked to multiple genes, as well as environmental factors that are less easily identified and manipulated. Personalized medicine, where drug treatments are targeted on the basis of genetic markers, has brought renewed hope for some patient populations (Hedgecoe, 2004). One recent example of success is the development of a new range of drugs expected to transform the lives of patients with the most common form of cystic fibrosis mutation. However, high treatment costs mean that they will not be accessible to all and thus contribute to health disparities.

Geneticization prompts sociologists to consider how genetic interventions become normalized – a process that is particularly evident within the field of reproductive technology. Population-level screening programmes routinely deploy prenatal genetic testing to help identify conditions such as Down's syndrome. These practices, coupled with specialized techniques such as in vitro fertilization (IVF) and pre-implantation genetic diagnosis (PGD), give rise to systems where the identification and (de)selection of embryos on the basis of disease, carrier and disease-susceptibility status has become deeply normalized. Whilst advanced diagnostic and selective technologies have mainly been limited to use within 'at-risk' populations, the recent advent of non-invasive prenatal testing (NIPT) promises to extend the diagnostic power of routine prenatal screening. NIPT exploits the presence of 'cell-free fetal DNA' in the maternal bloodstream; advances in genomic sequencing mean that small amounts of this fragmented genetic material are sufficient to enable accurate testing of fetal genetic makeup. The rapid development and diversification of NIPT – catalysed by significant public and commercial investment – means that the breadth and depth of testing continues to develop: tests become increasingly accurate and the range of conditions tested for grows (Strange, 2018). The diffusion of NIPT into routine prenatal care introduces the possibility that testing for rare and complex conditions, as well as non-disease traits, may also become normalized.

Critics show how reproductive technologies reinforce problematic cultural norms, such as ableism and gender preference; for example, widespread sex-selection has led to the 'gendercide' of female embryos in India and China (Sharma, 2008). Lower fertility rates and a shift toward late motherhood in some countries have resulted in high demand for technical solutions to fertility issues, such as IVF and surrogacy. Pressure to meet societal expectations may constrain individual choice regarding the use of reproductive technologies and questions about commercialization and equity of access are raised. Particular concerns are voiced about the potential for 'designer babies'. The creation of 'saviour siblings', embryos selected as genetically-identical matches (and potential tissue donors) for seriously ill children, has been extensively contested. Likewise, positive selection for deafness, supported by some sections of the deaf community, raises concerns regarding rights of the unborn child and highlights societal understandings of illness and disability (Scully, 2008). In 2021 a large-scale study of autism, Spectrum 10K, was put on hold mid-data collection. Patients, families and publics raised concerns including the process of consent, use of the data and eugenic implications of seeking a genetic solution, and despite updated statements from the project team, the study would not have any impact on the material experience of those living with autism (Mette, 2021). As this recent example highlights, despite rapid expansion and the availability of funding, little global consensus exists regarding the use and regulation of genetic and genomic technologies.

Geneticization prompts a re-framing of historically and culturally dominant understandings of individual health and collective responsibility. Practices such as newborn screening, carrier testing and personal genomic testing have extended the patient population to include patients 'without symptoms'; that is, carriers of a genetic disorder and those 'at risk' of developing late onset genetic conditions. Diagnosis of a potentially serious and life-threatening condition (often made in the absence of physical symptoms), or being 'at risk', has implications for self-identity and stigma, disclosure practices, insurance and access to employment. The 'genetically responsible patient' is expected to assimilate new knowledge to make informed and responsible decisions that benefit others. Sociological enquiries focus on negotiation of guilt and blame, understandings of genetic risk and familial communication strategies within 'webs of genetic connectedness' (Novas and Rose, 2000). Routine disclosure of individual genetic profiles to 'at-risk' family members has been fiercely contested, raising questions of ownership, confidentiality, the right to know and not to know. 'Genetic citizenship' encapsulates a movement from patient to active citizen, whereby individuals express 'biosociality' by influencing the direction of scientific work, and becoming contributors to and partners in the production of biomedical knowledge.

Technologies, which have brought genetic thinking to the fore, include mitochondrial donation and gene editing. In 2015, the UK became the first country to legalize mitochondrial donation (MD), an assisted reproductive technology for women with maternally-inherited mitochondrial disease. MD was widely celebrated as the only option that would enable at-risk women to have healthy, *genetically related* children; but it raised critical questions about the meaning of genetic material and whether a mitochondrial donor should be considered a parent (Dimond and Stephens, 2018). Concerns have been expressed regarding the possibility that individuals, groups and society as a whole may be adversely affected by (mis)use of gene-editing tools. The rapid development, low cost and ease of access of Crispr/Cas-9 – a new gene-editing technology with widespread applications in human health, animal husbandry, environment and warfare – have brought significant, global regulatory challenges (see Suggested Further Reading on Nuffield Council on Bioethics).

A narrow focus on the power and significance of genetic knowledge ignores the complex realities of diagnostic negotiations, diverse patient experiences and possibilities for resistance. The influence of genetic technology on medicine has been characterized as a shift away from the 'clinical gaze', towards the 'molecular gaze', relocating the diagnostic process to the genetic laboratory rather than the clinic. Detailed empirical studies have, however, identified the clinic's continued significance (Latimer et al., 2006). Likewise, whilst it might appear that genetic screening programmes attract public support, uptake can be low. For instance, although tests for the Huntington's disease gene have been available since 1993, less than 20 per cent of the 'at risk' population choose testing. The genetic nature of disease is challenging at certain times, for example when planning to have children, or communicating genetic risk information to family members; yet it does not always dominate identity, experience and activity. Indeed, individuals may identify more strongly with aspects other than their genetic status, which was one of the arguments against the previously mentioned Spectrum 10K study. Similarly, the way a disease is defined and managed as 'genetic' (or not) depends on the demands of science and society. Huntington's disease is, for example, a prominent focus of neuroscience research. The movement of diseases between categories is described as 'lumping and splitting' (Hedgecoe, 2004). This process allows promissory aspects of medical science to be maintained via identification of alternative treatment routes rather than genetic redesign.

The 'new genetics' also raises fears concerning recurrence of eugenic policies, which began in the late-19th century and remained popular across

Europe and the USA until the 1940s. The disability movement, among others, highlights how the prevention of difference through genetic manipulation holds significant potential to devalue disabled people's lives. Although many issues arising from 'geneticization' and the 'new genetics' are indeed not new, contemporary events such as the COVID-19 pandemic highlight their continued relevance. For example, studies (such as Genetics of Susceptibility and Mortality in Critical Care) hope to identify the specific genes that cause some people and populations to be susceptible to the virus, with the potential to lead to further 'lumping and splitting' and simplification of causal attribution. The search for genetic explanations and solutions for ethnic disparities experienced during the pandemic will no doubt inform future sociological research. Yet, researchers should exercise caution and critical reflexivity. Many claim Lippman's (1991) initial concept was both overly simplistic and ambitious, ignoring the complex forms of knowledge with which it competes and placing too great an emphasis on the transformative power of genetics (Weiner et al., 2017). It has been argued that the allure of geneticization relates to a particular (and outdated) Western intellectual and political context, where concerns about rapidly-developing technologies and the power of biomedicine have been over-emphasized (Arribas-Ayllon, 2016). Further sociological research is therefore needed in order to understand how or whether the concept of geneticization remains a useful tool to understand broader changes within society. Rethinking 'geneticization' involves recognizing the historical, cultural and social contexts that give meaning to genetic material and genetic knowledge, including greater acknowledgment of the significance of social and political movements, such as Black Lives Matter, and macro-socioeconomic inequalities, particularly between the Global South and Global North.

See also: Disability; Medical Technologies; Medicalization; Reproduction; Stigma.

REFERENCES

Arribas-Ayllon, M. (2016) 'After geneticization', *Social Science & Medicine*, 159: 132–139.

Courbier, S., Dimond, R. and Bros-Facer, V. (2019) 'Share and protect our health data: an evidence-based approach to rare disease patients' perspectives on data sharing and data protection – quantitative survey and recommendations', *Orphanet Journal of Rare Diseases*, 14 (1): 175.

Dimond, R. and Stephens, N. (2018) *Legalising Mitochondrial Donation: Enacting Ethical Futures in UK Biomedical Politics*. London: Palgrave.

Feld, A. and Kreimer, P. (2019) 'Scientific co-operation and centre–periphery relations: attitudes and interests of European and Latin American scientists', *Tapuya: Latin American Science, Technology and Society*, 2 (1): 149–175.

Gibbon, S., Kilshaw, S. and Sleeboom-Faulkner, M. (2018) 'Genomics and genetic medicine: pathways to global health?' *Anthropology & Medicine*, 25 (1): 1–10.

Key Concepts in Medical Sociology

Hedgecoe, A. (2004) 'Lumping and splitting revisited: or what happens when the new genetics meets disease classification', in P. Glasner (ed.), *Reconfiguring Nature: Issues and Debates in the New Genetics*. Aldershot: Ashgate Publishing Limited.

Latimer, J., Featherstone, K., Atkinson, P. et al. (2006) 'Rebirthing the clinic: the interaction of clinical judgement and molecular technology in the production of genetic science', *Science, Technology & Human Values*, 31 (5): 599–630.

Lippman, A. (1991) 'Prenatal genetic testing and screening: constructing needs and reinforcing inequities', *American Journal of Law & Medicine*, 17 (1–2): 15–50.

Mette (2021) 'Spectrum 10k study: an #ActuallyAutistic response', *Learning Disability Today,* 1 September. Online: www.learningdisabilitytoday.co.uk/spectrum-10k-study-an-actually-autistic-response

Novas, C. and Rose, N. (2000) 'Genetic risk and the birth of the somatic individual', *Economy and Society*, 29 (4): 485–513.

Reidpath, D.D. and Allotey, P. (2019) 'The problem of "trickle-down science" from the Global North to the Global South', *BMJ Global Health*, 4 (4): p.e001719.

Scully, L.J. (2008) 'Disability and genetics in the era of genomic medicine', *Nature Reviews Genetics*, 9 (10): 797–802.

Sharma, M. (2008) 'Twenty-first century pink or blue: how sex selection technology facilitates gendercide and what we can do about it', *Family Court Review*, 46 (1): 198–215.

Strange, H. (2018) 'The fetus as a patient: professional and patient discourse', in D. Schmitz, A. Clarke and W. Dondorp (eds), *The Fetus as a Patient: A Contested Concept and Its Normative Implications*. London: Routledge.

Weiner, K., Martin, P., Richards, M. and Tutton, R. (2017) 'Have we seen the geneticisation of society? Expectations and evidence', *Sociology of Health & Illness*, 39 (7): 989–1004.

SUGGESTED FURTHER READING

- Nuffield Council on Bioethics (2018) *Genome Editing and Human Reproduction*. London: Nuffield Council on Bioethics. Online: www.nuffieldbioethics.org/publications/genome-editing-and-human-reproduction

The Nuffield Council on Bioethics is an influential UK-based charitable organization, which explores the social and ethical implications of new and sometimes controversial developments in medical research. As a follow up to the Council's 2016 review on genome editing in human health, farming and the environment, the 2018 report identified ethical issues raised by genome editing as a reproductive technology. It concluded that genome editing would be ethical as long as it was safe, did not increase divisions or discrimination in society, there was broad public consensus about its use and it was strictly regulated.

- www.bionews.org.uk/

Bionews is a free resource, publishing short and accessible commentaries on genetics and related topics. Bionews is published by Progress Educational Trust (PET), a charity that aims to support public and professional understanding and encourage debate.

- Wahlberg, A. and Gammeltoft, T. (eds) (2018) *Selective Reproduction in the 21st Century*. London: Palgrave Macmillan.

This book explores how global human reproduction is changed by the impact of Selective Reproductive Technologies (SRTs), providing unique ethnographic insights on how SRTs are made available, used and perceived within different cultural, socio-economic and regulatory settings. Topics include sex-selective abortions, termination of pregnancy following prenatal screening, preimplantation genetic diagnosis and the genetic screening of egg and sperm donors.

38

Bioethics

Gabrielle Samuel and Bobbie Farsides

'Bioethics is the philosophical study of the ethical controversies brought about by advances in biology and medicine. The modern field of bioethics emerged when medical/scientific/technical advances in morally contested areas, including organ transplantation and end-of-life care, began posing new and novel questions' (Williams and Wainwright, 2013: 140). The field has expanded to include topics such as digital health, global health and the environment.

Bioethics came to prominence in the mid-1980s, originally emerging as a branch of academic moral philosophy and applied ethics. Since its inception, however, bioethics has moved from the philosophy department into medical and law schools, specialist research institutes, regulatory bodies and the front-line of the healthcare sector. It has also moved from the confines of a narrow Anglo-American model of moral philosophy, focusing on individual notions of autonomy and respect, to consider wider global issues. Bioethicists now work with partners in medical sociology to address profoundly ethical issues about our society, the environment and the world we will bequeath to future generations. Medical sociologists have proven adept at unpacking the social complexities and meanings associated with what can, in the hands of some philosophical bioethicists, seem like a set of unproblematic ideas. Sociological work associated with bioethics has been conveniently divided into two main areas: sociology *of* bioethics, and sociology *in* bioethics. While this division is blurry, with much sociological work contributing to both categories, or sitting at the boundary between the two, the division offers a useful heuristic and we will largely draw on this below. We address each in turn, particularly focusing on the latter, and using digital health as a case example.

Sociology *of* bioethics takes bioethics as a valid subject for research and theorization, and charts the social forces that have helped shape particular (dominant) varieties of philosophical bioethics (for example, principlism, utilitarianism, etc.). It examines the ways in which certain kinds of ethical questions are privileged, promoted and funded within bioethics whilst other questions and approaches tend to be marginalized (Williams and Wainwright, 2013). From this perspective, the professional field of bioethics can be seen as constraining the types of questions that can legitimately be asked and researched (Hedgecoe, 2010). In fact, by exploring how ethical issues are framed in public domains and health-related institutions, such as biobanks, sociologists have stressed the need to pose critical questions – or even meta-questions. As indicated by Petersen (2005: 305), the latter might include questioning 'the socio-political implications of applying the predominant "principle"-based approach to normative questions'. By doing so, sociologists have criticized early and still influential approaches to bioethics for being too narrow culturally, with practitioners adopting moral norms that are embedded within very specific socio-cultural models which need to be recognized, articulated and, where necessary, challenged (Petersen, 2005). Sociologists have shown how philosophical debates on informed consent, for example, can be inadequate when they run up against the complexities of real social worlds (Corrigan, 2003). In so doing, sociologists attempt to shift ethics debates away from those that are otherwise narrowly focused on formalized concerns (such as autonomy and privacy), and singular discourses which de-emphasize controversies (Poort et al., 2013).

Sociology *in* bioethics, also described as 'empirical bioethics' by philosophers, elucidates the social processes that frame ethical issues, analysing the ways in which ethical problems are identified, managed and resolved. By doing so, it aims to ground more abstract philosophical ethical debates in empirical case studies, exploring the embodied ethics of 'real actors' in particular social worlds (Williams and Wainwright, 2013). Sociological research, and the case studies it draws upon, are viewed as crucial components of any bioethics scholarship. For example, sociological research on the experience of people living with illness or disability has helped bioethicists understand how these issues, and others, such as those pertaining to parenting and identity, frame the ethical nature of an individual health encounter. One can point here to Boardman's (2020) empirical work exploring those who currently live with genetic conditions and Shakespeare (2017) on the social model of disability. In short, sociologists have expanded the methodologies and approaches used in bioethics. They have done so by framing the scope of inquiry beyond the clinic, practitioners and biomedical research, to encompass broader issues relating to healthcare systems, digital health, global health, public health, research ethics and the environment.

For some philosopher bioethicists (McMillan, 2016), it is important to ensure that medical sociology research explicitly embraces a normative dimension, such that it not only describes the complexities of ethical issues but also offers guidance on what ought to be done given this analysis. At the same time, it is increasingly felt that bioethicists must be able to defend themselves against any claim that philosophical analysis is of little value in helping 'real people in real settings' make ethical judgements due to a disconnect with the understanding provided by social science. It is clearly important to understand if and how the complexities of the social world undermine the premises and assumptions of philosophical arguments. For this reason, a mutual understanding and respect across disciplinary boundaries is needed, and bioethicists and sociologists must avoid the danger of talking at each other rather than with one another. Fortunately, as interdisciplinarity has become a valued hallmark for contemporary academic research, bioethicists and sociologists are beginning to foster more productive relationships. Furthermore, these relationships have extended to include scholars working in the fields of anthropology, science and technology studies (STS), gender studies, media studies, law and more recently economics. For example, sociologists have explored how bio-samples produce bio-value through economic markets because of the implicit assumption that research conducted on them will eventually lead to health (and economic) benefit (the 'bioeconomy'). In doing so, they have exposed how this process often obscures other values, such as experiential health benefit (what is the actual health benefit from this research?), as well as ethical and social value (Datta Burton et al., 2021). In another example, medical sociologists have worked with media studies scholars to contribute to bioethics by describing how different media (and, in particular, media discourses) shape people's understandings and beliefs about specific ethical issues (Williams et al., 2003).

The level of innovation and the challenges posed by new ways of working within the health and biomedical science sectors mean that medical sociologists working *in* bioethics will never be short of new issues to consider. Rapid technological development and the accompanying ambitions to pool and utilize health data for 'societal benefit', whilst also personalizing the delivery of healthcare, is a case in point. This process has shifted the bioethical gaze towards questions related to the collection and analysis of large and potentially sensitive data sets. The growing area of work associated with the impact of the digital turn (or 'big data' revolution) in healthcare, health research and health behaviours therefore offers a useful case example of the different ways medical sociologists understand how new innovations construct, shape and/or frame health values (Lupton, 2020).

Within 'digital health ethics', sociologically informed work questions the appropriateness of old ethical tools and concepts, such as consent and privacy, mentioned above, asking whether, and if so how, they need to be reimagined. Together, bioethicists and sociologists work to understand how online activities, social media, apps, etc., frame health knowledge and beliefs. Close attention has been paid to the burgeoning of digital health research methods (social media analysis, artificial intelligence) and how (or whether) these raise novel ethical issues that need to be negotiated (Vayena et al., 2012). Scholars have also paid close attention to the ethical issues raised by the use of digital technologies in both public health and clinical practice (for example, genomics, digital phenotyping, e-health). Further questions have also been asked with regard to the storage of health data, which nowadays includes written clinical data, bodily samples and genetic test results. These questions have led to a growing area of bioethical research that has focused on defining and refining the ethical principles guiding the establishment and ongoing governance of health data repositories and biobanks. Here there have been calls for appropriate ethical governance frameworks that go beyond a prescriptive list of 'dos and don'ts' to incorporate values of solidarity, trustworthiness, openness, transparency and accountability (Prainsack and Buyx, 2013).

The significant financial and reputational investment in the digital landscape of health and medicine has coincided with economic pressure on many long-standing elements of healthcare budgets. In studying the implications of this, bioethicists and medical sociologists in the UK have together highlighted issues relating to health inequalities, digital poverty and discrimination. They have also made clear the risks of these problems being perpetuated or exacerbated by any move that threatens the egalitarian foundations of the National Health Service. At the same time, the increasingly digital landscape has brought to the fore a growing appreciation of the importance of engaging with public health ethics, particularly those drawing on big data and technologies. Here, sociologists, together with bioethicists, have challenged those working in public health when they seek to compel citizens to undertake or refrain from practices for 'the general' or 'common good' – nationally and/or globally (Dawson, 2015).

Old issues do not disappear. Around the world reproductive rights remain under threat despite welcome and sometimes successful challenges to authority in which those working in bioethics have played their part. The debate around assisted dying has translated into democratically endorsed policies in some countries and bitter divides in others. People in too many places are too easily denied basic healthcare for a host of reasons, and clinicians and policy-makers turn to those working in the arena of bioethics – including sociologists – to ask how they should deal with this challenge. In global terms, bioethicists increasingly understand and acknowledge how concepts like justice, fairness, discrimination and solidarity bolster or threaten the geo-political environments in which they seek to establish and pursue their bioethical goals and projects. This understanding, in turn, informs their normative claims about what needs to be done to make the world a better place.

Currently, bioethics focuses on a wide range of subjects, in different geographical areas and under various political regimes across the world. Bioethics is also diversifying, casting its gaze more widely into areas previously considered under the remit of medical sociology. For example, bioethicists consider how social, political and economic factors come to construct values in health, healthcare and health systems. As such, there are growing opportunities for working together, paralleling recent proposals for a sociology *with* and not simply *of* or *in* public health (Mykhalovskiy et al., 2019). Space has also been created by organizations such as the UK-based Nuffield Council on Bioethics within which sociologists can work with bioethicists, as well as those from other disciplines such as law and anthropology. Here they can bring sociological concepts and ideas to ethical debate as they anticipate, and where possible address, ethical issues related to their area of inquiry. It seems clear that, at the time of writing, myriad issues demand the attention of medical sociologists working on bioethical matters. Pressing areas of concern include the COVID-19 pandemic and associated responses (such as mitigation policies), a late awakening to the urgency of acknowledging that Black Lives Matter, and a fracturing and polarization of views and practices around sex and gender.

In sum, since its origins, bioethics has expanded far beyond the original confines of a narrow Anglo-American model of moral philosophy. In working with others to acknowledge and understand the realities of health practices and inequalities based on intersecting factors such as disability, ethnicity, class and gender, bioethicists have been able to engage in a much more diverse and illuminating discourse around issues of justice, fairness and non-discrimination. But bioethics could and should move further, and it is difficult to argue that there is not an ethical imperative to do so. With greater visibility and influence comes greater responsibility to contribute to global issues, highlight and address injustice and participate in the pursuit of ethical progress. Medical sociologists working *in* bioethics can help with this by focusing case studies on analyses of these wider global issues and, in doing so, drawing attention to them. Meanwhile, the sociology *of* bioethics can help by continuing to shine a light on how certain ethics discussions become prioritized at the expense of others. Understanding what is missing from bioethical inquiry allows these underrepresented areas to be opened up for future inquiry and, indeed, points towards the possibility of a sociology *with* bioethics.

See also: Digital Health; Geneticization; Medicalization

REFERENCES

Boardman, F. (2020) 'Whose life is worth preserving? Disabled people and the expressivist objection to neonatology', *Acta Paediatrica*, 110 (2): 391–393.

Corrigan, O. (2003) 'Empty ethics: the problem with informed consent', *Sociology of Health & Illness*, 25 (7): 768–792.

Datta Burton, S., Kieslich, K., Paul, K.T. et al. (2021) 'Rethinking value construction in biomedicine and healthcare', *BioSocieties*. https://doi.org/10.1057/s41292-020-00220-6

Dawson, A.J. (2015) 'Ebola: what it tells us about medical ethics', *Journal of Medical Ethics*, 41 (1): 107–110.

Hedgecoe, A. (2010) 'Bioethics and the reinforcement of socio-technical expectations', *Social Studies of Science*, 40 (2): 163–186.

Lupton, D. (2020) 'A more-than-human approach to bioethics: the example of digital health', *Bioethics*, 34 (9): 969–976.

McMillan, J. (2016) 'Empirical bioethics and the fact/value distinction', in J. Ives, M. Dunn and A. Cribb (eds), *Empirical Bioethics: Theoretical and Practical Perspectives*. Cambridge: Cambridge University Press.

Mykhalovskiy, E., Frohlich, K.L, Poland, B. et al. (2019) 'Critical social science with public health: agonism, critique and engagement', *Critical Public Health*, 29 (5): 522–533.

Petersen, A. (2005) 'Biobanks: challenges for "ethics"', *Critical Public Health*, 15 (4): 303–310.

Poort, L., Holmberg, T. and Ideland, M. (2013) 'Bringing in the controversy: re-politicizing the de-politicized strategy of ethics committees', *Life Sciences, Society and Policy*, 9 (11). https://doi.org/10.1186/2195-7819-9-11

Prainsack, B. and Buyx, A. (2013) 'A solidarity-based approach to the governance of research biobanks', *Medical Law Review*, 21 (1): 71–91.

Shakespeare, T. (2017) 'The social model of disability', in L.J. Davis (ed.), *The Disability Studies Reader*, 5th edn. New York: Routledge.

Vayena, E., Mastroianni, A. and Kahn, J. (2012) 'Ethical issues in health research with novel online sources', *American Journal of Public Health*, 102 (12): 2225–2230.

Williams, C., Kitzinger, J. and Henderson, L. (2003) 'Envisaging the embryo in stem cell research: rhetorical strategies and media reporting of the ethical debates', *Sociology of Health & Illness*, 25 (7): 793–814.

Williams, C. and Wainwright, S. (2013) 'Bioethics', in J. Gabe and L.F. Monaghan (eds), *Key Concepts in Medical Sociology*, 2nd edn. London: SAGE.

SUGGESTED FURTHER READING

- Brisbois, B. and Plamondon, K. (2018) 'The possible worlds of global health research: an ethics-focused discourse analysis', *Social Science & Medicine*, 196: 142–149.

This article offers a very nice example of the sociology *of* bioethics in practice. The authors explore how global health narratives framed in ethics documents imply a 'discourse of development' that assumes technological innovation is the most appropriate approach to addressing the needs of the Global South. Such a discourse, argue the authors, hides messy legacies of colonialism and low-technological solutions.

- Cribb, A. (2020) 'Managing ethical uncertainty: implicit normativity and the sociology of ethics', *Sociology of Health & Illness*, 42 (S1): 21–34.

An exceptional example of sociology *of* ethics research, which undoubtedly sits right at the intersection of medical sociology and philosophy. This author has written numerous other articles in this area that are also worth exploring.

- Prainsack, B. and Buyx, A. (2011) *Solidarity: Reflections on an Emerging Concept in Bioethics*. Nuffield Council on Bioethics. Online: www.nuffieldbioethics.org/publications/solidarity

This report provides an example of sociology *in* bioethics. It explores the various historical iterations of 'solidarity', with the authors providing their own definition of the term and a description of how it can be usefully applied to the bioethical literature.

- Kerr, A., Chekar, C.K., Ross, E. et al. (2021) *Personalised Cancer Medicine: Future Crafting in the Genomic Era*. Manchester: Manchester University Press.

A great example of a sociological research project which seeks to shed light on many issues relevant to bioethicists working in the area of genomics, personalized medicine and patient experience.

39

Surveillance and Health Promotion

Sarah Nettleton

Within the context of health promotion, medical sociologists use the term 'surveillance' to refer to activities such as surveys, screening and public health campaigns, which are designed to monitor, regulate and induce good health practices in both individuals and the population in general.

Health promotion refers to those planned activities that are designed to prevent illness and improve the health of the population. Such activities comprise: assessing health needs; developing and evaluating interventions which aim to facilitate the improvement of people's health status; and supporting health professionals and the public by providing information on putatively the most effective means to achieve good health. The goal of health promotion is to effect change at both an individual level (by encouraging people to lead 'healthy' lives) and a societal level (by bringing about institutional changes which will facilitate healthier social and physical environments). An upstream/downstream metaphor is deployed to highlight the relative merits of *structural and individual level interventions*. The former address housing, employment, poverty, social exclusion and discrimination whereas the latter entail providing individuals with information and advice about health (Ingleby, 2019). Health promotion is aligned to a branch of medicine called 'public health', which deploys the disciplines of social science, biology, epidemiology, immunology and environmental science to deal with complex health matters such as, *inter alia*, improving access to services, handling environmental hazards and reducing the prevalence of threats to health. Such threats might include substance misuse, unhealthy eating, poverty, accidents and injury and emergent and infectious diseases such as, SARS and COVID-19.

This concept of surveillance in medical sociology is informed by Foucault (1979), in particular his notion of 'disciplinary power'. Disciplinary power refers to the way in which bodies are regulated, trained, understood and empowered and is most evident in social institutions such as schools, prisons and hospitals, though it also permeates throughout society. It is within social institutions that knowledge of bodies is produced. For example, the observation of bodies in prisons yielded criminology, the clinical 'gaze' upon bodies in hospitals contributed to medical science and the observation of people in social settings forms the basis of sociology. Foucault (1979) refers to this as power/knowledge. Foucault maintains disciplinary power works at two levels: individual bodies are trained and observed through an anatomo-politics of the human body; and concurrently, populations are monitored through the collection of data through a 'bio-politics' of the population. The examination of individuals and populations in tandem gives rise to epidemiological norms; a correlative is that those who deviate are deemed to need treatment, rehabilitation or correction. This can lead to a moral adjudication or 'victim blaming' (Crawford, 1977) of those who do not lead what are purportedly 'healthy' lives.

Health promotion and public health form the policy manifestations of what is conceptualized as 'surveillance medicine'. A 'cardinal feature of surveillance medicine', writes Armstrong (1995), 'is its targeting of everyone' (p. 395); health care is concerned not just with those who are ill but with those who are well. It is not just orientated towards treating the symptoms of disease but the identification and monitoring of a burgeoning or epidemic of risk factors, which serve as markers of potential disease. Skolbekken (1995: 296) argues that, 'through the ideological frame of health promotion we get a glimpse of some of the functions served by the risk epidemic'. French and Smith (2013) suggest that, analytically, health surveillance is bound up with wider social processes such as: 'subjectivity formation', 'actuarialism' and 'social control'. In other words, health promotion and surveillance 'function' to generate risky identities, calculate probabilistic risks and regulate populations. Writing on the COVID-19 pandemic, French and Monahan (2020) outline 'evidence of surveillance dynamics at play with how bodies and pathogens are being measured, tracked, predicted, and regulated' (p. 1).

Sociologists have pointed to the fact that late modern society is characterized by a 'politics of anxiety', indeed, that it is a 'risk society' (Beck, 1992). Risks associated with modern-day living are person-made. While in the 19th century health risks were associated with the 'natural' environment and dangers lurked within water, soil, air, food and climate, today the environmental factors that impinge on health – such as global warming, flooding and pollution – are the (unintended) consequence of human actions. Of course, not all contemporary health risks are 'purely' human products. AIDS, for example, is caused by a virus (HIV) and the 2020 global COVID-19 pandemic is caused by a variant of the coronavirus. Nevertheless, HIV and the coronavirus necessitate conceptualization within social matrices and are envisaged in terms of complex social interactions in concert with the global and local interdependencies of populations. Their spread and impact are socially patterned and subjected to differential forms of monitoring and regulation. For instance, amongst relatively wealthy regions where people living with HIV are able to access treatment, their viral load is then monitored as one of many 'risk factors' used to subject individuals to enhanced biological surveillance (Guta et al., 2016).

Research techniques deployed in the scrutinization of 'risk factors' within the context of public health and health promotion are primarily: screening for signs and symptoms and collecting information on patients through epidemiological research, social surveys and qualitative studies. Once a 'risk factor' such as eating 'fatty foods' is found to be statistically associated with an indicator of ill-health, such as cholesterol level, it is deemed to be a further 'risk factor'. The social aspects of eating fatty foods may then be explored by sociologists who aim to answer questions such as: Why do people eat fat? What meanings are associated with eating fatty foods? What is the symbolic significance of this, perhaps shared, practice? The findings are considered to be crucial to the development of socially sensitive health promotion interventions. However, despite research evidence that it is the socio-economic affordances and cultural contexts of eating that are critical to effective health promotion, the dominant 'policy scripts' are those of individual interventions which seek to encourage people to eat fewer fatty foods rather than address the upstream issues (Ingleby, 2019). Governments keep an eye on the population's fat consumption and set nutritional targets.

In the 21st century, technologies to identify genetic influences and other biomarkers associated with biological bodies add a further twist to individual risk identities and give rise to what Rose (2009) terms 'biological citizenship'. For example, in a bid to regulate and reduce risk, individuals who are identified as 'carriers' of genetic conditions may be encouraged to opt for testing so as to limit inherited diseases. Individuals who are at risk are informed that such testing is their 'choice'. However, this can raise the spectre of discrimination in the absence of nuanced understandings of how people navigate and reflect upon risks (see Berghs et al., 2017). In relation to genetic testing for the vast majority of diseases, diagnostically clear-cut genetic information is very rare. As Rose (2009: 74) puts it, 'there is no normal genome; variation is the norm'.

The digitalization, commercialization and marketization of genetic testing has far-reaching consequences. Commercial agencies harvest tissue from individuals who submit their biological data and, in return, companies provide them with a genetic analysis of their increased risk of developing particular morbidities. This harvesting of data, combined with smart technologies – where individuals can monitor their heart rate, step count, sleep patterns, and so on – render populations subject to increasingly profound modes of (self-)surveillance.

Such comprehensive data monitoring and tracking has, in turn, been conceptualized in interesting ways. For Prainsack (2017), the 'tablet computer', which is continuously on standby even when not being used, is 'a powerful metaphor for how people increasingly operate in the domains of health and medicine' (p. 48). The 'digital patient', Prainsack adds, is 'always on' within the 'assemblage' of 'contemporary digital health surveillance' (p. 51), with the concept of assemblage pointing to a complex and contradictory configuration of practices, motives and experiences that might include but are also irreducible to oppression.

Of course, none of the above rules out oppressive effects. Profiling populations leads to the classification of groups who are deemed to be at higher or lower risk of contracting diseases. Such practices can give rise to a vilification of groups who are judged as irresponsible and burdensome, such as 'the lazy', 'the overweight', 'the poor' or 'migrants' (Ingleby, 2019; Monaghan et al., 2019; Tyler, 2015). In short, surveillance can lead to the valorization and demonization of groups, with health promotion strategies 'targeting' the latter to induce them to change their ways of living. Mason's (2016) study of the transformation of public health in China following the severe acute respiratory syndrome (SARS) epidemic in 2003 found how those groups who migrated back and forth between rural and urban regions became known as the 'floating population' and were portrayed as a 'backward migrant population to be governed' (p. 41). By contrast 'immigrant populations' were imagined as those who had secure employment and lived settled lives in urban areas and who were considered to be worthy of healthcare services. Mason calls this the 'bifurcation of service and governance' (p. 4).

The concept of surveillance and the related notion of risk provide valuable analytic tools with which to make sense of developments within health promotion in particular (French and Smith, 2013; Petersen and Lupton, 1996). The concepts of surveillance and risk are useful in contributing to an appreciation of the ways in which collective, societal levels of intervention (for example, screening or education campaigns) can have an impact upon individuals in terms of the development of their 'risk identities'. These notions, when applied to the analysis of public health campaigns, can also help us to recognize how values are perpetuated when we categorize objects, people and places as more-or-less risky (Brown, 2020). Through the lens of surveillance, we can also decipher how values are embedded and inequalities are reproduced during interactions with health professionals – see for example how, in Brazil, community healthcare workers who deploy biomedical assumptions during one-to-one interactions to change behaviours can reproduce inequalities (Nunes and Lotta, 2019). Finally, the concept of surveillance can enable health practitioners and health researchers to gain an analytic appreciation of some of the societal implications of the routine day-to-day practices of health promotion.

See also: Digital Health; Geneticization; Medicalization; Risk.

REFERENCES

Armstrong, D. (1995) 'The rise of surveillance medicine', *Sociology of Health & Illness*, 17 (3): 343–404.

Beck, U. (1992) *Risk Society: Towards a New Modernity*. London: SAGE.

Berghs, M., Dyson, S.M. and Atkin, K. (2017) 'Resignifying the sickle cell gene: narratives of genetic risk, impairment and repair', *Health*, 21 (2): 171–188.

Brown, P. (2020) 'Studying COVID-19 in light of critical approaches to risk and uncertainty: research pathways, conceptual tools, and some magic from Mary Douglas', *Health, Risk & Society*, 22 (1): 1–14.

Crawford, R. (1977) 'You are dangerous to your health: the ideology and politics of victim blaming', *International Journal of Health Services*, 7 (4): 663–680.

Foucault, M. (1979) *Discipline and Punish: The Birth of the Prison*. Harmondsworth: Penguin Books.

French, M. and Monahan, T. (2020) 'Dis-ease surveillance: how might surveillance studies address COVID-19?' *Surveillance & Society*, 18 (1): 1–11.

French, M. and Smith, G. (2013) '"Health" surveillance: new modes of monitoring bodies, populations, and polities', *Critical Public Health*, 23 (4): 383–392.

Guta, A., Murray, S.J. and Gagnon, M. (2016) 'HIV, viral suppression and new technologies of surveillance and control', *Body & Society*, 22 (2): 82–107.

Ingleby, D. (2019) 'Moving upstream: changing policy scripts on migrant and ethnic minority health', *Health Policy*, 123 (9): 809–817.

Mason, K. (2016) *Infectious Change: Reinventing Chinese Public Health after an Epidemic*. Stanford: Stanford University Press.

Monaghan, L.F., Rich, E. and Bombak, A.E. (2019) 'Media, "fat panic" and public pedagogy: mapping contested terrain', *Sociology Compass*, 13 (1): e12651.

Nunes, J. and Lotta, G. (2019) 'Discretion, power and the reproduction of inequality in health policy implementation: practices, discursive styles and classifications of Brazil's community health workers', *Social Science & Medicine*, 242: 112551.

Petersen, A. and Lupton, D (1996) *The New Public Health: Health and Self in the Age of Risk*. London: SAGE.

Prainsack, B. (2017) *Personalised Medicine: Empowered Patients in the 21st Century?* New York: New York University Press.

Rose, N. (2009) 'Normality and pathology in a biomedical age', *Sociological Review*, 57 (s2): 66–83.

Skolbekken, J. (1995) 'The risk epidemic in medical journals', *Social Science & Medicine*, 40 (3): 291–305.

Tyler, I. (2015) 'Classificatory struggles: class, culture and inequality in neoliberal times', *The Sociological Review*, 63 (2): 493–511.

SUGGESTED FURTHER READING

- Green, J. (2018) 'Public health and health promotion', in G. Scambler (ed.), *Sociology as Applied to Health and Medicine*, 7th edn. Basingstoke: Macmillian.

This introductory yet comprehensive chapter is a great way to orientate yourself to the emergence of contemporary health promotion. It maps the theoretical terrain and gives a clear account of the central concepts.

- Jones, L. (2018) 'Pastoral power and the promotion of self-care', *Sociology of Health & Illness,* 40 (6): 988–1004.

An example of the links between policy and day-to-day clinical practice, where surveillance medicine is played out in doctor–patient consultations.

- Reubi, D. (2018) 'A genealogy of epidemiological reason: saving lives, social surveys and global population', *BioSocieties*, 13 (1): 81–102.

A case study of a philanthropic project – the 'Bloomberg Initiative to Reduce Tobacco Use in Developing Countries' – analysed through the lens of epidemiological logic and surveillance medicine. A compelling and illuminating read.

PART 4

HEALTH WORK AND THE DIVISION OF LABOUR

40

Medical Autonomy, Dominance and Decline

Jonathan Gabe and Mary Ann Elston

Medical autonomy is the publicly accepted control that the medical profession exercises over the terms and conditions of its work. Medical dominance is a relative concept, indicating the authority that the medical profession can exercise over other occupations within the healthcare division of labour, patients or society, through its cultural authority in matters relating to health. Since the 1980s, many medical sociologists have suggested that these characteristic expressions of professional power have been reduced by external challenges.

The concepts of autonomy and dominance inform sociological discussions of professional power, especially in relation to the medical profession. Indeed, they have often been used as if they were interchangeable. Clearly, they are very closely related, logically and empirically. In a complex division of labour, only an occupation able to exercise dominance over others can have very high levels of publicly accepted or legitimated autonomy and vice versa. But keeping an analytic distinction between the two is useful when analysing professional power – a recurrent theme within medical sociology over the past 60 years. Although the theme has recurred, the emphasis has changed. From the 1960s to the 1980s, medical sociologists' primary interest was in the origins and persistence of medical autonomy and in its social consequences. By the 1990s, the questions medical sociologists asked were more concerned with the possible decline of medical autonomy and dominance and, to some extent, with the possible negative consequences of this.

The American sociologist Eliot Freidson made a major contribution to this debate. In a landmark book on the American medical profession published in 1970, he argued that only certain professions, like medicine, have been *'deliberately* granted autonomy, including the exclusive right to determine who can legitimately do its work and how the work should be done' (1970: 72, emphasis in the original). For Freidson, possession of a high level of state-sanctioned autonomy, and, by implication, institutionalized expectations of societal trust in the occupation's claims, are the defining characteristics of a true profession. This autonomy had been achieved, he argued, through an essentially political process of professionalization; through the profession having convinced, over time, the public, or at least socially powerful groups, that its services were of value and then obtained legal sanction for its autonomy. The latter was expressed in the establishment of statutorily defined, self-regulating professional licensing and disciplinary systems, such as the UK's General Medical Council, first established in 1858 as an entirely medical institution.

Sociologists have proposed various typologies of autonomy. However, three main categories are usually identified: (1) clinical or technical autonomy – the right of the medical profession to set standards and evaluate clinical performance; (2) political autonomy – the right to make policy decisions as the legitimate experts on health and medicine; and (3) economic autonomy – the right to determine levels of personal remuneration or the level of resources available for their work (Elston, 1991: 61). Historical and comparative analysis suggests that these different aspects of autonomy can, to some extent, vary independently of each other. For example, hospital doctors in the USA enjoyed a much higher level of economic autonomy compared to their UK counterparts during the latter part of the 20th century. While doctors in the USA could charge a fee for services, doctors working in the UK's National Health Service (NHS) hospitals were salaried. However, the experience of doctors working for the UK state did not reflect a marked diminution in other aspects of their autonomy. For example, they had more clinical autonomy to decide how resources were spent and allocated than their US counterparts because they were not constrained by patients' varying ability to pay directly. It is also important to recognize that not all segments of the medical profession within the same society are likely to enjoy equal levels of autonomy. There may be differences between specialisms and positions in occupational structures and these can be related to social group membership. When discussing whether medical autonomy is increasing or diminishing, these complexities need to be recognized.

Medical dominance is also a concept that has been applied in a variety of contexts and to refer to different aspects of medical power. Three aspects have been particularly important within medical sociology: (1) medical dominance within society generally, for example the profession's cultural authority to determine what is to be counted as sickness; (2) medical dominance over patients; and (3) medical dominance over other occupations in the increasingly complex division of healthcare labour and in the policy-making process. The first of these aspects can be subsumed, for present purposes, under the concept of medicalization and the second under 'the doctor–patient relationship'. It is the third aspect, medicine's state-sanctioned dominance over other health occupations, that is closely associated with claims about medical autonomy, particularly in Freidson's work. For Freidson (1970), a crucial part of the professionalization process for medicine (that is, its achievement of autonomy) was the gradual subordination of other occupations, such as nursing, to medical control. As a result, although nursing in the mid-20th century had considerable control over some aspects of its work, it was suggested that it still lacked full professional status because its work was subject to 'doctors' orders' – a state of affairs that was likely to continue as medicine would seek to defend its autonomy from nursing's encroachment.

Since the late 1980s a substantial literature has been published assessing the future of medical autonomy and, more generally, professional power and authority (Kelleher et al., 2006; Timmermans and Oh, 2010). As outlined below, contributors to this literature have employed a variety of concepts, drawn from different theoretical perspectives. Before these are discussed, some preliminary points need to be made to set the context in which these concepts have been put forward.

The first, self-evident point is that to speak of the decline of medical or professional autonomy implies that there is or was autonomy to lose. Some have argued that the extent of medical power and its imperialistic tendencies over society or other occupations may have been overstated in the 1970s. However, few would dispute that, compared with most other occupations, the social and cultural authority exercised by the medical profession has been considerable and remains so. Even those who would argue that major change is taking place see this as a process that is underway, not a completed transformation. Moreover, in most cases, those who argue for a decline in medical autonomy are linking this to transformations that affect society generally and hence most, or even all, occupations. In this way, medical autonomy could decline while the relative dominance and advantage of medicine over other occupations would remain unchanged. Furthermore, there is relatively little agreement among contributors to these debates about what would count as firm evidence for or against decline, or how much decline would mark a significant change.

So, this is currently a very lively but somewhat speculative area of debate. Sociologists agree that medicine in the early part of the 21st century has been challenged on a number of fronts. The debate is over which, if any, of these are significant and how they can be explained theoretically. The challenges discussed in the literature can be categorized as arising from three main sources. The first is the growing and changing form of involvement of third parties in the funding or organizing of healthcare. Thus, in the UK, the major reforms to the NHS that have been introduced since the 1980s, including a more market-driven ethos and structure (although note the proposed shift from competition to collaboration in 2021), have been seen by many as constituting an attack on producer dominance and professional exemption from external scrutiny. In the USA, the expansion of for-profit healthcare corporations, the move to managed care and associated new financial management of medical practice have been widely hailed as representing an encroachment on professional prerogative, by those organized interests who increasingly buy medical services on behalf of patients.

A second type of challenge comes directly from the users of healthcare, the public. On the one hand, there is the apparent rise of consumerism with individual users rejecting, or being encouraged to reject, passive trust in medical expertise and medical reputations: a rejection expressed in increased complaints and malpractice allegations and in a more active involvement in clinical decision-making, or in an increased resort to alternative medicines. There is also a more collective consumerist challenge in the form of critical self-help groups and social movements, such as the women's health movement or patient advocacy groups for targeted cancer therapies

The third form of challenge identified is that from other healthcare occupations. For example, there have been many recent developments in nursing practice, such as the move to develop nurses' clinical skills and expand their role into areas previously regarded as medical responsibilities. Similar developments have occurred in some of the other occupations characterized as 'professions allied to medicine', such as physiotherapy or pharmacy. These have been seen by some commentators as moves in a professionalizing strategy on the part of these occupations. That there are new areas of inter-professional boundary blurring in delivering care involving medicine and nursing, and other fields, is clear. However, it is probably most helpful to follow Witz and Annandale (2006) and see many of these changes as being themselves related to the first kind of challenge – that from third parties, such as the state in the UK.

Different concepts, drawing on various broad theoretical approaches, have been used to elaborate and explain these types of challenge. Here, there is space to outline only the concepts particularly associated with third party and user/public consumer challenges, and two critical alternative positions.

According to some early American contributors to the debate (notably McKinlay and Arches, 1985) the effect of third party commercial purchasers of medical services on doctors' ability to determine their terms and conditions of work was tantamount to the incipient proletarianization of the medical profession. Drawing explicitly on Marxist theories of the logic of capitalist development, it was argued that the reduction in professional prerogatives such as the right to set remuneration was evidence that medicine was being incorporated into the class of those who produced surplus value for capital. Initial formulations of this position were controversial, not least because American doctors did not greatly resemble typical 'wage-slaves' and because the underlying Marxist theory is itself highly contested. Subsequent formulations from a similar perspective have tended to use the concept of corporatization as less contentious and more indicative of the putative cause of the changes than proletarianization (McKinlay and Marceau, 2002). Neither of these concepts can be unproblematically applied in societies where healthcare is mainly state-funded or provided but, arguably, some of the same rationalizing principles that underpin corporate managed care are in evidence here. Thus, in the UK, the concepts through which the changing fortune of medical autonomy in relation to the state has been considered include managerialism and privatization.

For those sociologists who see the challenge to medical autonomy as mainly arising from the public, either as individual users of services or collective groups, what is identified is a process of cultural change for which the term 'deprofessionalization' has been coined. On the one hand, exponents of this position argue that there is a more informed, critical public, less inclined to be deferent to experts and to express unconditional trust, a process fostered by the extensive media coverage given to specific incidents of gross medical malpractice. On the other hand, through increasing computerization and bureaucratic regulation (for example, in the form of performance indicators), expert knowledge is itself regarded as becoming more accessible to outsiders, enabling trust in doctors to be more informed. It is claimed, therefore, that there is a reduction in the knowledge gap between profession and public and in the areas of indeterminacy that support the exercise of professional discretion.

Both the corporatization and deprofessionalization theses have attracted considerable criticism. For example, they have been seen as insufficiently historically grounded and as generalizing too much from specific, short-term American developments. Freidson (1994) argued that both sets of claims tend to underplay the significance of the organized character of the medical profession. He suggested that, rather than external control of medicine being of growing significance, it was the increasing internal re-stratification of the profession that sociologists should attend to. Through enhanced disciplinary procedures, promulgation of clinical guidelines and protocols and the emergence of new cadres of medical managers, a professional elite is, according to Freidson (1994, 2001), becoming increasingly dominant over rank and file medical practitioners. This in itself may weaken the coherence and hence the autonomy of the profession over time.

Empirical applications of re-stratification include Calnan and Gabe (2009) who analysed the developments in the NHS primary care sector in England and suggested that we need to distinguish two levels of re-stratification in an increasingly complex division of labour – horizontal and vertical. Horizontal stratification refers to the development of divisions between paternalist and egalitarian general practitioners (GPs) and between them and salaried GPs, while vertical stratification relates to those GPs with managerial responsibilities compared to the remainder who are not involved in such activities. More recently Waring et al. (2020) report on re-stratification at the inter-organizational level and intra-professional dynamics. Focusing on structural changes which have resulted in the redistribution of hospital trauma care in the English NHS, they distinguish between specialist doctors working in regional hospital centres of excellence and rank-and-file doctors working in less prestigious district hospitals who have restricted involvement in trauma care. At an inter-organizational level parallel professional hierarchies have developed to co-ordinate specialist practices within and between organizations. These hierarchies have taken the form of senior 'elites', from the regional hospitals, whose influence depends on the status and reputation of professional figureheads (rather than any formal authority) and subordinate, second tier, leaders whose roles have been created to allay the resistance of doctors working in district hospitals.

Another alternative to corporatization and deprofessionalization is offered by Light (2010). His starting point is the assumption that modern societies (or at least the USA) are more pluralist than is envisaged by the neo-Marxism of the corporatization thesis. He suggests that rather than presume medical dominance as the starting point for analysis, the medical profession should be seen as only one of several major *countervailing powers* in society with interests in healthcare, with the other powers including the state, the healthcare industry, patient advocacy groups and consumers. Light depicts a system in which these different interests compete for power, influence and resources and, if one becomes predominant, a counter-movement will develop over time. The concept of countervailing powers has recently been applied by Speed and Gabe (2020) to explain the 2012 healthcare reforms of the English NHS, highlighting the ways in which the state asserted itself in the face of the historical dominance of the medical profession. They reveal how the processes of alliances and vested interests played out, with the various factions of the medical profession failing to unify against the proposed reforms. The profession's position was further restricted by the state's appeal to patient-centred medicine, juxtaposing this to a purported professional self-interest and making any concerted professional/patient alliance difficult. The model has the merit of including more than buyers and sellers of medical services; and the rise and putative fall of medical autonomy can be set in the same explanatory framework. What is less clear is how adequately the theory explains which interests predominate at particular times.

There is general recognition among medical sociologists that the accounts of medical power and autonomy that seemed appropriate to the 1970s are no longer so clearly applicable 50 years later. There are undoubtedly new challenges to medicine's authority, some of which have been discussed here. There is less consensus, however, on what their significance is for the future of medical autonomy and dominance. Time will tell whether medicine will retain its power and authority, by developing a new form of professionalism, based on active trust and partnership with patients, or whether its power has been irretrievably weakened by the challenges it is now facing.

See also: Consumerism; Medicalization; Practitioner–Client Relationships; Professions Allied to Medicine; Trust in Medicine.

REFERENCES

Calnan, M. and Gabe, J. (2009) 'The re-stratification of primary care in England? A sociological analysis', in J. Gabe and M. Calnan (eds), *The New Sociology of the Health Service*. London: Routledge.

Elston, M.A. (1991) 'The politics of professional power', in J. Gabe, M. Calnan and M. Bury (eds), *The Sociology of the Health Service*. London: Routledge.

Freidson, E. (1970) *Profession of Medicine*. New York: Dodds Mead.

Freidson, E. (1994) *Professionalism Reborn: Theory, Prophecy and Policy*. Cambridge: Polity Press.

Freidson, E. (2001) *Professionalism: The Third Logic*. Cambridge: Polity Press.

Kelleher, D., Gabe, J. and Williams, G. (eds) (2006) *Challenging Medicine*, 2nd edn. London: Routledge.

Light, D.W. (2010) 'Healthcare professions, markets and countervailing powers', in C.E. Bird, P. Conrad, A.M. Fremont and S. Timmermans (eds), *Handbook of Medical Sociology*, 6th edn. Nashville: Vanderbilt University Press.

McKinlay, J.B. and Arches, J. (1985) 'Toward the proletarianization of physicians', *International Journal of Health Services*, 15 (2): 161–195.

McKinlay, J.B. and Marceau, L. (2002) 'The end of the golden age of doctoring', *International Journal of Health Services*, 32 (2): 379–416.

Speed, E. and Gabe, J. (2020) 'The reform of the English National Health Service: professional dominance, countervailing powers and the buyers' revolt', *Social Theory & Health*, 18 (1): 33–49.

Timmermans, S. and Oh, H. (2010) 'The continued social transformation of the medical profession', *Journal of Health & Social Behaviour*, 51 (S): S94–S106.

Waring, J., Roe, B., Crompton, A. and Bishop, S. (2020) 'The contingencies of medical restratification across inter-organisational care networks', *Social Science & Medicine*, 263: 113277.

Witz, A. and Annandale, E. (2006) 'The challenge of nursing', in D. Kelleher, J. Gabe and G. Williams (eds), *Challenging Medicine*, 2nd edn. London: Routledge.

SUGGESTED FURTHER READING

- Calnan, M. (2015) 'Eliot Freidson: sociological narratives of professionalism and modern medicine', in F. Collyer (ed.), *The Palgrave Handbook of Social Theory in Health, Illness and Medicine*. Basingstoke: Palgrave Macmillan.

A useful assessment of the theoretical contribution of Eliot Freidson, focusing on some of his key concepts such as professional dominance, autonomy and re-stratification.

- Saks, M. (2015) *The Professions, the State and the Market*. London: Routledge.

This book explores the extent to which different socio-political philosophies have shaped the organization of medical work in the UK, USA and Russia. It also considers the development of medical professionalism and its implications for clients in these different socio-political contexts in the face of a series of challenges. The author pays particular attention to deprofessionalization, re-stratification, corporatization and medicine's relationship with allied health professions.

- Rozier, M.D., Willison, C.E, Anspach, R.R. et al. (2020) 'Paradoxes of professional autonomy: a qualitative study of U.S. neonatologists from 1978–2017', *Sociology of Health & Illness*, 42 (8): 1821–1836.

An interesting study of changes in professional autonomy of US neonatologists over time. Drawing on four waves of interviews with neonatologists, the authors discovered that while these doctors enjoyed high levels of professional discretion through the 1990s they were also constrained by bioethics and the law. By the 2010s parents were much more involved in decision-making, alongside other subspecialties, diffusing the burden felt by individual practitioners, but their professional autonomy was also diminished.

41

Trust in Medicine

Jonathan Gabe

> *Trust refers to a state of favourable expectations around people's actions and motives as embedded and constituted within social institutions and relationships.*

The concept of trust has been a prominent theme in both social theory and medical sociology for some years. From a sociological standpoint it is best seen as a form of social action (paying attention to the intentions of others), involving individuals or institutions in a social relationship, rather than a mental state. According to Sztompka (1999) it involves an optimistic bet about the future, which involves a degree of uncertainty.

Much of the work of social theorists (e.g. Beck, 1992; Giddens, 1990; Luhmann, 1984) has revolved around three themes (Elston, 2009). First, it has been argued that trust is becoming increasingly important for managing life in a world which is rapidly changing and becoming more risky. Second, while the increase in bureaucratic rationalization and an enhanced sense of risk in late modern society is generating more need for trust, the basis for trusting has become more precarious. People are becoming less deferential and more critical of experts, resulting in trust having to be actively earned in particular situations. Trust is now dependent on day-to-day experience providing reasons for trusting someone, but it is also dependent on a capacity to momentarily bracket-off uncertainty and the unknowable, in what Möllering (2001) describes as a 'leap of faith'. Such leaps of faith are common in decisions involving doctors and patients where there is uncertainty and a degree of risk regarding the doctor's competence and intentions (Calnan and Rowe, 2007). Third, in contemporary society there is a growing need to trust abstract systems alongside interpersonal trust (betting on the intentions of those who are known). Those who occupy 'key access points' for such abstract systems play a crucial role in developing trust. Doctors can be seen as being in such a position, representing the abstract system of biomedicine, but not being trusted automatically any more.

In the above account a distinction has been made between interpersonal trust and trust in a system. Interpersonal trust involves relations between individual patients and their clinician, and also between one clinician and another and between a clinician and a manager. This needs to be distinguished from trust in a particular healthcare organization or healthcare system (Calnan and Rowe, 2007, 2008a). These levels of trust are interconnected and may be mutually reinforcing (Stevenson and Scambler, 2005), although it is possible to trust one's doctor while distrusting the hospital in which she works and vice versa.

A distinction can also be made between embodied trust and informed trust. The former involves reliance on reputation, competence and empathy while the latter refers to new tools of bureaucratic regulation such as performance indicators which act as signifiers of quality (Kuhlman, 2006). Embedded in these two forms of trust is the distinction between affective and cognitive factors, with embodied trust relying on individual perceptions, desires and emotions and informed trust emphasizing 'rational', instrumental aspects (Kuhlman, 2006). It has been suggested that structural changes in the provision of care such as an increase in points of access to primary care (for example, through walk-in centres, National Health Service (NHS) 111 call centres and nurse triage clinics) has made embodied trust, based on an enduring relationship with a 'family doctor', less relevant than in the past. Faced with care being provided by an increasing variety of healthcare professionals, status, qualifications and reputation may now be an insufficient basis for trusting the quality of care on offer. Rather, trust may be contingent and based on the information provided with patients rationally weighing up the costs and benefits before accepting a proposed course of action.

Taylor-Gooby (2006) suggests that the decline in institutional trust may undermine welfare reform. He bases this assessment on the view that attempts to reinvigorate trust in institutions like the UK's NHS have been dependent on the introduction of policies based on rational choice, which may have the unintended effect of undermining non-rational/affective trust. For instance, the decision to disclose performance data about individual surgeons on the internet may have contradictory effects. Patients may view performance data as open to manipulation by managers. In a case study of the provision of care for elective hip surgery among patients in English hospitals, patients considered performance data to be unreliable and as likely to be massaged by managers to create as favourable an impression as possible (Calnan and Rowe, 2008a, 2008b). This lack of trust in the data may therefore have the effect of reinforcing interpersonal trust in doctors rather than increasing confidence in abstract systems, as claimed by Harrison and Smith (2004) in the context of discussing developments in clinical governance. As Calnan and Rowe (2008b: 202) put it, 'patients do not demand "proof" of trustworthiness, rather they assess for themselves the quality of service provision based on their personal experience of care'.

While much of the attention in medical sociology has been focused on the extent to which patients trust their doctor or the healthcare system, there has been rather less attention given to the extent to which doctors trust their patients and also the nature of trust relations between medicine and the state. Taking the issue of doctors' trust in patients first, Sousa-Duarte et al. (2020) argue that there needs to be a focus on how healthcare professionals interpret signs about the trustworthiness of their patients. These processes may be bound up with the way in which such professionals experience and understand their vulnerability and uncertainty, for example when making medical judgements about opioid prescriptions and addiction treatment. They also suggest that doctors' trust in patients needs to be understood in the context of shifting medico-legal and socio-political conditions of late modern healthcare. Shifting regulatory structures, a more market orientated approach to healthcare and changing interaction norms in the consultation may increase uncertainty and vulnerability among doctors and impact their trust in their patients.

As regards the nature of trust relations between medicine and the state, Elston (2009) argues that a series of medical malpractice scandals which came to light in the UK in the mid-to-late 1990s, including the conviction of the general practitioner Harold Shipman for murdering a large number of his elderly patients, resulted in medicine's regulatory institutions ceasing to be seen as trustworthy by the state. The response of the profession, or at least its leadership, has been to seek to craft a 'new professionalism'. This new position involves stressing patient partnership, accountability and transparency as the basis for renewed trust. Such a response can be seen as primarily a defensive move by the medical profession to head off challenges to their autonomy from the state against a background of growing distrust. But it can also be seen in part as an attempt by the profession to develop new disciplinary mechanisms through self-regulation at the individual level and through institutionalized procedures at the meso level (Elston, 2009).

Interestingly, medical sociologists too have come to the defence of the medical profession. Freidson (2001), for example, shifted from his earlier position of seeing professionalism as an ideology and professionalization as a competitive power struggle, to emphasizing the virtues of professionalism as a way of controlling the provision of expert services, rather than markets and bureaucratic mechanisms. Likewise Harrison and Smith (2004) have discussed the dangers of distrusting doctors and imposing excessive regulations on them. These authors reflect a shift among some sociologists from challenging medical power to acknowledging the importance of trusting the medical profession and the problems posed by its reported decline.

While such sociologists can be said to be basing their arguments on normative judgements about the benefits of trust for both patients and doctors, it is important to ask whether there is a dark side to trust. Some have suggested that it can lead to an abuse of power, as trust usually involves an asymmetrical relationship between the trustor (the subject) and the trustee (the object) (Calnan and Rowe, 2008b). In such circumstances trust may be used to legitimate the exercise of power and even to facilitate corrupt practices or cover up malpractice, as has allegedly been the case in the UK with the government said to have suppressed science by gagging scientists and cherry picking favourable research for political and financial gain (Abasi, 2020). These abuses of power may be less common, however, if trust now has to be constantly earned, whether at the micro level of the clinician–patient relationship, or the macro level of the relationship between the medical profession and the state.

While considerable progress has been made in studying trust, more studies are needed regarding the nature of the relationship between patients' interpersonal trust in clinicians and institutional trust in healthcare organizations and healthcare systems. The COVID-19 pandemic has been particularly significant in shining a light on such trust relations and how and why trust matters. As Calnan et al. (2020) argue, the extent to which people have trust in government, trust in the number of those said to have and to have died from COVID-19, the government's trust in the public and trust in COVID-related technologies (for example, around testing and tracing) all have a bearing on people's subsequent behaviour. Much more research is needed with regard to such trust relations following the COVID pandemic in particular and more generally as a result of changes in service delivery and its consequences for patient–clinician trust.

See also: Hospitals and Healthcare Organizations; Malpractice; Medical Autonomy, Dominance and Decline; Pandemics and Epidemics; Risk.

REFERENCES

Abasi, K. (2020) 'Covid-19: politicisation, "corruption", and suppression of science', *British Medical Journal*, 371: m4425.
Beck, U. (1992) *The Risk Society: Towards a New Modernity*. London: SAGE.
Calnan, M. and Rowe, R. (2007) 'Trust and health care', *Sociology Compass*, 1 (1): 1–26.
Calnan, M. and Rowe, R. (2008a) *Trust Matters in Health Care*. Maidenhead: Open University Press.
Calnan, M. and Rowe, R. (2008b) 'Trust, accountability and choice', *Health, Risk & Society*, 10 (3): 201–206.
Calnan, M., Williams, S.J. and Gabe, J. (2020) 'Uncertain times: trust matters during the pandemic', *Discover Society*, 2 June. Online: https://discoversociety.org/2020/06/01/uncertain-times-trust-matters-during-the-pandemic/
Elston, M. (2009) 'Remaking a trustworthy medical profession in twenty-first century Britain?' In J. Gabe and M. Calnan (eds), *The New Sociology of the Health Service*. London: Routledge.
Freidson, E. (2001) *Professionalism, the Third Logic*. Cambridge: Polity.
Giddens, A. (1990) *The Consequences of Modernity*. Cambridge: Polity.
Harrison, S. and Smith, C. (2004) 'Trust and moral motivation: redundant resources in health and social care?' *Policy & Politics*, 32 (3): 371–386.

Kuhlmann. E. (2006) *Modernising Health Care: Reinventing Professions, the State and the Public*. Bristol: Policy Press.

Luhmann, N. (1984) *Trust and Power: Two Works by Niklas Luhmann*. Chichester: John Wiley.

Möllering, G. (2001) 'The nature of trust: from Georg Simmel to a theory of expectations, interpretations and suspension', *Sociology*, 35 (2): 403–420.

Sousa-Duarte, F., Brown, P. and Mendes A.M. (2020) 'Healthcare professionals' trust in patients: a review of the empirical and theoretical literatures', *Sociology Compass*, 14 (10): 1–15.

Stevenson, F. and Scambler, G. (2005) 'The relationship between medicine and the public: the challenge of concordance', *Health*, 9 (1): 5–21.

Sztompka, P. (1999) *Trust: A Sociological Theory*. Cambridge: Cambridge University Press.

Taylor-Gooby, P. (2006) 'Trust, risk and health care reform', *Health, Risk & Society*, 8 (2): 97–103.

SUGGESTED FURTHER READING

- Brown, P. and Calnan, M. (2012) *Trusting on the Edge: Managing Uncertainty and Vulnerability in the Midst of Serious Mental Health Problems*. Bristol: Policy Press.

An important exploration of how trust develops or fails to develop in the context of severe mental illness, based on interviews with service users, practitioners and managers.

- Pedersen, I.K., Hansen, V.H. and Grunenberg, K. (2016) 'The emergence of trust in clinics of alternative medicine', *Sociology of Health & Illness*, 38 (1): 43–57.

An interesting account of how trust emerges in Danish alternative medicine clinics. Drawing on three separate qualitative studies, it shows how trust is situational and emerges through both clients' openness to work with practitioners and the latters' embodied practical skills and strategies.

- Ye, M. and Lyu, Z. (2020) 'Trust, risk perception, and COVID-19 infections: evidence from multilevel analyses of combined original data set in China', *Social Science & Medicine*, 265: 113517.

A study of how trust shapes risk perception towards infection from COVID-19 in China. On the basis of an analysis of big data, official data and surveys of residents from over 300 cities, it concludes that trust in local government and media helps reduce the infection rate of the disease but that generalized (unconditional) trust in other members of society promotes a higher rather than lower infection rate.

42

Professions Allied to Medicine

Ivy Lynn Bourgeault

Professions allied to medicine refers to all the different professions within the healthcare division of labour, which is hierarchical and tends to be dominated by physicians. Practised within and across various healthcare sectors, each profession claims a unique knowledge base whilst varying in their roles, relations and status.

The health workforce contains a range of health workers, defined by the World Health Organization (WHO, 2006: 1) as 'all people engaged in actions whose primary intent is to enhance health'. The health workforce can be described in more sociological terms as a healthcare division of labour. This division involves the various relationships between different types of personnel in the provision of healthcare and arrangements within and across healthcare settings (Storch, 2010). Diverse professions working within the healthcare division of labour have different roles, relations and status, and these have evolved over time. Gender, racial and other intersecting identities have influenced these different roles historically and continue to do so in the contemporary era. These dynamics not only change over time, they also differ across country contexts.

The health sector includes many different professions beyond those that typically come to mind: medicine and nursing. Some of these professions have historical roots that can be traced back to the emergence of the medical and nursing professions, such as midwifery, pharmacy and optometry. Other professions have emerged more recently as a result of the development of new healthcare technologies, like medical radiation therapy, or shortages of particular medical specialties, such as physician assistants/associates. There is also a somewhat separate dental division of labour ranging from dentists, dental specialists and surgeons to denturists and dental technicians to dental assistants, hygienists and, in some systems, dental therapists.

Historically, the professionalization of medicine preceded other healthcare roles and, as such, medicine emerged as the dominant profession by which most others in the formal healthcare sector relate; hence the term *allied to medicine*. A key element of dominance of the medical profession, historically entwined with White middle-class masculinity, is its control over other health professions within the healthcare division of labour. This dominance has also been described as *occupational imperialism*. As Larkin (1983) described it, occupational imperialism is 'an arena of tension and conflict between groups which is largely shaped in outcome by the differential access of each group to exterior power sources' (p. 17). It includes elements such as monopolizing particular skills and establishing advantageous relationships with allied groups, which can sometimes involve 'poaching' skills from other professions.

Similarly, Abbott (1988) described a system of professions as a complex, dynamic and interdependent structural network of various professions within a given domain of work, constantly struggling over areas of knowledge and skill expertise called jurisdictions. Professions develop within this system when jurisdictions are created or are vacated by other professions. These vacancies occur in response to external system disturbances, such as technological or organizational change, and/or because a previous tenant has abandoned it (Nancarrow and Borthwick, 2005). Subordination of one group by another occurs when a profession vacates a jurisdiction but maintains control over it through such strategies as supervising the new tenant.

Taking an explicit gender lens on the development of the healthcare division of labour, Witz (1992) described how the subordination of nursing and midwifery was the result of *demarcationary* efforts of the medical profession. These demarcationary strategies aim to create boundaries with adjacent professions in the division of labour and interprofessional control. As Davies (1996: 661) later remarked when describing this phenomenon, 'a key issue for consideration is not so much the exclusion of women from work defined as professional, but rather their routine inclusion in ill-defined support roles'.

Other professions allied to medicine have been described as having *limited* roles – specifically those professions that practise independently of medical supervision but with a more narrowly defined scope of practice, either in terms of the part of the body or range of treatment modalities (Willis, 1989). Examples include podiatry, which is limited to treatment of the foot, optometry to certain disorders of the eyes, and psychology, limited to the treatment of mental health issues. These specialties have been described as established allied health professions. Pharmacy is another example and it is worth discussing further with respect to history, competition and expansion in the context of further professionalization and, arguably, pharmaceuticalization.

The history of pharmacy and its relationship to the medical profession has been a quintessential story of professional competition. Prior to any strict form of regulation, pharmacists used to diagnose minor disorders for which they stocked the 'cure' and physicians used to regularly dispense similar 'cures' from their clinics following diagnosis. It is in part due to potential economic conflicts of interest that there was a division of the act of prescribing (following diagnosis) from dispensing of medicines. The task of prescribing fell within the domain of medicine whereas that of dispensing was within the domain of pharmacy. Pharmacists have always 'prescribed' over-the-counter medication within the context of their community-based pharmacies but were limited to dispensing those drugs that were restricted by prescription (Muzzin et al., 1994). In recent years the scope of pharmacy practice has expanded to include prescribing beyond over-the-counter medications as well as medication management. This expansion could be regarded as a contemporary dimension of their continued professionalization. There has been a consequent revamping of pharmacy educational programmes to reflect this more clinical dimension to pharmacy, which has been coined 'pharmaceutical care' or 'social pharmacy' (Hassali et al., 2011). The new curriculum focuses on a more patient- or client-oriented approach to the provision of pharmaceutical services. As the scope of pharmacy practice evolves, it has created new support roles such as pharmacy technicians, a similar dynamic that occurred for support roles to the medical profession. It has also brought a new dimension to the relationship between pharmacists and physicians (Bradley et al., 2018). Furthermore, pharmacists have had to manage the consequences of pharmaceuticalization, especially in jurisdictions that allow Direct to Consumer Advertising (DCA) through mass media. DCA has arguably encouraged viewers to request medicines directly from pharmacists.

Other limited professions include the rehabilitation professions of physiotherapy and occupational therapy. These emerged not so much out of the historical dynamic vis-à-vis the profession of medicine, but rather as a response to the increasing complexity of hospital-based healthcare in the early 20th century. This complexity included attending to the long-term treatment of those hospitalized for tuberculous, as well as the rehabilitative treatment of soldiers in the First and Second World Wars. Specifically with respect to the treatment of wounded war veterans, physiotherapists focused on their physical rehabilitation whilst occupational therapists focused on ways to accommodate them into the workforce. The practices of these professions have expanded, commensurate with the aging of the population, which in turn have sparked the development of allied support roles, including physiotherapy and occupational therapy assistants.

Techno-scientific advances have spurred on the development of the professions of medical laboratory and medical radiation technologists. These professions have evolved from playing more assistive roles to physician specialists (pathologist and radiologists) to having more independent roles coordinating laboratory, testing and screening facilities. The dietetics profession also has a unique history, emerging from the home economics and food science professions. Now playing a key role in the healthcare division of labour, dietetics has evolved to address the increasingly prevalent chronic conditions commonly related to diet and lifestyle factors. It is worth adding, however, that 'radical dieticians' also challenge such healthism. Indeed, some favour a 'relational-cultural' approach that is especially critical of weight-centric discourses and practices amidst medicalized calls to tackle obesity (Brady et al., 2013).

The status of these traditionally subordinate and limited professions within the healthcare division of labour is dynamic. For example, although midwifery was historically subordinated to the medical profession, it has evolved into a more limited profession focused on what is defined as normal pregnancy and childbirth. Also emerging from the nursing profession are specialized roles, including nurse practitioners, which can be more aptly described as a limited role. Similarly, many of the traditionally limited professions have recently expanded their scope of practice to include other tasks, including a strictly demarcated form of prescribing. This was noted above in the case of pharmacy, a profession which overlaps even more fully with the traditional domain of medicine. Nancarrow and Borthwick (2005) describe this movement of allied professional roles to take on tasks that are normally performed by other health professionals as a form of *vertical substitution*. For the most part, the medical profession has accepted this substitution which enables them to focus on more complex and higher status activities.

As interprofessional or team-based initiatives take hold, where there is a greater integration of professions working together, these categorizations will continue to evolve. The healthcare division of labour, and the allied health professional roles within it, have also shifted in response to rising consumerism as well as neoliberal managerial principles that redistribute resources on the basis of professional accomplishment rather than the historical workforce hierarchies (Nancarrow and Borthwick, 2005). Nevertheless interprofessional integration has been limited given the structural embeddedness of medical dominance in healthcare settings, as well as in legislative and financial systems (Bourgeault and Mulvale, 2006).

Gender dynamics have not only influenced the emergence of these roles traditionally, but their impact also continues in the contemporary era. Many of the allied professional roles are dominated by women and many of the traditionally masculine allied professions have become feminized. Indeed, the healthcare division of labour is one of the most gendered female sectors, where internationally over 70 per cent of the health workforce is composed of those who identify as women. A trend towards more independence of traditionally subordinated feminine roles of nursing and midwifery is buoyed by broader feminist efforts to push back against the gendered division of labour in healthcare (Bourgeault, 2006). Similar dynamics are also evidenced in dietetics amidst calls for politicized practice and challenges to the status quo (Aphramor and Gingras, 2011).

Finally, although much of the focus on formal health workers during the COVID-19 pandemic has been on the traditional roles of medicine and nursing, it has become clear that different roles within the healthcare division of labour vary in their level of exposure to the virus. Allied health professional roles in older adult care and in respiratory therapy have been particularly exposed. At present, more of the responses to the pandemic have focused on shoring up resources within rather than expanding scope across health professional roles, but the long-term impact of the pandemic on the healthcare division of labour remains to be seen (Bourgeault et al., 2020).

See also: Consumerism; Medical Autonomy, Dominance and Decline; Nursing and Midwifery as Occupations; Pharmaceuticalization; Social Divisions in Formal Healthcare.

REFERENCES

Abbott, A. (1988) *The System of Professions – A Study of the Division of Expert Labour*. Chicago: University of Chicago Press.

Aphramor, L. and Gingras, J. (2011) 'Helping people change: promoting politicised practice in the health care professions', in E. Rich, L.F. Monaghan and L. Aphramor (eds), *Debating Obesity: Critical Perspectives*. Basingstoke: Palgrave Macmillan.

Bourgeault, I.L. (2006) *Push!: The Struggle for Midwifery in Ontario* (Vol. 25). Montreal: McGill-Queen's Press-MQUP.

Bourgeault, I.L. and Mulvale, G. (2006) 'Collaborative health care teams in Canada and the U.S.: confronting the structural embeddedness of medical dominance', *Health Sociology Review*, 15 (5): 481–495.

Bourgeault, I.L., Maier, C.B., Dieleman, M. et al. (2020) 'The COVID-19 pandemic presents an opportunity to develop more sustainable health workforces', *Human Resources for Health*, 18 (1): 1–8.

Bradley, F., Ashcroft, D.M. and Crossley, B. (2018) 'Negotiating interprofessional interaction: playing the general practitioner–pharmacist game', *Sociology of Health & Illness*, 40 (3): 426–444.

Brady, J., Gingras, J. and Aphramor, A. (2013) 'Theorizing health at every size as a relational–cultural endeavour', *Critical Public Health*, 23 (3): 345–355.

Davies, C. (1996) 'The sociology of professions and the profession of gender', *Sociology*, 30 (4): 661–678.

Hassali, M.A., Shafie, A.A., Sa'di Al-Haddad, M. et al. (2011) 'Social pharmacy as a field of study: the needs and challenges in global pharmacy education', *Research in Social and Administrative Pharmacy*, 7 (4): 415–420.

Larkin, G.V. (1983) *Occupational Monopoly and Modern Medicine*. London: Tavistock.

Muzzin, L.J., Brown, G.P. and Hornosty, R.W. (1994) 'Consequences of feminization of a profession: the case of Canadian pharmacy', *Women & Health*, 21 (2–3): 39–56.

Nancarrow, S.A. and Borthwick, A.M. (2005) 'Dynamic professional boundaries in the healthcare workforce', *Sociology of Health & Illness*, 27 (7): 897–919.

Storch, J. (2010) 'Division of labour in health care', *Humane Medicine*, 10 (4). Online: www.humanehealthcare.com/Article.asp?art_id=543

WHO (2006) *World Health Report 2006: Working Together for Health*. World Health Organization. Online: www.who.int/whr/2006/en/

Willis, E. (1989) *Medical Dominance*, 2nd edn. Sydney: Allen and Unwin Australia.

Witz, A. (1992) *Professions and Patriarchy*. London: Routledge.

SUGGESTED FURTHER READING

- Bourgeault, I.L. (ed.) (2021) *Introduction to the Health Workforce in Canada.* Ottawa: Canadian Health Workforce Network.

This is the first text that offers a history of over 20 different health occupations and professions working in the Canadian health system that covers their history, education, scopes of practice, regulation, demographics and topical issues.

- Nancarrow, S. and Borthwick, A. (2021) *The Allied Health Professions: A Sociological Perspective.* Bristol: Policy Press.

This book helps to address a critical gap in our knowledge of who are the allied health professions – individually or collectively – how they have developed historically and their role and relationship to the other health professions within health systems.

- Saks, M. (ed.) (2020) *Support Workers and the Health Professions in International Perspective.* Bristol: Policy Press.

Drawing from a range of country exemplars from the UK, Japan, Australia, Brazil, Canada, Portugal, Sweden and The Netherlands, this edited text addresses the often neglected and invisible health and social care support workforces.

43

Nursing and Midwifery as Occupations

Abbey Hyde and Orla McDonnell

Nursing is an occupation involving the provision of care to facilitate the maintenance of, or improvement in, health and/or recovery from illness and the maximum quality of life until death. Midwifery as an occupation aspires to provide independent woman-centred care to healthy parturient women.

Sociological interest in nursing and midwifery as occupations has centred on issues of gender and professional power, and, in particular, on the complex historical relationship each occupation has with the medical profession, which affects its relative autonomy and authority in clinical settings. The professional autonomy of nurses and midwives has been enhanced by the extension of occupational roles to include technical tasks that previously belonged to the jurisdiction of medicine and the creation of specialist roles within particular domains of practice along with clinical management roles. At times, these new roles have been seen as a threat to the professional dominance of medicine. As well as making them powerful actors in the formation of healthcare policy, the control that doctors exercise over diagnosis, prescribing and referral has collectively afforded the medical profession considerable scope to direct the work of nurses and midwives. Hence, the extent to which nursing and midwifery have gained professional autonomy and the possible challenges that this poses to medical dominance is an issue that has been of enduring sociological interest. The direction that professionalization takes is also subject to ongoing debate within nursing and midwifery. Central to that debate is the self-image of nurses and midwives as 'new' professions, characterized by patient-centred and woman-centred care respectively (Porter et al., 2007). Let us first consider nursing before turning to midwifery.

Feminist scholarship on the gendering of health professions, referred to in the second edition of *Key Concepts in Medical Sociology*, highlights the particular challenges that nurses encounter in terms of how their occupation was distinguished from and held to be inferior to medicine. Early attempts to professionalize nursing in Britain and the USA included the regulation of training, culminating in nurse registration in the first quarter of the 20th century. Nurse registration enabled occupational closure (Witz, 1992), a key professionalizing strategy to control entry to the profession. Since the 1980s, the creation of a unique body of nursing knowledge has been key to the professionalization of nursing as an autonomous occupation. Nursing research has since acquired a new currency given the requirement of evidence-based practice. Nursing diagnosis – the idea that nursing-specific problems can be identified and mapped onto particular interventions for which a registered nurse is accountable – potentially offers the occupation formal autonomy to control a realm of patient care. However, a key challenge is gaining autonomy from medicine in the use of nursing knowledge.

While nurses have made strides in terms of clinical autonomy, and there is evidence of collaborative alliances between nurses and doctors, the prevailing order is of doctor domination (Carmel, 2006), particularly in acute settings (Nugus et al., 2010). For example, senior nurses tend to be assertive in decision-making about patient treatment and care, but this power is largely informal as doctors may overrule nurses' decisions when it comes to medical diagnosis; furthermore, the criteria specifying formal nursing jurisdiction over decision-making are highly restrictive. Doctors see themselves as the key decision-makers about patient care and this is legally, culturally and organizationally sanctioned. While doctors have formal responsibility for patient care, a key point of contention is whether this medico-legal responsibility also encompasses the power to determine the input of nurses working within their own jurisdictions.

In a recent Irish study, Hyde et al. (2016) found that despite objective evidence of the safety of nurses prescribing X-rays (similar to findings for the prescribing of medicine), doctors and radiographers expressed less confidence in the nurses' professional competence to prescribe safely. The authors argue that this perception of other healthcare workers arises from the power/knowledge dynamics of inter-professional relations. While radiographers are not licenced to prescribe, nurse prescribing is nonetheless an incursion into the radiographers' knowledge domain and thus potentially threatens a core aspect of their professional authority. The medical profession has generally conceded ground to nurses by accepting extending roles such as prescribing; however, physicians retain jurisdiction over their core clinical skills by governing the parameters of new nursing roles that have the potential to impinge on their clinical autonomy through, for example, the supervision of prescribing. The implication of this for healthcare systems is that nurses cannot maximize their full skill set as advanced practitioners if they do not have medical supervision. In the absence of objective evidence to support perceptions that nursing prescribing is less safe than if it were carried out by a doctor, Hyde et al. (2016) conclude that professional ideologies shape perceptions of risk. The extent to which those ideological preferences, in turn, shape healthcare policy is contingent on wider social, economic and cultural factors. Within the negotiated order of intra- and inter-professional boundaries, different interests are played out and the success of an initiative in shifting health policy agendas depends on the alignment of those interests.

Such multi-level social processes are evidenced in Drennan et al.'s (2017) study on the introduction of physician associates (PAs) as a new healthcare occupational group into general practice in England to address staff shortages. Their research shows that support varied across policy, professional organizations and service delivery levels within medicine and nursing. On the perceived threat that PAs pose to nursing, the authors note a division between nurse managers, professional leaders for advanced nurse practitioners, and practice nurses working in general practice. Interestingly, from the perspective of the professional autonomy of nurses, general practitioners and practice managers viewed PAs – whose roles are curtailed because of lack of formal, statutory recognition – as nonetheless having a wider range of competencies and greater autonomy in practice than nurses. Not surprisingly, those advocating for the professionalization of nurses were the most resistant to the introduction of PAs.

In turning attention to the occupational status of midwifery, we see some rather different issues emerging compared with nursing, as well as some shared concerns. The greatest difference is that midwifery stakes its claim over pregnancy and childbirth as normal life events. It is the aspiration of 'new midwifery' – a movement that first emerged in the mid - to late -1970s to reclaim traditional midwifery by promoting woman-centred practice – that trained midwives should exercise exclusive control over the care of healthy pregnant women and the process of normal childbirth. Indeed, the 'normal' and 'abnormal' distinction is understood by midwives as the boundary marker between the role of the midwife and that of the obstetrician (Prowse and Prowse, 2008). According to new midwifery discourse, obstetricians would only be needed to manage the relatively small number of pregnancies and births that midwives have assessed as abnormal. Central to the discourse of new midwifery is woman-centeredness, framed in terms of choice, autonomy and partnership between the midwife and woman.

The second edition of *Key Concepts in Medical Sociology* refers to seminal feminist texts that challenged the biomedical model of childbirth in the 1970s. New midwifery discourse has since become central to the critique of the over-medicalization of pregnancy and childbirth and emphasizes international evidence supporting the quality and safety of midwife-led care (Renfrew et al., 2014). There is growing evidence supporting an emerging international policy consensus that challenges obstetric-led care as the norm in high-income countries. The decline in 'normal' or non-invasive births is linked to the overuse of technological interventions (Seijmonsbergen-Schermers et al., 2020). The clearest evidence of the overuse of childbirth interventions is that countries with the highest levels do not have better outcomes. The policy implication of this is that finite resources are diverted to unnecessary, expensive and potentially harmful care when applied in a routine fashion. The shift to hospital-based care in low- and middle-income countries to address high maternal and neonatal mortality is leading to a similar pattern of over-medicalization coupled with inequality of access for the poorest women (Miller et al., 2016).

While many midwives embrace the ideology of new midwifery, there is a gap between the rhetorical consensus on woman-centred care and clinical practice (Porter et al., 2007; Prowse and Prowse, 2008). The policy legacy of obstetric domination continues to be a relevant factor. For example, the culture of risk that primarily defines birth as 'risky' impacts on women's choices in pregnancy and childbirth and midwifery practices (Healy et al., 2016). The medical profession has also been found to dominate midwifery to varying degrees, regulating its work practices and, in some contexts, prohibiting it from legal practice (Bourgeault et al., 2004). However, it is not merely the dominance of obstetrics that constrains midwives' autonomy. Benoit et al. (2005) observed definitive variations in the social organization of maternity care across four high-income countries: the UK, the Netherlands, Finland and Canada. They argued that the extent to which states were positively disposed both to women as workers (for example, midwives) and women as recipients of care (parturient women), often fuelled by consumer support and market principles, accounted for a good deal of the variation. In the Netherlands, for example, 'woman-friendly' state support for midwifery is high, as evidenced in laws and regulations, the education of midwives and research into midwifery outcomes. In contrast, in counties such as Finland, a gender-neutral emphasis and the politics of playing down differences between men and women rather than promoting 'woman-friendliness' have served to undermine midwives' professional interests.

While changes in state policies and legislation in many countries have seen extended roles for nurses and midwives that cross over into medicine's traditional jurisdiction, this has not necessarily entailed greater professional autonomy. Extending the midwife's role to include routine technical tasks that were previously carried out by junior doctors competes with time needed to provide individualized, woman-centred care. At the same time, the loss of traditional midwifery skills to maternity support workers and the possible erosion of those skills through the development of specialized roles undermines the professional identity of the new midwifery as the 'custodian' of normal pregnancy and natural childbirth (Prowse and Prowse, 2008).

The year 2020 was designated as the International Year of the Nurse and Midwife by the World Health Organization as a way of building policy consensus about the role of both occupations in enhancing universal healthcare. Commenting on the *Lancet* Midwifery Series on the efficacy of midwifery-led care, Judith Shamian (2014) of the International Council of Nurses suggests that the issue is no longer about inter-professional 'turf wars', but the absence from policy dialogue of those with the most to offer health. While there has been much research evaluating the clinical autonomy of nursing and midwifery as a marker of professional autonomy vis-à-vis medical hegemony, there has been less focus on their political autonomy to influence healthcare policy. In the context of COVID-19, future research in the sociology of professions might focus on the political autonomy of nurses and midwives as leaders in translating health policies into actions that reconfigure how services are delivered so that universal care is a perquisite for epidemic 'preparedness'. Writing just a few months after the pandemic erupted, McDonald (2020: 13) asserted: 'it is time nurses involved themselves in revisioning public policies and reforming health systems that could, if not guided, return nurses to hazardous work environments and trivialize foreseeable risks to us all'.

See also: Reproduction; Risk; Social Divisions in Formal Healthcare; The Medical Model.

REFERENCES

Benoit, C., Wrede, S., Bourgeault, I. et al. (2005) 'Understanding the social organisation of maternity care systems: midwifery as touchstone', *Sociology of Health & Illness*, 27 (6): 722–737.

Bourgeault, I.L., Benoit, C. and Davis-Floyd, R.E. (eds) (2004) *Reconceiving Midwifery: The New Canadian Model of Care*. Kingston, Montreal: McGill-Queen's University Press.

Carmel, S. (2006) 'Boundaries obscured and boundaries reinforced: incorporation as a strategy of occupational enhancement for intensive care', *Sociology of Health & Illness*, 28 (2): 154–177.

Drennan, V.M., Gabe, J., Halter, M. et al. (2017) 'Physician associates in primary health care in England: a challenge to professional boundaries?' *Social Science & Medicine*, 81: 9–16.

Healy, S., Humphreys, E. and Kennedy, C. (2016) 'Midwives' and obstetricians' perceptions of risk and its impact on clinical practice and decision-making in labour: an integrative review', *Women and Birth*, 29 (2): 107–116.

Hyde, A., Coughlan, B., Naughton, C. et al. (2016) 'Nurses', physicians' and radiographers' perceptions of the safety of a nurse prescribing of ionising radiation initiative: a cross-sectional survey', *International Journal of Nursing Studies*, 58: 21–30.

McDonald, T. (2020) 'Getting the COVID-19 pandemic into perspective: a nursing imperative', *International Nursing Review*, 67 (3): 1–13.

Miller, S., Abalos, E., Chamillard, M. et al. (2016) 'Beyond too little, too late and too much, too soon: a pathway towards evidence-based, respectful maternity care worldwide', *The Lancet*, 388: 2176–2192.

Nugus, P., Greenfield, D., Travaglia, J. et al. (2010) 'How and where clinicians exercise power: interprofessional relations in health care', *Social Science & Medicine*, 71 (5): 898–909.

Porter, S., Crozier, K., Sinclair, M. and Kernohan, W.G. (2007) 'New midwifery? A qualitative analysis of midwives' decision-making strategies', *Journal of Advanced Nursing*, 60 (5): 525–534.

Prowse, J. and Prowse, P. (2008) 'Role redesign in the National Health Service: the effects on midwives' work and professional boundaries', *Work, Employment and Society*, 22 (4): 695–712.

Renfrew, M.J., McFadden, A., Bastos, M.H. et al. (2014) 'Midwifery and quality care: findings from a new evidence-informed framework for maternal and newborn care', *Lancet*, 384: 1129–1145.

Seijmonsbergen-Schermers, A.E., van den Akker, T., Rydahl, E. et al. (2020) 'Variations in use of childbirth interventions in 13 high-income countries: a multinational cross-sectional study', *PLoS Medicine*, 17(5): e1003013.

Shamian, J. (2014) 'Interpersonal collaboration, the only way to Save Every Woman and Every Child', *Lancet*, 384 (9948): e41–e42.

Witz, A. (1992) *Professions and Patriarchy*. London: Routledge.

SUGGESTED FURTHER READING

- Allen, D. (2014) 'Lost in translation? "Evidence" and the articulation of institutional logics in integrated care pathways: from positive to negative boundary object?' *Sociology of Health & Illness*, 36 (6): 807–822.

Allen revisits earlier work on 'integrated clinical pathways' for which nurses in the UK have become clinical leaders. In the original analysis she theorized that clinical pathways function as 'boundary objects' by creating a shared language by which multidisciplinary teams can deliver quality care to patients in ways that cut through organizational hierarchies and potential jurisdictional disputes. In this article, she emphasizes how changing institutional practices require enrolling the support of the medical profession.

- Hunter, B. and Segrott, J. (2014) 'Renegotiating inter-professional boundaries in maternity care: implementing a clinical pathway for normal labour', *Sociology of Health & Illness*, 36 (5): 719–737.

Drawing on qualitative research, this article examines maternity care strategies in Wales, in light of the growing international policy support for midwifery-led models of care. Contra the potential of clinical pathways to dissolve inter-professional boundaries and enhance collaboration, the authors argue that clinical pathways are not ideologically neutral vis-à-vis competing interests. They also explore the implication of the deployment of risk discourse as a strategy to demarcate the boundary between normal and abnormal labour.

- Witz, A. and Annandale, E. (2006) 'The challenge of nursing', in D. Kelleher, J. Gabe and G. Williams (eds), *Challenging Medicine*, 2nd edn. London: Routledge.

The chapter charts the debate within nursing about the directions that professionalization has taken and the tensions between 'extended' roles (crossing over into medicine's jurisdiction) and 'expanded roles' (enhancing the role of nursing beyond routine, task-oriented care via the philosophy of the nursing process).

44

Social Divisions in Formal Healthcare

Catherine Theodosius

Social divisions in formal healthcare include professional status, power, gender, ethnicity and socio-economic status. Such divisions represent and perpetuate socio-cultural inequalities, nationally and globally, and can generate inter-professional conflict or 'boundary struggles'.

Social class, gender and ethnicity are typically divisive because of differences in the degree of social status and power accorded to them. Social status, usually conferred through birth or profession, is defined by Weber (1995: 155) as 'claims on positive or negative privileges in regard to social prestige' that are gained when they become part of everyday life, and when, through formal education, that way of life becomes assimilated. Social divisions occur when such privileges are unequally distributed between all groups of people. This process generates social stratification between class, gender and ethnic groups. In formal healthcare, social divisions between and within different groups of workers, incorporate the prestige of the medical profession that elevates science over care (thus reproducing masculine domination) and the intersectionality of gender with class and ethnicity. Despite the allied healthcare professions being interdependent, the vast difference in professional status and accompanying privileges is a source of ongoing conflict and dispute. These struggles reflect and reproduce historically transmitted divisions within global society and the healthcare division of labour.

Compared to other health professions, medicine enjoys higher social prestige and greater autonomy in practice and dominance in the development, maintenance and delivery of formal healthcare. Medical dominance is historical.

Arguably significant socio-economic, gender and ethnic divisions have become formalized over time, and represented within current and potentially contentious inter- and intra-professional boundaries. For example, in the Global North, members of the medical profession were historically upper-middle-class White men. Whilst ethnic and gender diversity within medicine has significantly increased, The Social Mobility Commission (2016) in the UK reported that there was little change in socio-economic representation in the medical profession, with only 4 per cent of doctors coming from working-class backgrounds. The dominance of medicine, however, is constantly being challenged due to the need to provide modern, flexible healthcare services that meet current demand, and due to new advanced roles within nursing and allied healthcare professions (Nancarrow and Borthwick, 2005). These challenges have resulted in a new literature base exploring social divisions using the developing field of boundary struggles (e.g. Ernst, 2020); that is, conflict between professions across boundaries as members seek to expand their scope of practice.

Boundary struggles between and within medicine and nursing are indicative of social class and gender divisions and intersections between the two. Arguably the intersection between gender and social class in the conflict between medicine and nursing lies in the symbolism attached to their respective knowledge bases and the professional capital each accrues. 'Professional capital materialises as advantageous wages (economic capital), the use of specialised knowledge (cultural capital) in practice and the possession and use of power' (Ernst, 2020: 1730). Ernst argues that the symbolism attached to medical knowledge supports medicine's high professional capital. For example, the unassailability of medical knowledge is taken as a self-evident truth. Medical knowledge is predicated on evidence-based medicine, defined as 'the conscientious, explicit, and judicious use of current best evidence in making decisions about the care of individual patients' (Sackett et al., 1996: 71). Although a contentious term, evidence-based medicine is 'perceived as scientific, neutral and objective' (Ernst, 2020: 1729).

In contrast, the symbolism attached to nursing represents further social divisions linked to gender disparities between and within healthcare professions, socially constructed around the dirty and caring nature of nursing. The social construction of 'care' as a 'natural' feminine quality, indicative of women's supposedly 'innate' nurturing ability, is perceived as inherently emotional and therefore irrational. This construction is in contrast to science, denoted as masculine and reasoned; the social difference being one of increased status and prestige for science over care. Because caring is feminized and deemed vocational, the satisfaction in undertaking this kind of work is typically considered a reward in itself and deemed a valid reason for why carers need not be overly financially rewarded. In response, the nursing profession has worked hard to move away from its gendered image, attempting to raise its status by asserting that nursing is a science. In doing so, nursing has also adopted evidence-based medicine, subtly developing its applicability to their profession by making the patient central to its definition and naming it 'evidence-based practice'. This practice, according to its advocates, entails nurses drawing on the best available research evidence, their clinical expertise and patients' preferences and needs when making clinical decisions and delivering care. Boundary theorists, such as Ernst (2020), argue that nursing has used evidence-based practice in support of their attempt to renegotiate their professional boundary, appealing to the symbolic capital of evidence-based medicine enjoyed by the medical profession. The nurses' assertion of professionalization is based on a real shift in the content of their work with the establishment of new roles, such as advanced practitioners and acute care practice nurses. These roles have expanded nursing knowledge and research, as well as skills such as prescribing and treating patients for minor procedures, using delegated medical skills and knowledge. However, many within nursing argue that professional legitimacy should be obtained by gaining status recognition for care – including hands-on-care (or so-called dirty work) – as it represents the nurse's relationship and proximity to the patient and requires knowledge and skill. Despite the medical profession's resistance, nursing has the potential to successfully challenge medical dominance because the reality is that nursing work encompasses medical and nursing knowledge, clinical skill *and* care.

Boundary struggles incorporate conflicting strategies. Roitenberg (2020) argues that it is difficult for groups to acknowledge both differences and hierarchy at the same time, thus they can both simultaneously deny and assert the same differences (such as role) and similarities (such as shared purpose). This conflict often occurs when there are shared and different co-existing identities, such as shared identity as healthcare workers providing evidence-based practice and different identities as nurses and doctors. Roitenberg, in her study examining ethno-national boundaries of care workers undertaking 'dirty work' in Israel, argues that these contradictory strategies support the contraction of difference and expansion of similarity in moral boundaries. She suggests that a way forward in supporting diversity in healthcare is to focus more on a shared vocation rather than stigmatized differences, such as class, ethnicity or gender.

Conflicting strategies concerned with the feminization of medicine and the gender pay gap are also evident within that profession. Because there are more women in the profession, medical practice is purported by some to have been feminized, developing a more therapeutic, preventative and communicative focus at the expense of a scientific and rational process (Levinson and Lurie, 2004). Levinson and Lurie identify several debates regarding the increased number of women in medicine. For example, medicine's inflexible structural inequalities are considered by some to alienate its female members whilst protecting male supremacy and prestige. Others, they note, argue that the impact of medical training actually neutralizes gender differences, inhibiting the positive values and skills that women bring to the profession. Nevertheless, gender inequalities within medicine appear to be widening. An independent review conducted in the UK, exploring the gender pay gap in medicine, found 'basic gender pay-gaps of 24.4% for HCHS [Hospital and Community Health Service] doctors, 33.5% for GPs and 21.4% for clinical academics. These gaps are considerable for a single occupational group' (Department of Health and Social

Care [DHSC], 2020: v). Similarly, Pelley and Carnes (2020), in a US-based study, found that certain medical specialties have become gender heavy, with women physicians gravitating towards predominately female specialties and men towards those that are predominantly male. This gravitation corresponds to a decline in earnings for doctors in female-dominated specialties accounting for '64% of the variation in salaries among the medical specialties' (p. 1499). They argue that female doctors face constant bias and fall behind their male colleagues in 'leadership attainment, academic advancement and earnings' (p. 1499). These differences have been further highlighted during the COVID-19 pandemic, with some arguing that women physicians are being disproportionately affected due to pre-existing inequalities (Narayana et al., 2020).

The inter-relationships between gender and social class, and gender and professional dominance are well established. It is only recently that research has examined the intersections between ethnicity, class and gender as encountered by formal healthcare providers. Focusing on the trajectories of Malawian-born women, who became nurses in the USA, Semu (2020) offers an insightful qualitative study on the intersections of race, gender and discrimination. She found that despite most nurses coming from middle class, educated backgrounds in their home country, they experienced downward social and occupational mobility once in the USA. Indeed, as a condition of migration, they already had degree level education in, for example, Education, Biology, Computer Programming and Agriculture, but once in the USA were unable to secure employment in those professions due to gender and ethnic discrimination. Forced to switch to nursing, on average it took between 5 to 12 years to retrain and gain employment as a registered nurse, a role seen as more acceptable for women. Furthermore, once employed as nurses, they experienced discrimination via excessive scrutiny of their work and preclusion to job advancement. These nurses even encountered racist stereotyping and rejection from patients and their families who questioned the validity of their professional position and knowledge base. Thus, Semu found that being African, immigrant and female predisposed them to face discrimination from multiple groups. Indeed, Black and Asian healthcare workers are often found in more lowly-paid, disadvantaged positions in formal healthcare. The NHS Workforce Race Equality Standard Report (2019) found that despite an increase in ethnic diversity, white candidates were more likely than other ethnic groups to be appointed to healthcare positions. Further, healthcare professionals from Black and Asian backgrounds were more likely to experience discrimination and bullying and be involved in formal disciplinary processes and were less likely to be promoted.

The need for greater diversity in the healthcare workforce is increasingly acknowledged and actively promoted in some countries because healthcare organizations have been tasked with tackling health inequalities. The link between health disparities in Black and Asian people has been connected to poor representation of such groups in the workforce. This disparity has become a more pressing need in the USA, where the number of white Americans is projected to fall from 78 per cent to 69 per cent, and the number of Hispanics, African Americans, Asian Americans and Native Americans is set to rise from 22 per cent to 31 per cent by 2060 (Wilbur et al., 2020). Wilbur et al. suggest that diversity in the healthcare workforce has increased over the last 10 years, exceeding that of the general population. However, most of the increase is in jobs with lower educational entrance requirements, such as nursing, nursing aides and social care aides.

These existing socio-economic, gender and ethnic divisions within healthcare are also being reinforced by the increasing global movement of migrant workers. The World Health Organization (WHO, 2016) has predicted that the global shortfall of nurses by 2030 will be approximately 7.6 million. Adhikari and Melia (2015: 359) state that the 'maldistribution of the nursing workforce' is a consequence of more affluent countries recruiting nurses and social care workers from low-income countries. They argue this process is due to a declining desirability of nursing as an acceptable career choice, alongside a lack of capacity to educate sufficient numbers of nurses, in more affluent nations. In lower-income countries there is both a lack of capacity to educate and a lack of employment opportunities due to inadequately resourced healthcare systems. The declining desirability of nursing is due in part to its symbolic status that marks nursing as dirty work. Migrants are used to fill less desirable positions, such as caring for older adults or adults with learning disabilities. Further, migrating nurses tend to be those who are the most educated, skilled and specialized (a requirement of immigration), seeking further career advantages elsewhere. Thus, as Adhikari and Melia note, using migrants to fill less desirable positions is a gross misuse of their abilities that results in them quickly becoming de-skilled. Indeed, these researchers found that migrant nurses refer ironically to such work as British Bottom Care (BBC), reflecting the lack of professional developmental opportunities and their frustration with the situation.

The migration of healthcare workers also reflects and reinforces global social divisions and inequalities. Populations in the Global South are left with fewer skilled healthcare workers, contributing further to poorer health outcomes and the ongoing disparity between a currently rich West and the rest of the world. Further, the COVID-19 pandemic has uncomfortably revealed the impact of social and health inequalities in the West. Otu et al. (2020: 1) report that in the first few months of the pandemic the mortality rate among those of Black African descent in English Hospitals was 3.5 times higher than the white British population. Indeed, 'people of BAME backgrounds accounted for 63% of all COVID-19 related deaths among NHS staff' (p. 2). Yet, there is no known genetic reason for the increased mortality rates among Black or Asian people. Rather, Black and Asian healthcare workers are over-represented in frontline roles. They are disproportionately exposed to higher risks within NHS workspaces and have less access to socio-economic resources that attenuate risks (Otu et al., 2020).

In conclusion, social divisions in formal healthcare constitute an important topic for medical sociology, as well as for policy and practice. The complexity of patients' needs necessitates the interdependent and integrated provision of care within and across occupational groups. Inter-professional collaboration and therefore shared responsibility and accountability are requisites. However, tensions and conflicts between and within formal healthcare reflect and reproduce persistent social divisions, including socio-economic, gender, and ethnic inequalities and their intersections. These divisions are also perpetuated by socio-cultural norms predicated in the recruitment, education and organization of service delivery. Social divisions within formal healthcare, therefore, significantly reduce the capacity of workers to draw on the talent of individuals dispersed across all sections of society. This process, which is international, perpetuates and compounds wider social inequalities that directly impact patient/client need. Indeed, in order to address the shortfall in the global healthcare workforce future research should be undertaken with a view to informing efforts to bridge and attenuate social divisions. Such a need has become all too apparent given the social divisions that have been exposed and amplified during the COVID-19 pandemic.

See also: Ethnicity; Health Professional Migration and Integration; Informal Care; Medical Autonomy, Dominance and Decline; Nursing and Midwifery as Occupations; Professions Allied to Medicine.

REFERENCES

Adhikari, R. and Melia, K. (2015) 'The (mis)management of migrant nurses in the UK: a sociological study', *Journal of Nursing Management*, 23: 359–367.

DHSC (2020) *Mend the Gap: The Independent Review into Gender Pay Gaps in Medicine in England*. Online: https://assets.publishing.service.gov.uk/government/uploads/system/uploads/attachment_data/file/944246/Gender_pay_gap_in_medicine_review.pdf

Ernst, J. (2020) 'Professional boundary struggles in the context of healthcare change: the relational and symbolic constitution of nursing ethos in the space of possible professionalisation', *Sociology of Health & Illness*, 42 (7): 1727–1741.

Levinson, W. and Lurie, N. (2004) 'When most doctors are women: what lies ahead?' *Annals of Internal Medicine*, 141 (6): 471–474.

Nancarrow, S. and Borthwick, A. (2005) 'Dynamic professional boundaries in the healthcare workforce', *Sociology of Health & Illness*, 27 (7): 987–919.

Narayana, S., Roy. B., Merriam, S. et al. (2020) 'Minding the gap: organizational strategies to promote gender equity in academic medicine during the COVID-19 pandemic', *Journal of General Internal Medicine*, 34 (12): 3681–3684.

NHS Workforce Race Equality Standard Report (2019) *2018 Data Analysis Reports for the NHS Trusts*. The WRES Implementation team, Publication Gateway Reference Number: 08735.

Otu, A., Ahinkorah, B.O., Ameyaw, E.K. et al. (2020) 'One country, two crises: what Covid-19 reveals about health inequalities among BAME communities in the United Kingdom and the sustainability of its health system?' *International Journal for Equity in Health*, 19: 189. https://doi.org/10.1186/s12939-020-01307-z

Pelley, E. and Carnes, M. (2020) 'When a specialty becomes women's work: trends and implications of specialty gender segregation in medicine', *Academic Medicine*, 95 (10): 1499–1506.

Roitenberg, N. (2020) 'Ethno-national boundaries in the construction of "dirty work" occupational identity: the case of nursing care workers in diversified workplaces', *International Journal of Intercultural Relations*, 76: 1–12.

Sackett, D., Rosenberg, W., Gray, J.A. et al. (1996) 'Evidence based medicine: what it is and what it isn't', *British Medical Journal*, 321: 71.

Semu, L.L. (2020) 'The intersectionality of race and trajectories of African women into the nursing career in the United States', *Behavioral Sciences*, 10 (4): 69. https://doi.org/10.3390/bs10040069

Social Mobility Commission (2016) *The State of the Nation 2016: Social Mobility in Great Britain*. Online: https://assets.publishing.service.gov.uk/government/uploads/system/uploads/attachment_data/file/569410/Social_Mobility_Commission_2016_REPORT_WEB__1__.pdf

Weber, M. (1995) 'Basic concepts of stratification', *Sociological Studies*, 5: 155.

WHO (2016) *Global Strategic Directions for Strengthening Nursing and Midwifery 2016–2020*. World Health Organization. Online: www.who.int/hrh/nursing_midwifery/global-strategic-midwifery2016-2020.pdf?ua=1

Wilbur, K., Snyder, C., Essary, A. et al. (2020) 'Developing workforce diversity in the health professions: a social justice perspective', *Health Professions Education*, 6 (2): 222–229.

SUGGESTED FURTHER READING

- Badejo, O., Sagay, H., Abimbolam S. and Van Belle, S. (2020) 'Confronting power in low places: historical analysis of medical dominance and role-boundary negotiation between health professions in Nigeria', *BMJ Global Health*, 5 (9): e003349.

An interesting article examining medical dominance in Nigeria. The authors advocate carrying out a historical analysis of interprofessional interactions and role-boundary negotiations in order to 'navigate the swampy lowland of professional rivalry and power' (p. 14), moving beyond typical social divisions of social class, gender and ethnicity.

- Cottingham, M. (2019) 'The missing and needed male: discursive hybridization in professional nursing texts', *Gender, Work & Organization*, 26 (2): 197–213.

This article takes a critical approach to the rhetoric regarding the need for men in nursing found in the nursing literature. Cottingham argues that the advantages men have in nursing are ignored, in favour of encouraging men into nursing.

- Nancarrow, S. and Borthwick, A. (2021) *The Allied Health Professions: A Sociological Perspective*. Bristol: Policy Press

This book explores the developing roles of the allied healthcare professions, focusing on the relationship between professional legitimacy and evidence-based practice.

It considers how these professions have been shaped by the socio-political context, offering a comparison between Australia and the UK.

- WHO (2019) *Delivered by Women, Led by Men, a Gender and Equity Analysis of the Global Health and Social Workforce.* World Health Organization Human Resources for Health Observer Series No. 24.

An interesting report arguing that unless gender disparity is addressed, the mismatch between supply and demand in the global healthcare workforce will continue.

45

Health Professional Migration and Integration

Ivy Lynn Bourgeault

Health professional migration typically involves moving from one's country of origin and training to another country to practise. Integration involves the attainment of a license and ability to practise one's profession but also inclusion into the local culture of the host health system and society. These dynamics have implications for the migrating health professional, their source and destination countries.

Health professional migration refers to all forms of temporary and permanent movement across borders, encapsulating emigration – the migration out of countries – and immigration – migration into countries. Such movement sometimes entails transiting through other countries. The integration of health professionals into a host health system involves the attainment of a licence to enable them to practise locally, which often requires bridging or re-training. After providing some recent descriptive data on health professionals' international mobility, the following will focus on the drivers of migration (including colonial legacies), the experiences of migrating and the social, political and economic implications of these dynamic flows.

The migration and integration of health professionals are not new phenomena, but the pace of their migration has accelerated as well as the breadth of countries involved. The healthcare labour market is increasingly global in scope, in part because international trade agreements and globalization policies facilitate labour mobility across national borders. A snapshot of the flow of health professionals into and out of key destination and source countries is instructive. A recent report from the Organisation for Economic Co-operation and Development (OECD, 2019), drawing upon data for doctors and nurses, reveals that migrating health professionals have contributed significantly to the increased growth in overall numbers of clinicians in the past decade. Among OECD countries, approximately one quarter of the medical workforce is *foreign born*. The average percentage is lower for foreign-born registered nurses (RNs) – 16 per cent – but numerically, foreign-born RNs constitute a larger group than foreign-born physicians (MDs). In absolute terms, the USA is the primary destination for the foreign-born MDs and RNs, followed by the UK, Germany, Australia and Canada (OECD, 2019). The proportion of *foreign-trained* health workers is typically lower than for foreign-born, revealing the contribution of destination countries to health worker training. The most recent OECD average is 16 per cent for MDs and 7 per cent for RNs. Again, the USA has the greatest share of foreign-trained doctors and nurses, followed in both cases by the UK (OECD, 2019).

Other important trends include the source of foreign-trained health professionals. Across all OECD countries, the Philippines occupies first place for migrant nurses whilst India figures prominently for migrant doctors and nurses, occupying first and second place respectively, with China being the second highest for migrant doctors (OECD, 2020). These trends are heavily influenced by data from the US. The implications of these data for the sustainability of health systems in the Philippines, India and other source countries are critically important.

Migratory flows of health professionals are intricately linked to key health workforce planning and policy decisions in both destination and source countries. Much of this literature focuses on the factors that *push* health professionals from their country of origin and *pull* them to their destination country (OECD, 2019, 2020). Typical 'push' factors include low pay, poor working conditions, lack of resources to work effectively, limited career and educational opportunities, unstable or dangerous work environments and overall economic instability. Typical 'pull' factors include higher pay, improved working conditions, better-resourced health systems, career opportunities, the provision of post-basic education and opportunities to travel. As recently documented in Smith and Gillin's (2021) research on Filipino nurse migration to the UK, we might also add to this list shared understandings of underlying social structures, a sense of political stability and ontological security.

Whilst the focus on certain 'push' and 'pull' factors tends towards those at an individual level, many factors are influenced by broader structural forces (Bourgeault et al., 2016b). Destination countries such as Canada, the USA and Australia, for example, all draw upon foreign-trained doctors to help address shortages in underserviced, often rural or remote, areas. Foreign-trained nurses are also a critical resource in the older adult care sector in the USA, UK and Canada (Spencer et al., 2010). Decision-makers in these countries have relied on international recruitment as a short-term solution, rather than focusing on the underlying problems that have resulted in domestic shortages in health professionals, including inadequate workforce planning. Such practices and structural considerations should also be placed in a much larger historical context. The migration of health professionals reveals the legacies of colonialization linking source and destination countries, including systems of training in colonized countries reflecting those of their colonizer. McNeil-Walsh (2004), for example, describes how British colonial power shaped the structure of healthcare education in South Africa, which translated into an advantage for South African nurses wishing to migrate to the UK.

Other trends include '*chain migration*', which involves health professionals migrating through certain countries on their way to their ultimate destination. This phenomenon also needs to be more fully taken into consideration in both policy and the literature on health professional migration (Connell, 2010). Originating in countries such as India and the Philippines, health professionals can move through Gulf states like Saudi Arabia and the United Arab Emirates on their way to the UK, the USA and Canada. One must also consider that the situation is more complex than a simple dichotomy because some countries can be both source and destination; Canada and South Africa, for example, experience an outflow but also benefit from an inflow from other even more disadvantaged nations. Thus, it is important to highlight that migration streams are increasing in complexity beyond that depicted by the descriptors of source and destination countries. Nonetheless, these descriptors still reflect a general movement from low- and middle- to high-income countries (Connell, 2010).

International migration and recruitment of health professionals came under sharp criticism in the early 2000s for exacerbating shortages and threatening the sustainability of health systems in low- and middle-income source countries, particularly in sub-Saharan Africa (World Health Organization [WHO], 2006). The controversy focused on the consequences of health professional migration, particularly in terms of severe staff and skill shortages in health systems of many 'source' countries. So called '*brain drain*' issues are salient in source countries for obvious reasons but are not as simple as mapping out the consequences of emigration of their much-needed health professionals. In some source countries, most notably the Philippines and India, there seems to be a *bifurcation* of interests (Palaganas et al., 2017; Walton-Roberts et al., 2017). On the one hand, the migration of health professionals can be seen as a means of achieving development, because of the remittances that health professionals (and nurses in particular) provide to their families back home. On the other hand, there is legitimate concern among some stakeholders with the consequences of the massive migration of their health professionals. Although cited as a model of *managed migration*, basic health indicators in the Philippines have worsened since embarking on an active health labour 'export' policy (Palaganas et al., 2017).

In addition to historical considerations, relating to colonialism, the context for healthcare deficits in 'source' countries that affects health professional migration can be traced to neoliberal policies. These include Structural Adjustment Policies implemented in the 1980s and 1990s by the World Bank and International Monetary Fund in exchange for international loans to a number of low- and middle-income countries. These policies led to severe public sector cutbacks in healthcare systems and the acceptance of various forms of privatization as a condition of these loans. This led to significant underemployment and unemployment of health professionals in the public sector, through layoffs, leaving health professionals with few options other than to migrate for employment (Packer et al., 2008). Although remittances often provide crucial income for families in several 'source' countries, it is important to acknowledge that they remain largely as a private infusion of funds rather than public funds to sustain health systems.

The WHO adopted a Global Code of Practice for the International Recruitment of Health Personnel in 2010, a voluntary tool to better address concerns among source, destination and transit countries. It has three key objectives: (1) ensuring that migration flows do not disrupt health services in source countries; (2) protecting migrant personnel's rights, and (3) providing adequate workplace support for migrant personnel (Connell and Buchan, 2011). The Code also encourages countries to concentrate on health workforce planning to reduce the reliance on international recruitment to shore up shortages that often arise. Although the Code is a significant achievement in international relations, it has unfortunately had a muted impact on policy communities in both source and destination countries (Bourgeault et al., 2016a).

The WHO Code addresses the experience of migrating health professionals in destination countries as well as the implications for source countries. Experiences of deskilling, discrimination, as well as personal and professional isolation of migrant health professionals in their destination country are notable trends in the literature. Depending on their migration pathway – self-initiated versus recruited – the integration outcomes for migrating health professionals can differ dramatically. Research on doctors who self-initiate their migration has long revealed a lack of recognition of their professional training and experience (Bernstein and Shuval, 1998), in some cases barring them from practising in their destination country.

In Canada, where its points-based immigration system enables migration but not necessarily labour market integration into highly regulated professions, there has been a longstanding concern with '*brain waste*' (Bourgeault, 2007). In response, several policy initiatives have been undertaken to better inform migrating health professionals of the necessary steps in the integration process in Canada; to create specific programmes to bridge the competency gap between international and local requirements; and to address associated economic and linguistic barriers to professional integration (Bourgeault, 2007). Bridging or adaptation programs are a common policy response to health professional integration across destination countries, enabling what Neiterman and Bourgeault (2015) describe as a form of *professional resocialization* into local health systems.

Even when licensed in their destination country, migrating health professionals can experience significant discrimination. This problem is evidenced by their concentration in the lowest echelons of the profession and less prestigious practice settings, and assignment to more onerous tasks, all of which are particularly notable if professionals' migrant status intersects with their racialization (Semu,

2020). Such workers often feel prejudice from and alienated by their colleagues (Neiterman et al., 2015), but they are also subject to discrimination by patients, including having their authority questioned (Bernstein and Shuval, 1998; Semu, 2020). Migrating health professionals are often confronting an explicit 'othering' and a constant comparison with locally born and trained clinicians. These experiences, however, attenuate the longer they are in their destination country.

Finally, policies and interventions intended to fight the COVID-19 pandemic have translated into a remarkable geographic immobility, including that of migrating health professionals. The longstanding impact remains to be seen. It is clear, however, that the enormous strain that has been placed on health professionals during the pandemic causes concern for the sustainability of health workforces in source, transit and destination countries. As such, a rise in the international recruitment of health professionals to redress shortages is anticipated causing a greater imbalance of human resources for health. Going forward, the implications of the pandemic for the movement of health professionals globally is an area where medical sociology ought to focus its attention.

See also: Ethnicity; Informal Care; Nursing and Midwifery as Occupations; Social Divisions in Formal Healthcare.

REFERENCES

Bernstein, J. and Shuval, J.T. (1998) 'The occupational integration of former Soviet physicians in Israel', *Social Science & Medicine*, 47 (6): 809–819.

Bourgeault, I.L. (2007) 'Brain drain, brain gain and brain waste: programs aimed at integrating and retaining the best and the brightest in health care', Special Issue of *Canadian Issues/Thèmes canadiens*, Spring: 96–99.

Bourgeault, I.L., Labonte, R., Packer, C. et al. (2016a) 'Knowledge and potential impact of the WHO Global Code of Practice on the International Recruitment of Health Personnel: does it matter for source and destination country stakeholders?' *Human Resources for Health – special supplement on the WHO Code.* 14 (Supl. 1). Online: https://human-resources-health.biomedcentral.com/articles/10.1186/s12960-016-0128-5

Bourgeault, I.L., Wrede, S., Benoit, C. and Neiterman, E. (2016b) 'Professions and the migration of expert labour: towards an intersectional analysis of transnational mobility patterns and integration pathways of health professionals', in M. Dent, I.L. Bourgeault, E. Kuhlmann and J.L. Denis (eds), *The Routledge Handbook on Professions and Professionalism*. London: Routledge.

Connell, J. (2010) *Migration and the Globalisation of Health Care: The Health Worker Exodus?* Cheltenham: Edward Elgar Publishing.

Connell, J. and Buchan, J. (2011) 'The impossible dream? Codes of practice and the international migration of skilled health workers', *World Medical & Health Policy*, 3 (3): 1–17.

McNeil-Walsh, C. (2004) 'Widening the discourse: a case for the use of post-colonial theory in the analysis of South African nurse migration to Britain', *Feminist Review*, 77 (1): 120–124.

Neiterman, E. and Bourgeault, I.L. (2015) 'Professional integration as a process of professional resocialization: internationally educated health professionals in Canada', *Social Science & Medicine*, 131: 74–81.

Neiterman, E., Salmonsson, L. and Bourgeault, I.L. (2015) 'Navigating through otherness and belonging: a comparative case study of international medical graduates' professional integration in Canada and Sweden', *Ephemera: Theory & Politics in Organization*, 15 (4): 773–795.

OECD (2019) *Recent Trends in International Migration of Doctors, Nurses and Medical Students.* Paris: OECD Publishing.

OECD (2020) *Contributions of migrant doctors and nurses to tackling COVID-19 crisis in OECD countries*, 13 May. Online: www.oecd.org/coronavirus/policy-responses/contribution-of-migrant-doctors-and-nurses-to-tackling-covid-19-crisis-in-oecd-countries-2f7bace2/

Packer, C., Labonté, R. and Spitzer, D. (2008) *Globalization and Health Worker Migration.* Globalization Knowledge Network. WHO Commission on the Social Determinants of Health.

Palaganas, E., Spitzer, D., Kabamalan, M.M.M. et al. (2017) 'An examination of the causes, consequences, and policy responses to the migration of highly trained health personnel from the Philippines: the high cost of living/leaving – a mixed method study', *Human Resources for Health*, 15 (25). https://doi.org/10.1186/s12960-017-0198-z

Semu, L.L. (2020) 'The intersectionality of race and trajectories of African women into the nursing career in the United States', *Behavioral Sciences*, 10 (4): 69. Online: https://doi.org/10.3390/bs10040069

Smith, D.M. and Gillin, N. (2021) 'Filipino nurse migration to the UK: understanding migration choices from an ontological security-seeking perspective', *Social Science & Medicine*, 276: 113881.

Spencer, S., Martin, S., Bourgeault, I.L. and O'Shea, E., (2010) *The Role of Migrant Care Workers in Ageing Societies: Report on Research Findings in the U.K., Ireland, the U.S. and Canada.* IOM Migration Research Series No. 41. Online: http://publications.iom.int/bookstore/free/MRS41.pdf

Walton-Roberts, M., Runnels, V., Rajan, S.I. et al. (2017) 'Causes, consequences and policy responses to the migration of health workers: key findings from India', *Human Resources for Health*, 15 (28). https://doi.org/10.1186/s12960-017-0199-y

WHO (2006) *Working Together for Health. 2006 World Health Report.* Geneva: WHO.

WHO (2010) *WHO Global Code of Practice on the International Recruitment of Health Personnel.* Online: www.who.int/hrh/migration/code/WHO_global_code_of_practice_EN.pdf

SUGGESTED FURTHER READING

- Bourgeault, I.L., Runnels, V., Atanackovic, J. et al. (2021) 'Hiding in plain sight: gendered dimensions of health worker migration', *Human Resources for Health*, 19 (40): 1–12.

The literature on health worker migration from key source countries such as the Philippines, India and South Africa reveals that gender can mediate access to and participation in health worker training, employment and ultimately migration. Regardless of these underlying influences in migration decision-making, gender is rarely considered either as an important contextual influence or analytic category in the policy responses. In this paper, this lack of explicit attention is described as leading to inadequate policy responses.

- Hochschild, A.R. (2000) 'Global care chains and emotional surplus value', in W. Hutton and A. Giddens (eds), *On the Edge: Living with Global Capitalism*. London: Jonathan Cape.

Hochschild first coined the term 'global care chains' to denote how migrant care workers fill the care deficits left by women's increased labour force participation in destination countries, but this in turn creates care deficits in the migrants' countries of origin. These transfers of paid and unpaid care labour from women in low- and middle- to high-income countries impact children, families and countries across the globe. The care deficits in the migrant workers' countries are largely borne by grandmothers, aunts and daughters left at home, albeit often buoyed by the remittances that migrant care workers in high-income countries are able to provide.

- Yeates, N. (2004) 'A dialogue with "global care chain" analysis: nurse migration in the Irish context', *Feminist Review*, 77: 79–95.

Although Hochschild, cited above, discusses domestic workers and nannies when proposing the concept of 'global care chains', Yeates argues that it can apply equally to the highly-skilled nursing labour sector. This article focuses on the longstanding migration of Irish nurses to England and other destinations.

- Walton-Roberts, M. (2015) 'International migration of health professionals and the marketization and privatization of health education in India: from push–pull to global political economy', *Social Science & Medicine*, 124: 374–382.

Walton-Roberts explores the role of education systems in producing internationally oriented health professionals. She advocates for a global political economy perspective that highlights how educational investment and migration tendencies are increasingly interlinked. She draws this out through a case study of the globally oriented nature of Indian nurse training, and how it reflects wider marketization tendencies evident in India's education and health systems.

46

Complementary and Alternative Medicine

Sarah Cant

Complementary and alternative medicine (CAM) refers to a broad set of therapeutic theories and practices, distinct from those of biomedicine and allied therapies.

CAM is a convenient, if imperfect, shorthand used to describe a wide array of therapeutic knowledges that are largely practised by non-biomedically qualified practitioners, and which tend to be offered outside state-endorsed and state-financed healthcare. Despite this positioning, CAM constitutes a significant feature of global healthcare provision, with variations in usage patterns, access and status broadly, but not uniformly, linked to whether it is practised in the Global South or the Global North.

Ranging from complete medical systems such as acupuncture, to diagnostic and healing practices such as reflexology and meditation, and including specific interventions such as colonic irrigation, the modalities included in this category vary considerably in their histories, scope and therapeutic claims. It is estimated that there are over 200 CAMs available within the UK, although there operates a distinct, if politically shaped, hierarchy. The House of Lords (2000: 2.1) used a tripartite grouping that remains the only official form of classification. The most popular and well established 'big 5' (Acupuncture, Chiropractic, Herbalism, Homeopathy and Osteopathy) are categorized as 'Principal' and 'professionally organised'. In contrast, therapies such as Shiatsu and Yoga are defined as 'complementary without diagnostic capacity'. Finally, Ayurvedic medicine, Traditional Chinese Medicine, and Eastern Medicine (Unani Tibb) are acknowledged as long established, but are regarded as 'indifferent to scientific principles of conventional medicine'. Consequently, CAM is not a homogeneous entity: it encompasses a complex, contested and controversial terrain, unified only by its distinctiveness from modern biomedicine. Moreover, any discussion of CAM requires consideration of its relationship with biomedicine which limits its role in the medical marketplace, shapes its own professional projects, frames judgements about its status and efficacy, and goes some way to explain its attraction to consumers.

Porter's (1992) edited text details the diversity of therapeutic practices and techniques available in Britain from 1650 to 1850, sometimes simultaneously practised by 'scientific' medical doctors. However, the passing of the Medical Registration Act in 1858 underscored the emergence of a strongly coalesced biomedical identity and community, paved the way for a state-endorsed bio-medical monopoly in NHS delivery, and sounded the death-knell for most other therapeutic systems. By the 1970s, biomedical epistemological authority was secured across the globe, described as a 'tool of Empire' (Lock and Nguyen, 2010), and accentuated by claims of objectivity, efficacy and scientific authority.

However, this biomedical monopoly stands as an atypical historical moment: spiralling costs, the persistence of chronic and degenerative diseases, the recognition of the iatrogenic effects of some biomedical interventions, alongside new opportunities to (re)learn about other medical systems and an appetite to explore different conceptions of self and well-being, provided the context for CAM to regain some popularity. By the 1980s, a 'new' variant of 'Western' medical plural-ism – where differing medical traditions co-exist – had taken root (Cant, 2020). In the Global South, the World Health Organization concurrently recognized that it was important to support traditional, Indigenous medicines to secure healthcare in the face of unmet need and population growth. It was also acknowledged that local therapeutic modalities chimed with cultural traditions and preferences, as well as sponsored nationalistic sentiments. Consequently, many non-biomedical systems became state-endorsed. For instance, the Department of AYUSH (Ayur-veda, Yoga, Unani, Siddha and Homeopathy) is central in the Ministry of Health and Family Welfare in India (Sujatha and Abraham, 2012).

Despite this, the power of biomedicine to shape the practice and reach of CAM has remained strong. This is most apparent in its naming. Various nomen-clature, ranging from 'fringe' and 'quackery', through to 'unconventional' and 'non-orthodox' medicine have been applied, but the current preference – 'complementary' or 'alternative' – continues to situate and understand all 'oth-er' therapeutic modalities in terms of their relationship to biomedicine. As in all forms of binary othering, a status hierarchy is suggested. CAM implies that Western colonial biomedicine is the norm, the yardstick to be judged against. In turn, biomedical epistemologies and standards of evidence determine the legiti-macy and positioning of CAM in the marketplace. Biomedical influence is also illustrated through the internal professionalization strategies undertaken by CAM groups, and the limited success they have enjoyed in terms of integration into state-provided healthcare, especially in the Global North (Cant, 2020).

While the early renaissance of CAM in the UK was characterized by ad hoc, informal teaching and open access, perceived hostility from the powerful biomedical lobby prompted CAM groups to engage in their own professional projects (Cant, 2020; Gale, 2014). This involved mimicry of biomedicine through the establishment of training schools and the inclusion of biomedical syllabi. There were also clear attempts to temper knowledge claims. Within non-medical Homeopathy, for instance, there was a conscious distancing from the druidic foundations that had instigated the revival of this therapeutic practice in the 1970s, a careful re-framing of controversial aspects of their knowledge base (such as 'the vital force'), and an acceptance of the need to limit their therapeutic claims. However, the success of these changes has been limited because, with the exception of Osteopathy and Chiropractic, they have not resulted in the state regulation of CAM practice.

Nevertheless, there is some evidence of rapprochement with biomedicine. The British Medical Association issued a first report in 1986, unashamedly designed to discredit 'alternative' therapies on the grounds of their 'unscientificity', but followed this with a more conciliatory report seven years later, focused on 'complementary' practice, albeit with the preference that biomedical doctors supervise and/or practice CAM. However, hostility from biomedicine remains (Lewis, 2019), and where integration has been enabled it has tended to be associated with more residual medical arenas – those with lower status and where biomedical interventions have little success, or where there are limited curative opportunities (for example, end of life care). Research focused on operational practices within integrative clinics has also established that CAM remains symbolically, structurally, epistemologically and economically marginalized (see, for example, Cant et al., 2011). As such, the positioning of CAM can be described as mainstream but marginal – widely used, but structurally disadvantaged in the medical marketplace.

CAM's popularity is evidenced through numerous surveys which suggest that between a quarter and a third of people in the UK and USA have consulted a CAM practitioner (for a review, see Cant and Watts, 2019). Nevertheless, users, in the main, come from a discrete demographic (middle-class, middle-aged and women), continue to use biomedicine, and tend to turn to CAM for limited or intractable conditions. Taken together, the popularity of CAM and its socio-demographic profile suggest a number of sociological questions, and throw some light on the dissatisfactions with biomedicine.

The revival of CAM in the Global North has been variously understood as emblematic of the postmodern condition, a radical and new social movement, and an inevitable product of neoliberal capitalism and consumerism, as well as an agent of change (Brosnan et al., 2018). Its popularity is linked to the rise of individualism with its concomitant emphasis on self-improvement and increased scepticism towards experts. Additionally, users are described as being drawn towards ideas of holism and harmony with nature, and the desire to have a more active role in defining and maintaining their health and healthcare needs, based on collaborative relationships with healthcare providers (Gale, 2014).

The correlation between use and gender has prompted sociologists to posit an association between CAM and feminist campaigns, seeing the former as an alternative space to develop gender-sensitive healthcare (Cant and Watts, 2012). While it should be remembered that women are also the primary consumers of biomedicine, various studies have shown that women turn to CAM for female-specific events or conditions such as pregnancy and menopause – areas heavily critiqued as sites of (bio)medicalization. CAM is described as empowering, providing an internalized 'power from within' (Keshet and Simchai, 2014: 77), a means to resist dominant biomedical definitions, assert ownership and self-responsibility over health, and offering opportunities to navigate new forms of self-hood (see Suggested Further Reading).

Whilst insightful, it is important to introduce some caution into these analyses. First, the research tends to be ethnocentric, focused on privileged, middle-class women in the Global North who can afford to use CAM and who, in so doing, reinforce dominant ideologies that emphasize individual responsibility and support the commercialization of therapies. In contrast, in India, for instance, it is women and the poor who tend to use Homeopathy, as it is a cheaper option compared to biomedical care (see Suggested Further Reading). Second, the focus on women's engagement has diverted attention away from understanding usage patterns by men and by ethnicity. Cant and Watts (2019) have shown that men's use of CAM is far from insignificant. Men also tend to consult CAM practitioners for male-specific health conditions such as impotency and prostate cancer, or conditions with a higher prevalence, such as HIV/AIDs. These are health conditions that arguably position men in a marginal relationship to the dominant discourse of masculinity, and where the biomedical emphasis on restoration of function can be experienced as disempowering and alienating.

It may be contended that marginal positioning is also a defining feature of use amongst minority ethnic groups, linked to racial discrimination. Migration is central to understanding the renaissance of CAM in the UK: mobile populations brought their therapeutic modalities with them, and migratory experiences help explain the attraction of using CAM alongside biomedicine. Traditional healing, especially recourse to the Hakim (that is, a 'wise man' who practices Unani medicine), has been shown to be commonly used by British Asians to assert cultural identity. And migrant Chinese women often turn to CAM when discrimination or communication difficulties block their access to biomedicine (see Cant and Watts, 2012; Cant, 2020, for a review).

The sociology of CAM has provided significant insight on consumer motivations, but has also tended to have been rather uncritical. To remedy this emphasis, sociologists have also explored how CAM is implicated in processes of medicalization and surveillance (see Suggested Further Reading). It has been suggested that there is a tendency in CAM practice towards a moralistic promotion of self-care which, in turn, reproduces neoliberal forms of governance and individualized conceptions of health. Scott (1999) describes the focus upon wider self-holism (as opposed to wider world-holism) as having the unintended consequence of elevating individual responsibility and failing to question how social and environmental structures might account for ill-health. It is also the case that the sociological study of the relationship between biomedicine and CAM has largely ignored the impact of colonialism (Gale, 2014), and it is important to understand the long history of appropriation and assimilation of Indigenous knowledges by drawing on post/anti-colonial theory (Cant, 2020).

CAM is a mainstream component of healthcare in most societies, and this historically contingent social phenomenon is worthy of, and should be subject to, ongoing sociological analyses. The sociology of CAM provides a rich seam of research opportunities and remains central to medical and generic sociology, providing insight on the operation of inequality, power and empowerment, patriarchy, governance, neoliberalism, capitalism, (post) colonialism and individualization.

See also: Consumerism; The Medical Model; Trust in Medicine.

REFERENCES

Brosnan, C., Vuolanto, P. and Brodin Danell, J-A. (2018) *Complementary and Alternative Medicine: Knowledge Production and Social Transformation*. London: Palgrave Macmillan.

Cant, S. (2020) 'Medical pluralism, mainstream marginality or subaltern therapeutics? Globalisation and the integration of "Asian" medicines and biomedicine in the UK', *Society and Culture in South Asia*, 6 (1): 32–51.

Cant, S. and Watts, P. (2012) 'Complementary and alternative medicine: gender and marginality', in E. Kuhlmann and E. Annandale (eds), *The Palgrave Handbook of Gender and Healthcare*. London: Palgrave Macmillan.

Cant, S. and Watts, P. (2019) 'Hidden in plain sight: exploring men's use of complementary and alternative medicine', *The Journal of Men's Studies*, 27 (1): 45–65.

Cant, S., Watts, P. and Ruston, A. (2011) 'Negotiating competency, professionalism and risk: the integration of complementary and alternative medicine by nurses and midwives in NHS hospitals', *Social Science & Medicine*, 72 (4): 529–536.

Gale, N.K. (2014) 'The sociology of traditional, complementary and alternative medicine', *Sociology Compass*, 8 (6): 805–822.

House of Lords Select Committee on Science and Technology (2000) *Report on Complementary and Alternative Medicine*. London: Stationary Office.

Keshet, Y. and Simchai, D. (2014) 'The "gender puzzle" of alternative medicine and holistic spirituality: a literature review', *Social Science & Medicine*, 113: 77–86.

Lewis, M. (2019) 'De-legitimising complementary medicine: framings of the Friends of Science in Medicine-CAM debate in Australian media reports', *Sociology of Health & Illness*, 41 (5): 831–851.

Lock, M. and Nguyen, V.K. (2010) *An Anthropology of Biomedicine*. Chichester: Wiley Blackwell.

Porter, R. (ed.) (1992) *The Popularisation of Medicine, 1650–1850*. London: Routledge.

Scott, A.L. (1999) 'Paradoxes of holism: some problems in developing an anti-oppressive medical practice', *Health*, 3 (2): 131–149.

Sujatha, V. and Abraham, L. (2012) *Medical Pluralism in Contemporary India*. Hyderabad: Orient BlackSwan.

SUGGESTED FURTHER READING

- Sointu, E. (2011) 'Detraditionalisation, gender and alternative and complementary medicines', *Sociology of Health & Illness*, 33 (3): 356–371.

This article reveals the variable appeal of CAM among men and women in the UK, drawing from 44 qualitative interviews. Although the findings reflect specific cultural and economic hierarchies and are by no means universal, the study usefully explores how modern selfhood, traditional gender roles and life trajectories are renegotiated through CAM use.

- Broom, A., Doron, A. and Tovey, P. (2009) 'The inequalities of medical pluralism: hierarchies of health, the politics of tradition and the economies of care in Indian oncology', *Social Science & Medicine*, 69 (5): 698–706.

Broom and colleagues found that women with cancer in India were likely to employ traditional medicines because their lack of status and value to the family meant they were denied access to biomedical treatment. The authors caution against generic explanations for the attraction of CAM, suggesting the advocacy of medical pluralism can conceal important forms of social inequality and cultural divides.

- Fries, C.J. (2008) 'Governing the health of the hybrid self: integrative medicine, neoliberalism, and the shifting biopolitics of subjectivity', *Health Sociology Review*, 17 (4): 353–367.

Drawing on Foucauldian analyses, Fries contemplates how CAM's holistic focus permits surveillance into all aspects of human life and constitutes a pervasive form of biopower – operating to analyse, control, regulate and define human subjectivity and behaviour. Fries suggests that integrative medicine is 'fashioned as a technology for the neoliberal governance of "body, mind, heart, and soul"' (p. 363). This provides an interesting contrast to Sointu's (2011) work, above, with CAM seen here as a mechanism of power rather than being empowering.

- Sered, S. and Agigian, A. (2008) 'Holistic sickening: breast cancer and the discursive worlds of complementary and alternative practitioners', *Sociology of Health & Illness*, 30 (4): 616–631.

Drawing on 46 interviews with CAM practitioners, this article shows how holistic explanations for disease (in this case breast cancer) move beyond biology to encompass all aspects of human life. In this way, CAM practitioners, when compared to biomedical doctors, ascribe greater individual responsibility for illness. The authors refer to this as 'holistic sickening' – a 'discursive process' that extends from a discrete disease entity to myriad aspects of life that are deemed problematic, ranging from character to the environment.

47

Emotional Labour

Catherine Theodosius

Emotional labour (EL) is the induction or suppression of feeling in order to sustain
an outward appearance that produces an emotion in others. EL is controlled by
employers and can be seen as a commodity that has exchange value, even though it
draws on a deep sense of self that is integral to the individual.

American sociologist Arlie Russell Hochschild developed the term EL during
the 1970s. She was interested in how emotion was used as a commercial commodity to sell products, images and organizations. She drew on the work of
Goffman, Dewey, Gerth, C. Wright Mills, Freud and Darwin to create a bio-
psycho-social interactionist approach towards emotion and how it is managed.
She suggested that through socialization individuals learn how to manage their
emotions based on feeling rules. Feeling rules are moral social values that act
as internal and external constraints on what emotions should be displayed and
exchanged in differing social situations. For example, it is acceptable to laugh
at a party and cry at a funeral irrespective of one's actual feelings. Hochschild
termed this 'emotion work', because the management of emotions takes work
to achieve.

Socially appropriate emotions are displayed through surface or deep acting.
Surface acting is where an individual pretends to feel an emotion they do not
really feel for the benefit of the social group, for example, laughing at a joke
they do not find funny. In deep acting, the individual draws on feelings they
have learnt through their emotion memory or imagination to generate feelings
that they experience as real. For example, by remembering what it felt like

when one fell over, it is possible to generate a feeling of sympathy for a friend who has just fallen.

Hochschild maintained that private emotion work is exploited in the workplace, where it undergoes transmutation into emotional labour, a saleable commodity that is subject to the supply and demand of market forces. EL therefore is sold for a wage and has exchange value. Drawing on empirical data on the EL of flight attendants and bill collectors, Hochschild argued that commercial companies train their workers in what emotions they can or cannot display. Their EL requires them to 'induce or suppress feeling in order to sustain the outward countenance that produces the proper state of mind in others' (1983: 7). This proper state of mind in others is used to deliver the product the company is selling. In the case of the flight industry this has traditionally been a pleasant, predictable and efficient travel experience that encourages contented customers to re-use the airline. Irrespective of their actual feelings, therefore, flight attendants are not allowed to display anger, frustration or anxiety towards customers, but are expected to display geniality and hospitality. The flight attendants' EL is taught and monitored by the company. However, when the flight industry expanded with the arrival of budget airlines, 'speed up' occurred in service delivery. With a massive increase in passenger numbers the time and consideration spent on EL was significantly reduced. Whilst EL consequently became less valuable to airlines, they still expected flight attendants to carry it out, resulting in the attendants experiencing emotional inauthenticity and alienation of self.

EL also occurs in other forms of employment, including health and social care where practitioners have to be attentive to and/or produce an emotional state in their patients or clients. Thus, Hochschild's theory has wider relevance, particularly in respect to the capitalist exploitation of workers, social inequalities such as gender and alienation or loss of self-authenticity. However, the application of the EL concept to the caring professions is not straightforward and practical considerations warrant careful consideration, especially among nurse educators. For Theodosius (2008), nurses perform EL though it is not the same as that of flight attendants due to the recipients' vulnerability and the type of bodywork performed. Also mindful that nurses, like flight attendants, risk exploitation and the devaluation of labour largely performed by women, she makes several recommendations. In particular, nurses should be taught about EL with an eye on how their sense of self-worth tends to be connected to caring and how this needs to be facilitated and constantly developed. In so doing, nurses would be better able to practise EL without fear of exposing their private self and respond more effectively to changes in the division of labour and increasingly consumer-orientated patients' needs. Further, the various ways in which nurses carry out EL need to be defined and contextualized with reference to different nursing roles. When advancing her argument, Theodosius developed a typology of EL that connects its purpose in nursing practice to the relationships that nurses form and how they draw on their sense of self in the process. She defines *therapeutic EL* as pertaining to the patient/relatives' emotional and psychological well-being and connected to the nurse's sense of self-worth. *Instrumental EL* concerns the patient's physical well-being and is connected to the nurse's self-worth and practical competency. *Collegial EL* relates to emotion interactions between healthcare professionals in order to collectively meet their patients' multiple, complex healthcare needs. Collegial EL is linked to the nurse's self-worth and their place in the social organization's hierarchy.

Others argue that EL in nursing is in fact similar to emotion *work* rather than emotional *labour*, which is controlled by employers for commercial gain. For Bolton (2000: 584), 'the emotion work nurses offer to patients is given with little or no expectation of a return on their investment' and, as such, it is a gift. As a gift, emotion work can be given freely or not at all. The choice to give EL implies it is not an accountable requirement of nursing work. However, nurses are held accountable for their EL by their employer, their professional body *and* by those they care for. Such accountability may ultimately result in the loss of their professional registration, precluding them from finding similar employment elsewhere. Further, Theodosius (2008) argues that Bolton's position is to misunderstand the reciprocal exchange of emotion that takes place in the giving of care and receiving of thanks between nurses, patients and their relatives. Seeing emotion work as a gift also fails to acknowledge that patients are vulnerable and have no choice but to trust those who care for them and effectively have power over them. By acknowledging EL as a component of nursing practice, nurses are made accountable for that care.

Bolton (2000) also asserts that the autonomy healthcare professionals have over their 'emotion work' means it is not sufficiently commodified to result in exploitation or alienation. In North America, however, sociologists interested in the relationship between EL and alienation have identified that repetitive faking of one's emotion in surface acting EL results in emotional dissonance. Brotheridge and Lee's (2003) work has been instrumental in developing a valid EL measure in which the intensity, frequency and variety of EL can be gauged. The availability of a validated measure has enabled researchers to establish a positive correlation between surface acting EL and burnout and intention to leave nursing (Theodosius et al., 2020). Critically, however, the sociological significance of status, power and gender embedded within organizational structure and feeling/display rules in Hochschild's (1983) theory are lost when EL is broken down into variables. Research examining the relationship between EL and burnout does not take into account the social causes of emotional dissonance or explain its relationship with professional autonomy. It is worth adding that the association between EL surface acting and burnout has been established across a plethora of work environments inclusive of the commercial workplace, the police and the legal and teaching professions, as well as amongst social workers and other healthcare professionals (Theodosius et al., 2020). Further, in nursing these studies span a wide range of healthcare systems and cultures such as Japan, Iran, the USA, Canada as well as the UK and Europe. Accordingly, it appears that the exploitative nature of EL is not limited to a particular healthcare system, nor the employee–employer relationship, nor can burnout be seen only from the perspective of those with burnout.

Other research is also noteworthy when conceptualizing the delivery of care for a wage as EL. Focusing on care workers in private residential homes, Johnson (2015) argues that the moral values embedded in feeling rules that shape EL are used to exploit these employees. She contends that because carers are predisposed and encouraged by the company to see their EL as being natural, altruistic and its own reward, this makes them vulnerable to economic exploitation. However, she argues that carers also draw on similar feeling rules 'to feel a sense of moral righteousness in defending the moral interests of the residents against the commercial interests of their employer' (p. 123). She argues that the contrasting use of these feeling rules constitutes a form of ersatz morality. Johnson's insight on the moral character of EL is significant when its gendered nature is underscored.

Hochschild's (1983) insight that EL is gendered and predominantly carried out by women is clearly evidenced in nursing. Men only constitute an average of 10 to 12 per cent of the nursing workforce in the UK and USA. This imbalance is largely due to the stereotypical image of nurses as kind, nurturing and caring women, representing gendered social norms and feeling rules about their presumed innate nature. Smith (2012) argues that the gendered image of nursing is central to the recruitment process, with decisions made on how well candidates can demonstrate caring attributes. The common belief that caring is innate is also crucial to patients' expectations of nursing and underpins public trust. Smith argues, however, that the nursing profession needs to challenge the belief that a nurse either is or is not caring; rather, as Hochschild (1983) demonstrates, EL is a skill that can be taught and refined. Indeed, whilst emotional skills are often considered inherent, they are also seen as less important than clinical skills. Smith (2012) suggests this is due to the low status accorded to emotion management skills underpinning care in contrast to more reasoned, evidence-based clinical and medical work. Yet, when performed by men who are nurses, EL is not necessarily devalued but is instead credited in various ways.

Simpson (2007) found that the gendered nature of EL can favour male nurses who accrue respect for being caring. Indeed, their EL might be considered philanthropic in contrast to women's supposedly innate and undervalued EL. More recently, researchers suggest that 'the rise of the male nurse' (Elliott, 2017: 1074) has increased the value placed upon EL by the public and medical profession. Indeed, Vinson and Underman (2020: 1) suggest clinical empathy practiced by physicians is an example of EL. Clinical empathy, a form of reason, is 'operationalized' by the physicians and 'used instrumentally to smooth' their work (p. 1). Clinical empathy here represents a more detached form of EL that serves the physicians' role, moving away from the feminized representation of EL in nursing. These authors also emphasize Hochschild's (1983) original point about the commercialization of EL. They argue that for physicians in the USA, it is about increasing patient satisfaction to support the 'increasingly consumer-driven and for-profit provision of healthcare' (Vinson and Underman, 2020: 7). Thus, they take EL in healthcare back to Hochschild's roots, but via a more masculinized route that makes EL instrumental and operationalized.

Whilst men who are nurses may garner greater respect for their individual EL practice than their female counterparts, this has not affected the overall status of EL in nursing as a profession. In the UK, for example, the appalling care uncovered at Mid Staffordshire NHS Trust and the subsequent Francis Report (2010) negatively impacted on the image of nurses as 'naturally kind'. Smith (2012: 34) notes that the Francis Report, published shortly after the introduction of all graduate nursing, resulted in nurses being accused of being 'too posh to wash'. This accusation led to the suggestion that 'equipping nurses with technical and academic expertise renders them less compassionate and able to care' (Smith, 2012: 34). The idea that having a degree renders somebody uncaring is illogical but is applied to nursing as a genuine concern. Indeed, the suggestion that kindness and intelligence are incompatible is an irrational argument not levelled at any other caring profession (Willis Commission, 2012). The hostility expressed towards nursing being an all-graduate profession reflects the strong societal belief that the ability to care is inherent and the desire to care vocationally motivated (Smith, 2012). Thus, graduate education in nursing is perceived to threaten the nurse's ability to genuinely care for their patients. Further, there are nurses who express similar beliefs. Thus Johnson's (2015) assertion that ersatz morality is being used by commercial organizations to exploit workers can arguably be seen in public nursing too.

In sum, despite some contestation and complexity when applied outside of her original research context, Hochschild's (1983) seminal concept of EL remains relevant to healthcare and particularly to nursing. It highlights sociological concerns with personal and social identity, power, exploitation, social stratification (such as gender and the division of labour) and alienation. There remains, however, a need to challenge the 'predominant organisation of health care as an institution governed by a masculine model of professionalism and the medical model of detached care' (Erickson and Grove, 2008: 722). Indeed, the COVID-19 pandemic has raised the import of EL in both public and professional domains (Hayes et al., 2020). The heightened significance of EL is due to its embodied and relational dimensions, which do not lend themselves to being 'separated by plastic sheeting, the anonymising of facial features and the homogenising of appearance in human interaction via the necessity for PPE [personal protective equipment]' (Hayes et al., 2020: 322). Arguably, however, PPE does obfuscate both gender and professional divisions of status and power, without lessening the requirement of healthcare workers' capacity, ability and accountability to carry out EL in highly dangerous and complex situations. How the concept of EL will evolve in light of the COVID-19 pandemic is yet to be revealed. It is nonetheless certain that EL remains both relevant and dynamic, highlighting significant societal challenges and social inequalities.

See also: Consumerism; Emotions; Informal Care; Nursing and Midwifery as Occupations.

REFERENCES

Bolton, S.C. (2000) 'Who cares? Offering emotion work as a "gift" in the nursing labour process', *Journal of Advanced Nursing*, 32 (3): 580–586.

Brotheridge, C.M. and Lee, R.T. (2003) 'Development and validation of the emotional labour scale', *Journal of Occupational Health Psychology*, 76 (3): 365–379.

Elliott, C. (2017) 'Emotional labour: learning from the past, understanding the present', *British Journal of Nursing*, 26 (19): 1070–1077.

Erickson, R.J. and Grove, W.J.C. (2008) 'Emotional labour and health care', *Sociology Compass*, 2 (2): 704–733.

Hayes, C., Corrie, I. and Graham, Y. (2020) 'Paramedic emotional labour during COVID-19', *Journal of Paramedic Practice*, 12 (18): 319–323.

Hochschild, A. (1983) *The Managed Heart*. Berkeley: University of California Press.

Johnson, E.K. (2015) 'The business of care: the moral labour of care workers', *Sociology of Health & Illness*, 37 (1): 112–126.

Simpson, R. (2007) 'Emotional labour and identity work of men in caring roles', in P. Lewis and R. Simpson (eds), *Gendering Emotions in Organisations*. Houndsmill: Palgrave.

Smith, P. (2012) *The Emotional Labour of Nursing Revisited*, 2nd edn. Basingstoke: Macmillan Press.

The Francis Report (2010) *Independent Inquiry into Care Provided by Mid Staffordshire NHS Foundation Trust January 2005 to March 2009*. Online: www.gov.uk/government/publications/independent-inquiry-into-care-provided-by-mid-staffordshire-nhs-foundation-trust-january-2001-to-march-2009

The Willis Commission (2012) *Quality with Compassion: The Future of Nursing Education*. Online: https://cdn.ps.emap.com/wp-content/uploads/sites/3/2012/11/Willis-Commission-report-2012.pdf

Theodosius, C. (2008) *Emotional Labour in Health Care: The Unmanaged Heart of Nursing*. London: Routledge.

Theodosius, C., Koulougliotti, C., Kersten, P. and Rosten, C. (2020) 'Collegial surface acting emotional labour, burnout and intention to leave in novice and pre-retirement nurses: a cross sectional study', *Nursing Open*, 7 (2): 642–649.

Vinson, A.H. and Underman, K. (2020) 'Clinical empathy as emotional labor in medical work', *Social Science & Medicine*, 25: 112904.

SUGGESTED FURTHER READING

- Bailey, S., Scales, K., Lloyd, J. et al. (2015) 'The emotional labour of health-care assistants in inpatient dementia care', *Ageing & Society*, 35 (2): 246–269.

An interesting article exploring feeling rules representing the balance between engagement and attachment in EL as performed by healthcare assistants in dementia care.

- James, N. (1992) 'Care = organisation + physical labour + emotional labour', *Sociology of Health & Illness*, 14 (4): 488–509.

A classic article showing how EL is a key component of care in hospice nursing.

- Ward, J. and McMurray, R. (2016) *The Darkside of Emotional Labour*. London: Routledge.

This book explores EL from the perspective of people managing emotions that are considered disturbing, upsetting and often stigmatizing yet necessary to the function of organizations, such as healthcare providers/systems.

48

Informal Care

Sue Hollinrake

Informal care is given by one person, such as a family member (child or adult), friend or neighbour on a regular basis to another person without financial payment, though such care does incur (in)visible costs.

Care is a social relational activity basic to the preservation of human life, which entails interdependency and vulnerability. The varying capacity of individuals to respond in a caring way to others, alongside how this work is divided in society, is very much shaped by social and cultural factors. Social constructionist arguments highlight how ideology influences cultural meanings of the value of care and associated need through discourse and social practices. Informal care is distinguished from formal care – the latter is paid and the former is unpaid.

Discussions about informal care evoke a multitude of meanings and practices, explored in a growing body of research and academic theorizing. Conradi (2020) distinguishes two strands to theorizing care (formal and informal) within academic literature. Firstly, the ethico-political strand is rooted in challenges to mainstream ethics, which focuses on the everyday, practical, dyadic situations of offering and receiving care. The second, welfare-resourcing strand, with its origins in sociology and critical theory, emphasizes the political aspects of care work, how and why it is undervalued, and its inequitable distribution in relation to gender. Moving from the personal to the social, structural and political, and focusing on both strands, Tronto (2013) analyses the nature and function of caring and critiques the power relations that lie behind how it is organized. She flags the political and policy meanings which focus on the role of the state in determining care relations, their gendered character and the boundaries between the private and public spheres, which feminist critiques had already highlighted, as explored below.

For the first strand, pertinent themes include the personal qualities of caring *about* someone, physical tasks, duties and the organization of these in direct engagement in caring *for* someone, modified by the degree of availability and sense of responsibility. As Noddings (2002) explains, emotional work is important here, offering moral insights, based on establishing empathy, trust and compassion. Such emotional work entails insightfully managing one's own feelings (e.g. pleasure, ambivalence, anger, vulnerability) and others' feelings, alongside changing patterns of demand relating to dependence and independence through the lifecourse, with likely increasing intensity during times of stress such as during the COVID-19 pandemic.

For the second strand, neoliberalism's championing of autonomy and independence constructs a myth of individuals as primarily economic actors, separate from others and self-reliant, eschewing dependence. The actual 'dependency' of the older or disabled person who needs care invites the expected sense of personal responsibility from those in their social circle, especially family members. This typically produces derivative dependency for the informal family carer who may become dependent on wider family and/or the state for support. Against the backdrop of prevailing norms, the informal carers' dependency work is unrecognized in the economy and so undervalued, as the unpaid labour is a subsidy for the rest of society reinforced by notions of filial duty. This social obligation is enshrined in law in some countries where the state expects practical and financial contributions from adult children, as in some Asian countries and some North American states, whilst elsewhere, as seen in some Southern European countries, and in many African countries, this expectation is based within culture and customs (see Suggested Further Reading).

The carer's sense of social responsibility, experienced particularly by women socialized into a female identity (a 'caring self' linked to virtue ethics), is highlighted in feminist literature (see Phillips, 2007: 73–78). This critique has informed a feminist 'ethic of care', part of the ethico-political strand of theorizing, and writers such as Tronto (2013) attempt to bridge the gap between carer and cared-for. Rather than independence as the basis of citizenship, these writers consider *interdependence* as the foundation for a caring relationship. This approach embraces diversity and an awareness of power relations between care-giver and care-receiver, from which notions of rights and citizenship are developed. Work in this area highlights how interdependence and reciprocity characterize all human interactions.

Feminists have significantly shaped debates around informal care. They have exposed gender ideologies and developed a critique of caring (informal/formal) as a gendered activity performed largely by women, which is undervalued and exploited in policy and practice. With women traditionally seen as being more suited to caring than men (essentialists see caring as a woman's natural disposition), care efforts in the privacy of the family home have been rendered invisible economically. Hegemonic masculinities support gender inequality in caregiving, reinforcing the moral responsibility for informal care as integrally female and private, whilst men fulfil their care obligations in the workplace based on 'economic achievement, power and public status' (Hanlon, 2009: 197). In the West, such thinking has a well-documented history and economic logic (see this entry in the second edition of this volume). Feminist economists (e.g. Nelson and England, 2002) have challenged the androcentric biases of traditional economics which treat women as invisible and reinforce policies that are oppressive to them. Marxist feminists, who highlight the reproductive function of family caring in nurturing the next generation of workers and in maintaining the working-age population, have also focused on tensions in this reproductive role which have provoked a 'crisis of care' (Fraser, 2017). For the informal carer, time poverty and isolation are often significant and invisible issues, as is a more visible care penalty in giving up work to care, so losing out on wealth accumulation and pension assets, risking hardship in later life. Equally, to remain in work and simultaneously to be an informal carer brings with it often invisible, psychological stresses (Starr and Szebehely, 2017), as does the experience of abuse from a cared-for individual (Isham et al., 2020).

As an activity that is inseparable from the privacy of the body, and bodily functions, informal 'care work' risks being undervalued as 'dirty work' (Fine, 2007), but care's enmeshment with gendered ideologies and configurations of practice can also provide an aura of respectability. The mother/child relationship is typically seen as the blueprint for caring relationships – often idealized and sentimentalized, but also vilified as the cause of personality and behavioural problems in adult life when it does not go well, with negative consequences for women's mental health (Henderson et al., 2016). Of course, it should be added that gender is not the only social division that has attracted critical attention within caring debates, which deepened, for example, with the involvement of the Disability Movement. In their critique of developing UK community care services, disabled feminists took issue with able-bodied feminists whom they saw as rigidly splitting user and carer interests into a false dichotomy, reinforcing constructions of disabled people as 'burdensome' and problems for others (see Erevelles, 2011).

In social policy terms, informal carers are now a significant 'stakeholder' group within the delivery of care in the community. Informal care has a distinct place in the welfare policy context of most European countries, including the UK, following formal legal recognition from the state over the last three decades. Western governments have sought to champion the dedication of informal carers, viewing them as an important resource for the state alongside professionals, as reflected in policy developments and legislation. The Care Act 2014 in England introduces new rights for informal carers and stresses that they must be treated with the same respect and parity of esteem as those they care for, though evidence from practice shows difficulties in the achievement of this (Larkin and Mitchell, 2016; Peters et al., 2019).

Recent explorations of caring by social policy commentators have noted new influences on informal caring in Western economies. These influences include changes in economy and society that have impacted on family structures/relationships and the gendered division of labour, alongside demographic factors, i.e. an ageing population with more complex care needs in later years (see, for example, Wittenberg et al., 2019). Economic changes have forced more women into full-time employment and the family unit has diversified. These changes have not necessarily lessened the demands on women, since women who work full-time often continue to carry the main caring and domestic responsibilities, unless they employ usually low-paid female substitute carers from immigrant populations. This type of employment highlights the global issue of female migrant workers from developing countries in the Global South, who move to wealthier economies to work in low-paid private domestic jobs in order to improve the work/life balance of women with disposable income in these countries. These 'global care chains' create care deficits in poor countries as they solve care deficits in wealthy ones (Ehrenreich and Hochschild, 2003).

The relationship between the public and private worlds of informal caring in welfare regimes continues to be an area of tension. Governments have reluctantly addressed this hitherto hidden, private aspect of the economy through policy and legislation as economic challenges and demographic changes expose informal caring. However, in practice, a consistent and enduring gender inequality persists as women continue to do the majority of informal (and formal) caregiving. This enduring inequality is supported by and reproduced in cultural systems that place primary responsibility for care firmly at the feet of women. Furthermore, the 'lockdowns' during the COVID-19 pandemic in 2020/21 have exposed just how demanding caring can be. Informal carers, who pre-pandemic often received insufficient support, have encountered further reductions in help thus increasing their levels of stress, exhaustion and isolation (Carers UK, 2021). In sum, whilst more men are becoming informal carers, this remains a social space that women are more generally expected to fill and particularly where high levels of care are required.

See also: Emotional Labour; Gender; Nursing and Midwifery as Occupations.

REFERENCES

Carers UK (2021) *Breaks or breakdown, Carers Week 2021 report,* 7 June. Online: www.carersuk.org/for-professionals/policy/policy-library/breaks-or-breakdown-carers-week-2021-report

Conradi, E. (2020) 'Theorising care: attentive interaction or distributive justice?' *International Journal of Care and Caring,* 4 (1): 25–42.

Ehrenreich, B. and Hochschild, A.R. (eds) (2003) *Global Woman: Nannies, Maids and Sex Workers in the New Economy.* London: Granta.

Erevelles, M. (2011) *Disability and Difference in Global Contexts: Enabling a Transformative Body Politic.* London: Palgrave Macmillan.

Fine, M.D. (2007) *A Caring Society? Care and the Dilemmas of Human Service in the 21st Century.* Basingstoke: Palgrave Macmillan.

Fraser, N. (2017) 'Crisis of care? On the social reproductive contradictions of contemporary capitalism', in T. Bhattacharya (ed.), *Social Reproduction Theory: Remapping Class, Recentering Oppression.* London: Pluto Press.

Hanlon, N. (2009) 'Caregiving masculinities: an exploratory analysis', in K. Lynch, J. Baker and M. Lyons (eds), *Affective Equality: Love, Care and Injustice.* Houndsmill: Palgrave Macmillan.

Henderson, A., Harmon, S. and Newman, H. (2016) 'The price mothers pay, even when they are not buying it: mental health consequences of idealized motherhood', *Sex Roles*, 74 (11–12): 512–526.

Isham, L., Bradbury-Jones, C. and Hewison, A. (2020) 'Female family carers' experiences of violent, abusive or harmful behaviour by the older person for whom they care: a case of epistemic injustice?' *Sociology of Health & Illness*, 42 (1): 80–94.

Larkin, M. and Mitchell, W. (2016) 'Carers, choice and personalisation: what do we know?' *Social Policy and Society*, 15 (2): 189–205.

Nelson, J.A. and England, P. (2002) 'Feminist philosophies of love and work', Special Issue of *Hypatia*, 17 (2): 1–19.

Noddings, N. (2002) *Starting at Home: Caring and Social Policy.* Berkeley: University of California Press.

Peters, M., Rand, S. and Fitzpatrick, R. (2019) 'Enhancing primary care support for informal carers: a scoping study with professional stakeholders', *Health and Social Care in the Community*, 28 (2): 642–650.

Phillips, J. (2007) *Care.* Cambridge: Polity Press.

Starr, M. and Szebehely, M. (2017) 'Working longer, caring harder – the impact of "ageing-in-place" policies on working carers in the UK and Sweden', *International Journal of Care and Caring*, 1 (1): 115–119.

Tronto, J.C. (2013) *Caring Democracy: Markets, Equality, and Justice.* New York: New York University Press.

Wittenberg, R., Hu, B., Barraza-Araiza, L. and Rehill, A. (2019) *Projections of Older People with Dementia and Costs of Dementia Care in the United Kingdom, 2019–2040.* London School of Economics and Political Science Care Policy and Evaluation Centre.

SUGGESTED FURTHER READING

- Calvó-Perxas, L., Vilalta-Franch, J., Litwin, H. et al. (2018) 'What seems to matter in public policy and the health of informal caregivers? A cross-sectional study in 12 European countries', *PLoS One*, 13 (3): 1–12.

This article reports on a research project that draws upon previous data on carers' experiences across 12 European countries, with differing cultural norms about caring, in relation to policies and systems of support, both financial and non-financial. It seeks to determine which supports had a more beneficial impact on carers. It seems that non-financial support, such as some free time from caring, emotional help with caregiving and skills development for their caring role, had a more protective impact on their health than financial support measures.

- Nortey, S.T., Aryeetey, G.C., Aikins, M., et al. (2017) 'Economic burden of family caregiving for elderly population in southern Ghana: the case of a peri-urban district', *International Journal for Equity in Health*, 16:16. https://doi.org/10.1186/s12939-016-0511-9

This retrospective, cross-sectional cost-of-care study of a community-based carers' support group in Ghana reveals the economic burden of family caregiving for the elderly, with women in particular reporting a high level of financial stress as a result of caring for their elderly and vulnerable relatives in a low-income country.

- Aboderin, I. and Hoffman, J. (2017) 'Research debate on "older carers and work" in sub-Saharan Africa? Current gaps and future frames', *Journal of Cross-Cultural Gerontology*, 32 (3): 387–393.

This article discusses the limited nature of African debate about older informal carers who may be in work as well as providing long-term care for younger people commonly with HIV/AIDS, as well as older more dependent adults, in a culture that emphasizes family solidarity. It reviews existing literature, identifies gaps in knowledge and suggests ways forward for progressing a research agenda to highlight the support needs and promote the well-being of this group of carers.

- Rand, S., Malley, J. and Forder, J. (2019) 'Are reasons for care-giving related to carers' care-related quality of life and strain? Evidence from a survey of carers in England', *Health & Social Care in the Community*, 27 (1): 151–160.

The increasing focus on quality of life for carers is explored in this study which surveys informal carer quality of life and subjective strain in relation to carer-reported reasons for caring. The study, conducted in England, concludes that where carers have more choice quality of life is better and the limiting of carers' choice about whether to provide care is related to worse outcomes. These findings may usefully inform policy and practice to improve carers' quality of life.

PART 5

HEALTHCARE ORGANIZATION AND POLICY

49

Hospitals and Healthcare Organizations

Per Måseide

Hospitals and healthcare organizations refer to institutions that provide professional medical services.

The term 'health system' signifies the wider organization of healthcare services for a given population. Such systems differ between nations with regard to organizing and financing and they may have unclear boundaries compared to other service providers. The organization of the healthcare system has significant implications for the role, staffing and organization of hospitals and other healthcare services. Historical observations in Europe are illustrative. In its early medieval version, the hospital was a 'shelter' and caring organization with religious orientations, staffed by nuns and monks. Its history as a formally institutionalized site dominated by professionals and scientifically-based medical knowledge and competence is relatively recent and dependent on the development of sciences within modern universities.

An early object of sociological interest was the mental hospital. Goffman (1961) conducted a study of a traditional North American state mental hospital and categorized it under the wider concept of 'total institution'. Such institutions had total control of their inmates; control was their primary function and inmates or 'patients' stayed for an indeterminate length of time. To establish and preserve a personal identity or self, following their hospital admission, patients engaged in informal and 'self-protecting' activities constituting what Goffman described as 'the underlife' of the total institution. To display a personal identity and resist mortification of the self, patients sought to resist the full incorporation of the total institution, though this kind of 'deviant behaviour' might be interpreted as a sign of mental illness by the hospital staff. Because of critical studies like this, as well as changing psychiatric ideologies and economic considerations, the organization of psychiatric hospitals and mental health services started to change during the 1960s in many Western countries.

These changes triggered several micro-sociological studies of psychiatric hospitals as organizations in the process of transformation. Strauss et al. (1963) developed the concept of 'the negotiated order' from such studies. The concept refers to social organizations, not as products of formal structures and rules, as might be inferred from a Parsonian functionalist perspective, but as resulting from emergent processes of bargaining and negotiations between organizational members concerning the division of work and the adequacy and functions of institutional roles. Roth (1963) described social life in a tuberculosis hospital and looked upon the organization of time in the hospital in terms of timetables. Patients spent long and indeterminate amounts of time in tuberculosis hospitals and while patients negotiated with staff members about a date for discharge, medical professionals used timetables to structure the patients' careers in ways that best suited the healthcare organization.

After the 1960s the sociological interest in hospital organizations gradually disappeared. What took over was an interest in medical work and the healthcare professions. Stimulated by pragmatism and symbolic interactionism, such studies concentrated on the treatment of chronic illnesses and the diversity of forms of medical work conducted in hospitals. Researchers employed terms like 'professional dominance', 'illness trajectory' and 'work trajectory'. Several studies focused on the routinized and ritual form of medical consultations, and the constitutive role formats that organizational members creatively employed. For instance, ceremonial, symbolic and constructive aspects of surgical work in hospitals were studied together with the ritual characteristics of physicians' talk that secured professional and institutional adequacy, when conducting 'information work' in hospital settings (Hirschauer, 1991).

A focus on the medical object as discursively generated and the production of medical knowledge has also been influenced by Foucault (1973), who wrote about the historical development of 'medical perception' as being fundamental for modern medical work. He has inspired sociological studies of the generation of medical knowledge and perception, and the social construction of medical objects and problems (Armstrong, 2002). Such studies have influenced and been influenced by recent work in the sociology of science and technology and various interactionist approaches. Talk and collaboration in hospital settings have received much attention recently from sociologists and various kinds of discourse analysts, including those from the humanities. The emphasis on medical talk and conversation in the context of medical problem-solving processes and on the generation of a professional medical vision has been part of these analyses (Måseide, 2016). These studies are generally restricted to limited areas of the hospital and focus on the details of work, the forms of talk and the interdisciplinary and collaborative nature of medical work, as parts of the 'work trajectory'.

Taking a perspective from Actor Network Theory (ANT), material semiotics or new materialism, Mol (2002) has focused on the nature of medical work in hospitals, the complexity of medical objects or problems and how this complexity is managed to reach a singular medical problem that can be institutionally dealt with. Other studies of medical work in hospitals have shown the general need for and use of support systems to generate routines, efficiency, standardization and institutional control of the various professionals involved in complex problem-solving tasks. The purpose has been to promote adequate medical work. However, research has documented resistance to the introduction of new technologies among health professionals in hospitals. It has been argued that development of the medical knowledge base and the introduction of new technologies from relatively early on have led to a reciprocal transformation of technology and hospital organization and to the constitution of a compartmentalized and expanded patient body, fitting the compartmentalized hospital organization (Berg and Harterink, 2004). The reason why medical sociological studies of hospitals to a large extent have been restricted to limited parts of the arc of medical work may be because of the increasing diversity and distribution of biomedical knowledge and competence, which again has affected the complexity of medical work and hospital organization.

Healthcare organizations have changed considerably in recent years alongside the content and practice of medicine itself. Much of the problem-solving work conducted in hospitals requires collaboration between different medical specialists or experts and different professions. Associated with this development is the emergence of what in organization studies is called 'the problem of many hands', a problem that has to be dealt with during the conduct and organization of medical work in hospitals. The use of sophisticated technological equipment is part of collaborative medical work: it produces representations or images, of what might be called 'virtual patients' that replace the actual patient in medical problem-solving. The organization and functions of hospitals and other healthcare systems have increasingly become influenced by the development of new medical knowledge, new technologies and new specialities and sub-specialities. The resulting distribution and compartmentalization of medical competence and work, of the patient's body and of medical problems require detailed studies of the practices that constitute healthcare organizations and their functions.

Information technology has become an essential and integrated part of medical work in healthcare organizations. The development and use of electronic patient records and their consequences for clinical work have been the topic of much sociological research. Lupton (2017) has introduced the term 'm-health', which is technology that has replaced or expanded healthcare systems. In its digitalized form it may move into the patient's home or body. The clinic may then be where the patient is and healthcare is outsourced from health professionals and hospitals to technology. Lupton calls this the 'digital cyborg assemblage', referring to Haraway's 'cyborg' concept, and suggests that this assemblage may not necessarily be only advantageous; it may also have suppressive functions and represents a new field of critical sociological research.

For medical, economic and technological reasons, the hospital's position and functions within the healthcare system have changed in many countries, a process that has been characterized as the decline of the hospital. More medical activities now take place outside the hospital or in out-patient clinics than was the case earlier. Patients are also discharged earlier from hospitals. This development reflects changing health policies, discourses of management and the development of medical technologies and competencies. In addition to the healthcare system becoming more complex, its functions are more widely distributed than previously. Hence, sociological attention should be paid to the relationship and collaboration between its diverse parts amidst changing hierarchical power relations. Hospitals were once sites or organizations characterized by professional medical dominance. However, this has changed in many countries with the development or introduction of what is termed 'new managerialism'. Studies from various countries indicate that medical doctors do not have the same authority within the health service organization as before (e.g. Scott, 2008). Not only do they have to share power with other health professions but they are also under governance of a management system that represents the owners of the health service organization and takes care of the owners' interests. The managers' duty is not only to improve the medical services of the hospital; they are also responsible for the hospital's financial situation. The economy of the hospital may be increasingly constrained under conditions of neoliberalism and, because of that, medical and economic interests may be conflicting. The new managerialism has introduced several systems to guide and control the medical work conducted on hospital wards. From this process, a contradiction has been described between managerial and professional logics in healthcare organizations. The development of hybrid logics has been a result of such contradictions (Exworthy et al., 2019) and new concepts have appeared, such as 'soft surveillance', 'collaborative professionalism' and 'mutating professions'. An important topic for sociological research is to study the processes and consequences of implementation of managerial control systems and other general 'support systems' for medical professionals and their contact with patients. Finally, emphasis has recently been placed on patients' roles as consumers of healthcare services, on the importance of partnership in healthcare and on patient empowerment. The latter should allow patients to regain control of their bodies, their health and health problems (Allen et al., 2016). This development demands critical research and analysis as part of a sociology *of*, rather than simply *for*, healthcare and organizations.

A recent branch of sociological research on healthcare organizations is a sociology of healthcare architecture. It is influenced by the spatial turn in the social sciences together with new materialism. Buildings are attributed a form of agency, and since architects design healthcare buildings that regulate how patient bodies are enacted, they are ascribed roles as body workers. Architects establish and reproduce ideals about medical objects, roles and practices. Concepts like 'materialities of care' and 'architectural care assemblage' (Nettleton et al., 2020) have been introduced to analyse these processes. The latter concept refers to the material used in architecture and architectural design as actors involved in the process of developing buildings for healthcare. It is suggested that 'materialities of care' and 'mundane materialities' can be used as a lens to study care practices (Buse et al., 2018). Architecture and buildings are seen to have implications for policies and practices of healthcare. This is a relatively new field of medical sociological research with relevance for studies of healthcare organizations.

With regard to staffing, necessary equipment and technological resources, hospitals seem in general to have been organized to handle other kinds of health problems than a pandemic like COVID-19. The consequences of this vary between countries. Many problems have been articulated about hospitals' preparedness for such a crisis; one of them concerns the priority of patients in need of intensive care, which belongs to one of medical sociology's topics, rationing of care. It may also be asked if the ill-preparedness of hospitals has contributed to reproducing social inequalities in disease outcomes. The question of how the pandemic has affected healthcare organizations will be an important topic for further medical sociological research.

See also: Consumerism; Digital Health; Managerialism; Neoliberalism.

REFERENCES

Allen, D., Braithwaite, J., Sandall, J. and Warring, J. (2016) 'Towards a sociology of healthcare safety and quality', *Sociology of Health & Illness*, 38 (2): 181–197.

Armstrong, D. (2002) 'Foucault and the sociology of health and illness: a prismatic reading', in A. Petersen and R. Bunton (eds), *Foucault, Health and Medicine*. London: Routledge.

Berg, M. and Harterink, P. (2004) 'Embodying the patient: records and bodies in early 20th-century US medical practice', *Body & Society*, 10 (2–3): 13–41.

Buse, C., Martin, D. and Nettleton, S. (2018) *Materialities of Care. Encountering Health and Illness Through Artefacts and Architecture*. Oxford: Wiley Blackwell.

Exworthy, M., Gabe, J., Jones, I.R. and Smith, G. (2019) 'Professional autonomy and surveillance: the case of public reporting in cardiac surgery', *Sociology of Health & Illness*, 41 (6): 1040–1055.

Foucault, M. (1973) *The Birth of the Clinic*. London: Tavistock.

Goffman, E. (1961) *Asylums*. Harmondsworth: Penguin.

Hirschauer, S. (1991) 'The manufacture of bodies in surgery', *Social Studies in Science*, 21 (2): 279–319.

Lupton, D. (2017) *Digital Health: Critical and Cross-Disciplinary Perspectives*. London: Routledge.

Måseide, P. (2016) 'Team talk and problem solving in thoracic medicine', *Communication & Medicine*, 13 (1): 9–22.

Mol, A. (2002) *The Body Multiple*. Durham: Duke University Press.

Nettleton, S., Daryl, M., Buse, C. and Prior, L. (2020) 'Materialising architecture for social care: brick walls and compromises in design for later life', *British Journal of Sociology*, 71 (1): 153–167.

Roth, J.A. (1963) *Timetables: Structuring the Passage of Time in hospital Treatment and Other Careers*. Indianapolis: Bobbs-Merrill.

Scott, W.R. (2008) 'Lords of the dance: professionals as institutional agents', *Organization Studies*, 29 (2): 219–230.

Strauss, A., Schatzman, L., Ehrlich, D. et al. (1963) 'The hospital and its negotiated order', in E. Freidson (ed.), *The Hospital in Modern Society*. New York: Free Press.

SUGGESTED FURTHER READING

- Atkinson, P. (1995) *Medical Talk and Medical Work*. London: SAGE.

Atkinson focuses on the discursive generation of professional skills among haematologists, such as professional vision. A discursive approach is combined with sociology of knowledge.

- Berg, M. (1997) *Rationalizing Medical Work*. Cambridge, MA: MIT Press.

This book is an early and comprehensive introduction to an important medical sociological issue: how modern medical work has become influenced by development of systems and technologies for support and rationalization.

- Strauss, A., Fagerhaugh, S., Suczek, B. and Wiener, C. (1985) *Social Organization of Medical Work*. Chicago: University of Chicago Press.

This text is a crucial introduction to the sociology of healthcare organizations. It is grounded in important qualitative empirical research in hospitals, which is still relevant, as is the comprehensive conceptual framework presented therein.

- Blaxter, M. (2009) 'The case of the vanishing patient', *Sociology of Health & Illness*, 31 (5): 762–778.

This is an autobiographical one-case study from a patient perspective, written by a major contributor to medical sociology. Blaxter closely observes and records processes of generating a diagnosis, which would not be available for ordinary researchers, and shows the socially distributed workings of a healthcare system.

50

Privatization

Jonathan Gabe

Privatization refers to a set of policies that aim to limit the role of public sector healthcare, increase the role of the private sector, while improving the performance of the remaining public sector.

The heath service in Britain, like those of other countries in the Global North, has long been pluralist in the sense that publicly funded (through taxation) and privately funded (through payment for a service in person or by private health insurance) healthcare have co-existed. However, the healthcare reforms from the 1980s onwards have shifted the balance profoundly in favour of greater private sector involvement. Below we consider the strategies employed to achieve this and the reasons for doing so, with particular reference to the private acute sector. The consequences of such restructuring for the National Health Service (NHS) and the principles on which it was founded will also be considered. As we will see, since political devolution in 1999, the shift in the balance between public and private has been particularly marked in England.

One strategy for shifting the balance between the public and private sector has involved the development of policies to encourage the growth of the private sector. In the 1980s planning controls were relaxed on the development of private hospitals and the power of local authorities to object to such developments was curtailed. In addition, NHS consultants' contracts were revised to enable them to undertake more private practice in addition to their NHS commitments and tax changes were introduced to encourage higher levels of private health cover. Together these changes created the climate for private hospital development with the number of private hospitals increasing by 35 per cent and the number of private beds by 40 per cent between 1980 and 2001. Many of these hospitals were located in the prosperous southeast of England, compounding rather than eliminating geographical inequalities in the distribution of resources. At the same time the level of private health insurance increased from 5 per cent of the population in 1979 to a peak of 13 per cent in 1989, with company-purchased schemes being particularly popular (Harley et al., 2011). Thereafter numbers covered fell again, in part because of the subsequent financial crisis, until 2015 when they increased sharply by over 2 per cent to 10.6 per cent. This rise has been attributed to fears about waiting times for operations, which have lengthened as a result of the funding crisis facing the NHS under the Conservative(-led) administration's austerity policies. Traditionally coverage has been concentrated in London and the southeast of England with policy holders tending to have professional and managerial jobs and to be male, though roughly equal numbers of both sexes are actually covered (Foubister et al., 2006).

A further strategy to shift the balance between the public and private sectors has involved the introduction of reforms that have facilitated greater collaboration between the two sectors. An early attempt was the Conservative government's policy of requiring NHS District Health Authorities (HAs) to introduce competitive tendering for domestic, catering and laundry services in the 1980s. The intention was to challenge the monopoly of in-house providers of services on the assumption that costs would be reduced and greater 'value for money' would be achieved. In practice the financial benefits proved relatively modest, at least to start with, and the savings achieved were said to be at the expense of quality of service (Mohan, 1995). More recently, the NHS has been encouraged to contract out-patient care to the private sector. These co-operative arrangements were initially undertaken on a voluntary basis by individual HAs that did not have in-house alternatives, for example as a result of capacity constraints. Subsequently Conservative and Labour governments have used private hospitals as a way of reducing NHS waiting lists for non-urgent cases and those waiting more than a year. For instance, Tony Blair's New Labour government instituted a 'concordat' between the NHS in England and the private sector in 2000. This allowed patients to be treated at NHS expense in the private sector if NHS hospitals were full. Labour also introduced Independent Treatment Centres as a way to expand private sector involvement in routine NHS work and allowed Primary Care Trusts to award contracts to private companies in addition to general practitioners. The subsequent Conservative-led government built on this policy in the 2012 Health and Social Care Act by allowing Clinical Commissioning Groups (which had replaced Primary Care Trusts) to contract with 'any qualified provider' (AQP), including private and third sector organizations as well as public sector bodies. The decision to introduce contracts to alternative providers was based on the assumption that diversification of providers would result in improved efficiency through market competition (Pollock and Price, 2011). The ability of private hospitals to compete with NHS hospitals for NHS patients has resulted in a considerable increase in spending on private facilities by NHS Commissioners (PCTs and subsequently Clinical Commissioning Groups). By 2012 this amounted to 28 per cent of inpatient income for private hospitals, and this spending has increased subsequently. In 2018–19 NHS Commissioners spent £9.2 billion on services delivered by the private sector (King's Fund, 2019). Moreover, during the COVID-19 pandemic, NHS England block booked 8,000 private beds because of insufficient predicted capacity in the NHS. This collaboration gave the NHS access to much needed beds but it also provided financial relief to the private sector at a time of considerable uncertainty as a result of non-urgent operations being cancelled.

Another example of collaboration has been the development of the Private Finance Initiative (PFI). Launched by the Conservatives in the early 1990s and subsequently continued by Labour and the Conservative(-led) administrations, the aim was to encourage private capital investment in the NHS, thereby increasing overall resources in the service while avoiding raising taxes or increasing public borrowing. Much of the investment was used to build new acute hospitals, with 101 of the 135 built in England between 1997 and 2009 being financed under this scheme (Pollock and Price, 2011). Under PFI, private companies designed, constructed, owned and operated services for a 25–30 year period, in return for an annual fee. While clinical services remained the responsibility of government, PFI was seen as permitting an element of risk to be transferred to the private sector, as building cost overruns were picked up by the private sector. Critics argued, however, that there were serious disadvantages associated with PFI-funded projects, including: reduced bed numbers (substantially in excess of what would be expected from long-term demand trends) – a problem which resurfaced during the 2020–21 COVID-19 pandemic; the need for a quicker throughput of patients; a significant reduction in spending on clinical staff, especially nurses; higher interest rate charges compared to the cost of government borrowing, thereby putting a severe strain on hospital Trust budgets; and the creation of substantial debt over time (Mohan, 2009). The Conservative government announced in 2018 that they had ended PFI, although there had been no new schemes since 2014, due to a squeeze on budgets which made it difficult for hospital Trusts to make repayments for existing PFI schemes.

The third strategy has been to encourage competition between the NHS and the private sector. This strategy is best illustrated by the Conservative government's willingness to encourage the NHS to expand its pay-bed provision, thereby sharpening competition for private patients and threatening the private providers' profit margins. Originally introduced when the NHS was established in 1948 as a concession to hospital consultants, pay-beds were in decline when the Conservatives came to power in 1979 and their number continued to decline subsequently. In the late 1980s, however, the Conservatives decided to revitalize this provision in the face of increasingly severe financial constraints. The policy was also in line with their belief in generating competition between providers in order to enhance consumer choice and maximize efficiency. In 1988 it therefore used the Health and Medicines Act to relax the rules governing pay bed charges so that hospitals could make a profit instead of simply covering costs. This propelled hospitals to upgrade their private wings or develop dedicated pay bed units, as well as increasing the number of pay beds on NHS wards. Under

Labour there was a strict cap on the number of private patients the NHS could treat. However, under recent Conservative(-led) administrations this has been relaxed, allowing the NHS in England to be a major provider of private healthcare. In 2016 it was estimated that there were 1,140 pay beds in the NHS. This compares with 8,900 beds in the private sector at that time (King's Fund, 2020).

These three strategies illustrate the shift to a new public/private mix of services and growing privatization – that is, the transfer of assets from the public to the private sector. The policy has been driven in large part by neo-liberalism with its emphasis on individuals exercising choice in the market and the need to maximize efficiency and get value for money from existing tax revenues.

Politicians may also have been encouraged to move towards what has been called a 'mixed economy of healthcare' by segments of the medical profession and by some users of healthcare. Certain members of the medical profession have stood to gain financially from the expansion of the private sector, as a result of an increase in fees for private medical practice, paid out by insurance companies, and from ownership of new private hospitals and private companies providing primary care services. An increase in 'consumer' demand for private healthcare could be said to explain the growth in private health insurance in the 1980s although, as noted earlier, this increase was primarily a result of the expansion of company-paid schemes rather than individual-paid schemes. There is also evidence of growing dissatisfaction with the NHS in social attitude surveys, which might have encouraged a greater willingness to use private healthcare. Historically, however, there has been strong loyalty to the NHS, even amongst those who have private health insurance, and this loyalty has acted as a break on those politicians who might otherwise have favoured a greater shift towards private healthcare on ideological grounds. In addition, the gratitude felt to the NHS as a result of the role that it has played in providing care during the COVID-19 pandemic, including to Prime Minister Boris Johnson, has arguably further limited the likelihood of an openly expressed move towards private healthcare.

Whatever the reasons for the development of the public–private mix, it can be argued that the shift towards a greater role for private medicine has undermined the egalitarian principles associated with the founding of the NHS and created a two-tier system. It is certainly the case that those with private health insurance can 'jump the queue' for elective surgery and that these people tend to be better off. However, there is little evidence to suggest that the quality of care provided in the private sector is superior to that offered by the NHS. While private care might be more comfortable and convenient, the levels of medical and technical care are similar. More significant, perhaps, is the impact of the introduction of commercial imperatives in the NHS and the increasing emphasis on healthcare as a commodity and patients as consumers. This cultural change is arguably as transformative as any of the other alterations to the public–vprivate mix and supports the claim that the NHS in England is being privatized from within. More research is needed to assess whether this is in fact the case, especially in light of the COVID-19 pandemic.

See also: Consumerism; Managerialism; Pandemics and Epidemics.

REFERENCES

Foubister, T., Thompson, S., Mossialos, E. and McGuire, A. (2006) *Private Medical Insurance in the United Kingdom*. European Observatory on Health Systems and Policies. Online: https://apps.who.int/iris/bitstream/handle/10665/107741/E88671. pdf?sequence=1&isAllowed=y

Harley, K., Willis, K., Gabe, J. et al. (2011) 'Constructing health consumers: private health insurance in Australia and the United Kingdom', *Health Sociology Review*, 20 (3): 306–320.

King's Fund (2019) *Is the NHS Being Privatised?* www.kingsfund.org.uk/publicati ons/articles/big-election-questions-nhs-privatised

King's Fund (2020) *NHS Hospital Bed Numbers: Past, Present and Future*. London: Kings Fund.

Mohan, J. (1995) *A National Health Service? The Restructuring of Health Care in Britain since 1979*. Basingstoke: Macmillan.

Mohan, J. (2009) 'Visions of privatisation. New Labour and the reconstruction of the NHS', in J. Gabe and M. Calnan (eds), *The New Sociology of the Health Service*. London: Routledge.

Pollock, A.M. and Price, D. (2011) 'The final frontier: the UK's new coalition government turns the English National Health Service over to the global health care market', *Health Sociology Review*, 20: 294–305.

SUGGESTED FURTHER READING

- Calnan, M., Cant, S. and Gabe, J. (1993) *Going Private. Why People Pay for Their Health Care*. Buckingham: Open University Press.

An old but still unique study of when and why people use private healthcare in the UK. Based on a survey of people likely to have private health insurance and in-depth interviews with those who hold private health insurance and those who do not, it also explores what people think of private healthcare compared with care provided by the NHS.

- Sheaff, R. and Allen, P. (2016) 'Provider plurality and supply-side reform', in M. Exworthy, R. Mannion and M. Powell (eds), *Dismantling the NHS? Evaluating the Impact of Health Reforms*. Bristol: Policy Press.

An important chapter which focuses on the spread of differently-owned organizations which now provide NHS care in England as a result of the neoliberal reforms which have fundamentally changed the NHS since 1979.

- Speed, E. and Gabe, J. (2013) 'The Health and Social Care Act for England 2012: the extension of "new professionalism"', *Critical Social Policy*, 33 (3): 564–674.

A critical assessment of the 2012 Health and Social Care Act, including how it was intended to attract private providers into statutory healthcare at the expense of public providers.

51

Managerialism

Jonathan Gabe

Managerialism refers to an ideology that reframes healthcare using managerial symbols and language and encourages healthcare professionals to accept managerialist thinking.

For more than three decades many countries in the Global North have turned to management in an attempt to contain healthcare costs, improve performance and outcomes and make their services more user-sensitive. In place of an administrative approach where managers 'oiled the wheels' in consultation with other healthcare workers, an industrial model of management has been introduced, regardless of its relevance or appropriateness for public services like healthcare. The emphasis now is on managers taking control, setting performance targets and imposing budgetary and workload ceilings. This approach has arguably set managers on a collision course with other healthcare professionals such as doctors because of the latter's claim to autonomy. In this entry the development of what has been called 'New Public Management' (NPM) in the UK's National Health Service (NHS) is briefly described and the implications for social relations in healthcare and, in particular, for relations between managers and doctors, are considered. Since political devolution in 1999 it has been claimed that the relationship between management and medicine in Wales, Scotland and Northern Ireland has been less fraught and adversarial than in England, so the impact of NPM will be considered only in relation to the latter (Hunter, 2006).

It is possible to see the development of NPM as involving two elements: challenging professionals in the health service and incorporating them (Harrison and Pollitt, 1994). Each will be considered in turn. *Challenging* health service professionals involves subordinating professional autonomy to managerial will, an approach first adopted in 1983 with the introduction of general managers into the NHS as recommended in the Griffiths Report.

Prior to this report NHS managers, or as they were then called, administrators, acted as diplomats, helping to organize the facilities and resources for professionals to get on with their work and reacting to problems as they arose. Decisions were made consensually by multidisciplinary teams that included doctors and nurses, as well as administrators. The Griffiths Report recommended altering the organizational culture of the service by introducing features of business management, along the lines suggested particularly by US management theorists. General managers were to be appointed who would proactively develop management plans, ensure quality of care, achieve cost improvements and monitor and reward staff. At the same time managers would be paid by performance as a spur to good management, as happened in the private sector.

These proposals, which were accepted wholesale by the Conservative government of the time, were designed to alter the balance of power in favour of managers at the expense of other professionals, especially doctors (Hunter, 2006). Before the Griffiths Report, doctors' clinical freedom to make decisions about patients regardless of cost had been seen as a major determinant of the level of expenditure. In the new system doctors were to be more accountable to managers, who had strict control over professional and labour costs through a system of management budgets that related workload objectives to the resources available. In practice, general managers were unable to challenge the medical domain, let alone make significant inroads into it. While they now found it easier to close hospital beds and make other changes to the service without long periods of consultation, in every other respect they were no more able to control doctors than their predecessors (Harrison and Pollitt, 1994). Consequently, doctors continued to exercise considerable autonomy and managers continued to lack real control over medical work.

Subsequently the Conservative government enacted the 1990 NHS and Community Care Act, which attempted, among other things, to shift the balance of power more forcefully in the direction of managers. Following the Act managers became more involved in the specification and policing of consultants' contracts, discussing consultants' job description with them on a yearly basis and helping to determine the merit awards which are given to some consultants to supplement their salaries. At the same time a plethora of new techniques of managerial evaluation were developed. Quality assurance and performance indicators, made possible by advances in information technology, increased opportunities for the managerial determination of work content, productivity, resource use and quality standards (Flynn, 1992).

Under the Labour government from 1997, managers were given further powers to challenge doctors' autonomy. The introduction of 'clinical governance' as a mechanism to control doctors resulted in hospital chief executives becoming responsible for clinical as well as financial performance. From 1999 these chief executives were expected to make sure that their clinicians restricted themselves to treatments recommended on grounds of clinical and cost effectiveness by the National Institute for Clinical Excellence (now the National Institute for Health and Care Excellence). They were also expected to see that clinicians complied with service guidelines for specified conditions under the National Service Frameworks. Furthermore, managers were required to provide evidence to demonstrate that doctors in their Trusts were complying with these guidelines for the rolling programme of inspections to be conducted by the Commission for Health Improvement (Harrison and Ahmad, 2000) and its successor (the Care Quality Commission). This focus on measuring service quality via metrics has been described as a shift from government to governance, because of the wider range of agencies and stakeholders involved in health service delivery (Dopson, 2009).

One such metric is that of surgical performance, where surgeons in England are required to report their post-operative mortality rates online to maximize transparency (Gabe et al., 2012). This practice has been labelled 'soft surveillance', following Foucault, where the logic of management discourse is internalized and physicians become involved in auditing their practice through public reporting.

It might be argued that these developments have given managers in England the opportunity to constrain doctors as never before, along the lines identified by the proletarianization/corporatization thesis. Advocates of this position argue that doctors are being deskilled, are losing their economic independence and are being required to work in bureaucratically organized institutions under the instruction of managers, in accordance with the requirements of advanced capitalism (McKinlay and Marceau, 2002). However, as Freidson (1989) indicated, the widespread adoption of new techniques for monitoring the efficiency of performance and resource allocation does not, on its own, illustrate reduced professional autonomy. What really matters is whose criteria for evaluation and appraisal are adopted and who controls which actions are taken. More recent work, undertaken in a range of countries within and outside of Europe (e.g. Sweden and the USA), illustrates how doctors often retain clinical autonomy by intervening in the process of creating rules and protocols or actively influencing their implementation (Weisz et al., 2007).

The more oblique approach to managerialism involves *the incorporation* of professionals into management activity on managers' terms. In England this approach pre-dated the 1990 NHS and Community Care Act, but was significantly enhanced by it. For example, under the Griffiths Report doctors were encouraged to become general managers and a few experiments were set up involving the delegation of budgetary responsibility to doctors. At the same time most doctors were reluctant to become managers and continued to exercise considerable autonomy. Following the 1990 Act, however, doctors were required to be involved in management at every level. They were forced to become part-time managers, integrated into the management structure, and could no longer ignore it. Thus doctors became part-time clinical directors who, while retaining their professional identity, became subordinate to managers and were expected to 'manage', using their position to control their medical colleagues. Although sometimes reluctant to take the role initially, they generally came to see it subsequently as a way of retaining control over the service.

Having learnt the language and values of management, or what has been called managerial logic (Martin et al., 2015), alongside their professional logic, doctors have been able to interpret and reframe problems, to adopt a clinical perspective on managerial issues and a managerial perspective on clinical matters (Thorne, 2002). Adopting what amounts to a 'hybrid' logic, they may be able to deflect or neutralize changes being required under the government's reform agenda, or may even attempt to reshape them (Hunter, 2006).

In contrast to arguments about proletarianization/corporatization, mentioned earlier, attempts to incorporate the medical profession by turning them into managers have arguably been used by doctors to enable them to re-professionalize. Creating new forms of expertise by assimilating management skills has enabled clinical directors to extend their jurisdiction and domain. The resulting differentiation between these clinical directors and other doctors may, however, lead to greater internal stratification and hence the fragmentation of the medical profession (Thorne, 2002). Others have pointed out that such internal stratification does not exclusively result in growing inequalities within the medical profession. It can also provide new opportunities for lower segments of the profession such as general practitioners, facilitating their re-positioning (Calnan and Gabe, 2009).

Whatever its impact on the medical profession, the growth of managerialism has been enhanced by a series of government policies, initiated first by the Conservatives and subsequently modified by New Labour and more recent Conservative(-led) governments. The introduction of an internal market in the 1990 NHS and Community Care Act, with the division of the NHS into providers and purchasers, has given managers a pivotal role. Likewise, the introduction of the Patient's Charter in 1991, involving the setting of rights and service standards that consumers could expect, and its modification by the Labour government on coming to power in 1997, has helped to enhance the power of managers who have been responsible for monitoring and enforcing these service standards. The passing of the Health and Social Care Act by the Coalition government (of Conservatives and Liberal Democrats) in 2012, which re-enforced the market for healthcare in England, has given further power to managers in the drawing up of contracts for suppliers and producers of services and in monitoring clinical performance through clinical and patient outcome data.

At the same time there are countervailing forces at work, which may restrain the advance of management (Harrison and Pollitt, 1994). We have already seen that doctors (and nurses) have taken up management posts, bringing a different set of priorities and values with them. In addition to this 'colonization of management' by healthcare professionals, managerial power and authority may be curtailed by the fragmentation of management itself. Thus, those working for Hospital Trusts providing services may have different interests to those involved in purchasing these services. And top management who are concerned with controlling the overall system may prioritize things differently to middle managers who are more interested in maximizing service provision. Moreover, managers may be constrained by consumer power, by having to take heed of surveys of consumer opinion that they are expected to undertake. Information about such preferences can be used by professionals seeking to defend their specialty as well as by middle managers seeking to convince top management that they need more resources. Furthermore, being concerned to reduce costs, the neoliberal state has more recently questioned the number of managers employed by the NHS. It has been claimed that the NHS has become too bureaucratized and that there are now too many managers. Subsequently the number of managers has indeed been reduced but overall the managerial discourse has continued, with an emphasis on entrepreneurialism (Hyde and Exworthy, 2016).

The march of NPM may therefore be constrained but its impact on professionalism has still been significant. While some have argued that doctors have been proletarianized or corporatized, others have suggested that they have responded by employing management skills to extend their jurisdiction and thus re-professionalize. Either way, the development of NPM has arguably transformed what used to be a high-trust relationship between managers and other healthcare workers, with all parties observing a diffuse pattern of shared obligations, into a low-trust relationship with mutual suspicion replacing the mutual honouring of trust (Calnan, 2020). The longer-term impact of such a transformation is yet to be fully researched.

See also: Consumerism; Medical Autonomy, Dominance and Decline.

REFERENCES

Calnan, M. (2020) *Health Policy, Power and Politics*. Bingley: Emerald.

Calnan, M. and Gabe, J. (2009) 'The restratification of primary care in England? A sociological analysis', in J. Gabe and M. Calnan (eds), *The New Sociology of the Health Service*. London: Routledge.

Dopson, S. (2009) 'Changing forms of managerialism in the NHS: hierarchies, markets and networks', in J. Gabe and M. Calnan (eds), *The New Sociology of the Health Service*. London: Routledge.

Flynn, R. (1992) *Structures of Control in Health Management*. London: Routledge.

Freidson, E. (1989) *Medical Work in America: Essays in Healthcare*. New Haven, CT: Yale University Press.

Gabe, J., Exworthy, M., Jones, I.R and Smith, G. (2012) 'Towards a sociology of disclosure: the case of surgical performance', *Sociology Compass*, 6 (11): 908–922.

Harrison, S. and Ahmad, W.I.U. (2000) 'Medical autonomy and the UK state', *Sociology*, 34 (1): 129–146.

Harrison, S. and Pollitt, C. (1994) *Controlling Health Professionals: The Future of Work and Organization in the NHS*. Buckingham: Open University Press.

Hunter, D.J. (2006) 'From tribalism to corporatism: the continuing managerial challenge to medical dominance', in D. Kelleher, J. Gabe and G. Williams (eds), *Challenging Medicine*, 2nd edn. London: Routledge.

Hyde, P. and Exworthy, M. (2016) 'Setting the workers free? Managers in the (once again) reformed NHS', in M. Exworthy, R. Mannion and M. Powell (eds), *Dismantling the NHS? Evaluating the Impact of Health Reforms.* Bristol: Policy Press.

Martin, G.P., Armstrong, N., Aveling, E-L. et al. (2015) 'Professionalisation redundant, reshaped or reinvigorated? Realizing the "third logic" in contemporary health care', *Journal of Health and Social Behaviour*, 56 (3): 378–397.

McKinlay, J.B. and Marceau, L.D. (2002) 'The end of the golden age of doctoring', *International Journal of Health Services*, 32 (2): 379–416.

Thorne, M.L. (2002) 'Colonizing the new world of NHS management: the shifting power of professionals', *Health Services Management Research*, 15 (1): 14–26.

Weisz, G., Cambrosio, A., Keating, P. et al. (2007) 'The emergence of clinical practice guidelines', *The Milbank Quarterly*, 85 (4): 691–727.

SUGGESTED FURTHER READING

- Cox, D. (1991) 'Health service management – a sociological view', in J. Gabe, M. Calnan and M. Bury (eds), *The Sociology of the Health Service*. London: Routledge.

A useful historical account of the shift from administration to management in the British NHS.

- Exworthy, M., Gabe, J., Jones, I.R. and Smith, G. (2019) 'Professional autonomy and surveillance: the case of public reporting in cardiac surgery', *Sociology of Health & Illness*, 41 (6): 1040–1055.

An illuminating study of cardiac surgeons and their response to the publication of their clinical performance, under the guise of transparency. The research shows how the collection of these data and the managerial gaze it enables are accomodated by this surgical specialty.

- Numerato, D., Salvatore, D. and Fattore, G. (2012) 'The impact of management on medical professionalism: a review', *Sociology of Health & Illness*, 34 (4): 626–644.

An insightful review of the literature on the relationship between clinicians and management at an organizational level, focusing on socio-cultural and task-related dimensions. Its authors argue for the need to overcome the hegemony/resistance framework in analyses of the impact of management on professionalism.

52

Consumerism

Jonathan Gabe

Consumerism, when applied to healthcare, suggests that users of services should and do play an active role in making informed choices about health.

The term 'consumer' has its origins in the world of private business and reflects recognition that producers should take account of the preferences of the purchasers of their goods in order to maximize their profits. Its use blossomed first in North America where market researchers were employed by manufacturers after the Second World War to establish consumer demand for their products and customer relations departments were set up to provide a service to customers and seek to meet their needs. In the UK context, which is the focus of this entry, consumers' rights were recognized with the founding of the Consumers' Association in 1957. This organization aimed to provide readers of its magazine with information about the quality of high-street products so that they could make an 'informed choice' when making purchasing decisions.

The language of consumerism is now commonplace in healthcare policies in many Western countries (Harris et al., 2010). It was first applied to users of UK public-sector services like healthcare in the early 1980s and was initially criticized on the grounds that the consumption of medical care is different from, say, the consumption of supermarket goods. For example, in the UK people do not pay directly for medical care provided by the National Health Service (NHS), but do so through taxation. And they can exercise more choice when buying from a shop, compared with deciding which doctor to see and which treatment to have. Furthermore, consumers of healthcare are at the same time producers of good health in that they are involved in the prevention of illness through health maintenance practices in contexts of everyday life, such as the home. From this standpoint the distinction between consumption and production is artificial. Despite these concerns consumerism has become a leitmotif of health policy and practice over the last 40 years in the UK, as will be seen below.

The influence of consumerist principles can be seen, first and foremost, in a range of policies introduced by Conservative governments during the 1980s and 1990s. An early example was the decision by the Thatcher administration in 1983 to follow the advice of the Griffiths Report and introduce managerialism into the NHS. In line with neoliberal thinking, with its emphasis on individuals exercising choice through the market (Gabe et al., 2020), Griffiths stated that managers should give pride of place to the preferences of 'patients', or as they were re-named 'consumers', and to use a range of market research techniques to find out their views. While the use of these techniques may have legitimated managers' knowledge claims about their customers and what they wanted, the kind of information collected seemed to be of limited use to patients, as the focus was on their views of hotel aspects of care (for example, cleanliness and food) rather than their assessment of clinical effectiveness (Calnan and Gabe, 2001).

The 1990s witnessed further policy initiatives intended to enhance 'consumer choice'. The 1990 NHS and Community Care Act turned the NHS into an internal market, with purchasers and providers of healthcare, while reaffirming the principle of healthcare free at the point of use. To make the market work, supply side providers such as large hospitals were given the opportunity to become self-governing trusts, with the promise of increased financial freedom and greater autonomy. On the demand side, general practitioners (GPs) were permitted to become fundholders, who could then place contracts for non-emergency care on behalf of their patients. A justification for the development of this market for healthcare was that it would shift the culture of the NHS from one determined by the preferences and decisions of professionals to one shaped by the views and wishes of users. GPs were, however, purchasing services on their patients' behalf, and were thus acting as proxy or surrogate consumers, with patients having no purchasing rights of their own. It was assumed that these fundholders had the incentive to fulfil this role effectively as otherwise their patients would simply switch to a competing practice. However, as patients lacked the necessary knowledge or inclination to shop around in the medical marketplace and often did not have much choice of alternative GPs with which to register, critics argued that there was little evidence that this aspect of the reforms markedly increased consumer choice (Calnan and Gabe, 2001).

Consumerism was also promoted by the introduction of the Patient's Charter in 1992, one of a number of charters planned by the Conservatives to transform the management of the public services. The Patient's Charter was designed to make the health service more responsive to consumers and raise quality overall at nil cost, by setting rights and service standards that consumers could expect. New rights were established such as the right for detailed information about quality standards and waiting lists and having any complaint investigated and dealt with promptly. Critics of the Patient's Charter agued that while it may have increased individual users' right to information, it was premised on the dubious assumption that making such information available to the public would in and of itself change the practices of clinicians and managers (Crinson, 1998). The problem with this assumption, however, was that the medical profession and management have a vested interest in maintaining the status quo and the Patient's Charter did nothing to challenge such interests.

When Labour regained power in 1997, the emphasis shifted from one of competition to that of partnership and co-operation, with Primary Care Trusts (PCTs) replacing fund holding. Central to these organizational arrangements was the requirement that users and local people were involved in decision-making. In the NHS Plan, published in 2000, it became a statutory duty for Strategic Health Authorities (responsible for the oversight of trusts), PCTs and NHS Trusts in England to involve users and the public in the planning and operation of services. The Plan, and subsequent policy developments discussed below, did not apply to Wales, Scotland and Northern Ireland, as these countries have followed an increasingly divergent path since administrative devolution in 1999. At a national level lay participation in policy-making in England was increased, with lay people invited to sit on bodies set up to enhance the governance of the NHS (for example, the National Institute for Clinical Excellence, now the National Institute for Health and Care Excellence, which is responsible for providing guidance on the cost effectiveness of treatments). In addition, citizens' juries were used to gauge views on issues such as the out-of-hours services provided by GPs. While these forms of collective involvement were welcomed, especially by health consumer groups, it was generally felt that the Department of Health in England still set the agenda and rules of engagement. Moreover, there was a danger that decision-makers and service providers would respond first and foremost to more articulate groups at the expense of those that were hidden or less well organized (Forster and Gabe, 2008).

Alongside this concern with public participation at the collective level, the Labour government also continued to talk about the individual consumer. Indeed, in the latter stages of their time in power, this individual level approach came to dominate, as it had done with their predecessors. Initially Labour revised the Conservative government's Patient's Charter, making it a contract between the NHS and its clients, and turning these clients into responsible consumers who had both rights (old Left) and responsibilities (New Right). As such, this change reflected Labour's preference for the 'third way', pragmatically drawing on values from both sides of the policy spectrum. At the same time Labour focused on ways to make patients more informed and more actively involved in their healthcare by introducing the Choose and Book computer system to give patients more choice about how, when and where to receive elective care.

Subsequently it was recognized that patients' awareness of the right to choose and GPs' willingness to offer choice were slow to grow (Coulter, 2005). However, where choice was offered, patients responded positively, even though most chose to remain at their local hospital (Dixon et al., 2010). More recently it has been shown that poor and minority group patients were much less likely to choose private hospitals and that choice was also affected by the geographical distribution of hospitals (Beckert and Kelly, 2017). (In 2015 Choose and Book was replaced by the NHS e-Referral service which continues to allow patients to choose appointments with NHS hospitals in England, and also private hospitals, as long as they provide NHS services.)

Labour also introduced the NHS Choices website to provide comparative information about a range of services provided by hospitals and GPs and their performance against quality indicators. How might patients have responded to such data? The first point is that patients vary in their 'information literacy' – the skills and competence to understand the context of the information provided and its interpretation (Henwood et al., 2003). Of course some patients with long-term conditions have become 'expert patients', or 'experts by experience' (Jones and Pietilä, 2020), with regard to their condition so may well be able to understand and find such data helpful. Others may, however, feel too ill to want to explore such information and thus ignore the sense of obligation to take responsibility for healthcare decisions that governments in England now apparently wish them to feel. And the patients' age may also be significant. Older patients may be less used to the internet and hence might not feel confident to use sites like NHS Choices (now known as the NHS website). Overall it seems that the publication of data on clinical performance has not led the majority of patients to shop around (Coulter, 2005).

Alongside these policy initiatives there is some evidence that patients wish to participate in decision-making in the consultation (Elwyn et al., 2010). And this consumerism has been further encouraged by the growth of the internet. As illustrated by the NHS website, the internet is now a major resource for those seeking health information, especially women and young people, alongside patient support platforms and social media (Lupton, 2018). It provides an easy source of information about medical services and general medical knowledge which helps patients to engage in consumerist behaviour. Patients are now more likely to search for information about illnesses and treatment options, enabling them to *self-diagnose* before they even book an appointment to see their doctor.

Since the Conservatives (and their Coalition partners the Liberal Democrats between 2010–15) came to power, consumer choice has remained an important discourse in English healthcare policy, with it being assumed that a 'more decisive market orientation will bring about more patient choice and hence better quality and more efficiency' (Asthana, 2011: 817). As a further initiative to develop choice, patients have been given the right to choose to register with any GP practice, without restriction in terms of where they live, effectively giving patients the right to choose their own commissioner of services. Concern has, however, been expressed that competition and choice might lead to fragmentation, and it appears that very recently there has been more of a focus in policy discourse on the need for integration, especially between health and social care.

Given the above, how is the popularity of consumerism and partnership in policy circles to be explained? One response is that the different government initiatives have been driven by ideology. Certainly the policies of the

Conservatives (and their Coalition partners) seem to have been heavily influenced by a neoliberal ideology based on a belief in the value of self-reliance, individual responsibility and the rule of the market, with sovereign consumers expressing demand on the basis of knowledge about the choices available. Yet the Conservatives have not followed this ideology to the letter, as the service remains free at the point of use. The last Labour government also seemed to accept elements of neoliberalism (increasing individual choice, and maximizing personal responsibility for healthcare), but combined this with a more collectivist approach, thus reflecting a preference for pragmatism.

An alternative explanation is that the emphasis on consumerism reflects more general socio-economic changes, encapsulated in the phrase 'post-Fordism' (Gabe, 2021). From this standpoint the health service reforms described above parallel a shift from Fordist principles (mass production, universalization of welfare, mass consumption) to those of post-Fordism (flexible production techniques designed to take account of rapid changes in consumer demand and fragmented market tastes). In a post-Fordist society it is the consumers rather than the producers that call the tune. While this approach has some value in placing the health policy changes mentioned above in a broader context, it fails to distinguish between surface changes in appearance and underlying social relations. While the rhetoric has been about enhanced consumer power or partnership, producers in the form of the medical profession and health service managers arguably continue to hold the upper hand over the users of services. Future research needs to consider whether this imbalance between producers and consumers has now changed, in the UK and other countries of the Global North, and how this compares with the Global South.

See also: Citizenship and Health; Managerialism; Practitioner–Client Relationships.

REFERENCES

Asthana, S. (2011) 'Liberating the NHS? A commentary on the Lansley White Paper, "Equity and Excellence"', *Social Science & Medicine*, 72 (6): 815–820.

Beckert, W. and Kelly, E. (2017) *Divided by Choice? Private Providers, Patient Choice and Hospital Sorting in the English National Health Service*. IFS Working Paper. London: School of Business, Economics and Informatics, Birkbeck College, University of London.

Calnan, M. and Gabe, J. (2001) 'From consumerism to partnership? Britain's National Health Service at the turn of the century', *International Journal of Health Services*, 31 (1): 119–131.

Coulter, A. (2005) 'Shared decision making: the debate continues', *Health Expectations*, 8 (2): 95–96.

Crinson, I. (1998) 'Putting patients first: the continuity of the consumerist discourse in health policy: from radical right to New Labour', *Critical Social Policy*, 18 (55): 227–239.

Dixon, A., Robertson, R., Appleby, J. et al. (2010) *Patient Choice: How Patients Choose and Providers Respond.* London: King's Fund.

Elwyn, G., Laitner, S., Coulter, A. et al. (2010) 'Implementing shared decision making in the NHS', *British Medical Journal*, 341: c5146.

Forster, R. and Gabe, J. (2008) 'Voice or choice? Patient and public involvement in the National Health Service in England under New Labour', *International Journal of Health Services*, 38 (2): 333–356.

Gabe, J. (2021) 'The British health care system', in W.C. Cockerham (ed.), *The Wiley Blackwell Companion to Medical Sociology*. Oxford/Malden, MA: Wiley-Blackwell.

Gabe, J., Cardano, M. and Genova, A. (eds) (2020) *Health and Illness in the Neoliberal Era in Europe.* Bingley: Emerald.

Harris, R., Wathen, N. and Wyatt, S. (eds) (2010) *Configuring Health Consumers. Health Work and the Imperative of Personal Responsibility.* Basingstoke: Palgrave Macmillan.

Henwood, F., Wyatt, S., Hart, A. and Smith, J. (2003) '"Ignorance is bliss sometimes": constraints on the emergence of the "informed patient" in the changing landscapes of health information', *Sociology of Health & Illness*, 25 (6): 589–607.

Jones, M. and Pietilä, I. (2020) 'Personal perspectives on patient and public involvement – stories about becoming and being an expert by experience', *Sociology of Health & Illness*, 42 (4): 809–824.

Lupton, D. (2018) *Digital Health: Critical and Cross-Disciplinary Perspectives*. London: Routledge.

SUGGESTED FURTHER READING

- Calnan, M. (2020) *Health Policy, Power and Politics*. Bingley: Emerald.

This text contains an illuminating chapter on patient choice and public involvement, with a focus on whether patients are now co-producers of their treatment and care.

- Gabe, J., Harley, K. and Calnan, M. (2015) 'Healthcare choice: discourses, perceptions experiences and practices', *Current Sociology*, 63 (5): 623–778.

An important special issue, which brings together papers on healthcare choice from the Global North and Global South.

- Milewa, T. (2009) 'Health care, consumerism and the politics of identity', in J. Gabe and M. Calnan (eds), *The New Sociology of the Health Service*. Abingdon: Routledge.

An interesting sociological assessment of consumerism. The author argues that this policy can only be understood with reference to wider social perceptions and motivations around ideas such as trust, expectations, obligations and responsibility, which help to cohere understandings of identity in relation to healthcare.

- Seale, C. (1993) 'The consumer voice', in B. Davey and J. Popay (eds), *Dilemmas in Health Care*. Buckingham: Open University Press.

A useful historical account of the development of consumerism in healthcare.

53

Citizenship and Health

Gareth H. Williams, Patrick Brown,
Eva Elliott and Jennie Popay

'Citizenship and health' refers to those aspects of health affected by the changing nature of the state, and the relationships between the state, institutions, professionals and the people they serve, under varying social and economic conditions.

For several decades social scientists have reflected critically on healthcare and health in terms of how these (re)configure relationships between the modern state and its citizens. Today, these reflections focus on the nature of citizenship, the appropriate balance of rights and responsibilities between a state and its citizens and how entitlements to the benefits of citizenship should be determined. In this entry we explore how these debates have evolved in relation to: public provision of healthcare; the emergence of the concept of 'active citizenship' and responsibility for health; and contemporary arguments about the need for a new social contract between citizens and the state. In doing so we offer a critical sociological reading of these debates, illuminating the contested nature of the concepts and processes involved and the power dynamics at work that reproduce intersecting social inequalities.

The shifting relationship between the state and citizens is evident in debates about entitlement to healthcare and other public services. In a celebrated essay on citizenship and social class the sociologist T.H. Marshall (1950) argued that rights to welfare, social security and a general share in the benefits of progress signified fully *social* citizenship and developed after *civil* rights (to freedom of speech, thought and belief) and *political* rights (to participate in the exercise of political power through voting and representation) were established. His developmental theory has been criticized for oversimplifying the processes involved and understating the importance of gender, ethnicity and religion (Walby, 1994). However, universal access to healthcare has now become an important signifier of 'fully social citizenship' in many countries and is enshrined in the UN Sustainable Development Goals.

Modern healthcare systems were the beneficiaries of what are now seen as the 'Golden Years' of 20th-century Western capitalism, stretching from the start of the 1950s to the OPEC oil crisis and economic turbulence of 1973 and after. Increasingly the only certainty in healthcare was that it was going to cost more. Much of the sociological analysis that emerged during the 1970s represented the beginnings of an extended examination of the relationship between citizens and professionally controlled health services. These analyses emerged in the context of growing evidence of the limited effectiveness of much modern medicine, persisting health inequalities in an era of neoliberal globalization, the perception that patients are disenfranchised in the organization and delivery of healthcare systems and, latterly, the unfolding consequences of new genetic knowledge and medical technologies.

From the 1980s onward the issue of the relationship between citizens and their health became increasingly debated as the UK and other high-income societies engaged in severe economic 'restructuring'. This restructuring involved a move away from the corporatist social contract between centralist political parties and the trades unions, on which public healthcare systems had hitherto been based, towards market-style expectations and relationships. Management systems were introduced to control health professionals' expenditure, and quasi-markets were employed to stimulate competition between providers. In the context of a severe squeeze on public services, debates about the roles and rights of 'consumers' in the planning and delivery of health services became more prominent (Calnan and Gabe, 2001). Knowledgeable and informed consumers making rational choices about treatment became the leitmotif of reform across Europe and North America. Developments during the 1990s such as the Patient's Charter in the UK – a list of rights (not legally binding) to certain standards of care – were designed to make services more responsive to 'consumers' and thereby improve quality at no extra cost.

In the UK there was also growing evidence that some groups, such as mental health service users, were having a range of citizenship rights threatened (Rogers and Pilgrim, 1989) and that basic needs of older people and people with learning disabilities in both National Health Service facilities and care homes were not being met. Critics began to argue against the consumer model of involvement in health service decision-making, and for a more radical citizenship approach. In response, the Labour government, elected in 1997, modified the emphasis on markets, toned down the language of consumerism and implemented a series of changes that aimed to 'bring patients and citizens into decision-making at every level of service' (Lewis and Gillam, 2001: 113). In a detailed and comprehensive analysis of these changes between 1997 and 2006, Forster and Gabe (2008: 348) concluded that there had been 'a significant extension of opportunities for individual patients and the public to communicate their views in more ways and on different levels'. Subsequent UK governments on the centre right and right have continued this emphasis on a strengthened role for citizens in healthcare decision-making. However, evidence of significant shifts in the power relationship between service users, health institutions and professionals remains limited.

More recently, sociologists have drawn attention to the emergence of the concept of 'active citizenship' in debates about, and policies for, health and welfare entitlement. Active citizenship, as we will discuss further below, is an ideological construct and practice that reproduces intersecting social inequalities (for example, through a behavioural focus on lifestyles in health policy). Tonkens and Duyvendak (2016) have linked this to the development of culturally grounded models of citizenship – alongside or as alternatives to civil, political and social citizenship – that are reconfiguring understandings about what it means to be a citizen and to be entitled to – or (un)deserving of – care. The increasing prominence of cultural citizenship models in public policy has also been linked to neoliberal governance and in particular the responses of economies shaken by the global financial crisis which began in 2007/8 and reverberated around the world.

These culturally grounded models of active citizenship give primacy to particular kinds of thinking, behaviour, participation and integration, leading to widespread notions of an incompatibility between certain cultures, groups and religions and 'good citizenship'. Within the Dutch context, for example, research points towards the emotional reconfiguring of various 'citizen regimes', whereby underlying policy models of welfare state provision require particular modes of behaving and feeling from 'good' citizens (Tonkens and Duyvendak, 2016). The same processes can be identified in many contemporary welfare regimes, not least across northern Europe, where citizens are now expected to be *active* in caring for themselves, relatives and neighbours in ways which complement, and are fostered by, health and social care systems and which compound existing social inequalities. Women, who provide disproportionate amounts of care in most societies, face a greater burden and pressure in these 'active' citizenship regimes. Other groups, including working-class people and cultural minorities, are also more likely to be judged negatively by professionals and in policy rhetoric for failing to meet the demands of good citizenship – to stay healthy and to care in the right manner. These groups are often the targets of interventions that aim to foster more 'appropriate' behaviours. For example, initiatives designed to develop 'good' parenting implicitly exert morally-loaded pressures to conform to White middle-class ideals of the healthy family and 'good' motherhood (Simmons, 2020).

Notions of active citizenship also focus on the thinking and behaviours of communities of interest and/or place. Initially, this focus emerged as the prominence of health inequalities in policy grew globally from the late 1990s. For example, in the UK during this period, national interventions such as the Healthy Living Centres programme and New Deal for Communities sought to galvanize communities of place to identify and address the determinants of health inequalities locally, albeit in partnership with public and third sector organizations. It was a contract between citizens and the state in which local people were the agents of change and not just the state or market forces. However, in response to the financial crisis, a new

Conservative–Liberal Coalition government implemented unprecedented cuts in public expenditure (austerity) in 2010. This led to reduced public service provision and compounded the shift in responsibility for health and welfare from the state to individuals and communities. In parallel, forms of place-based stigma evolved, labelling many disadvantaged places, and their residents, as worthless and failing to live responsible and, by implication, healthy lives. These stigmatizing processes have been linked to neoliberal governance and the use of weaponizing strategies to instil shame and apportion blame (Scambler, 2018).

The health and welfare provisions put in place in many high-income countries following the Second World War were a central pillar of an enduring *social contract* between the state and the people, in which basic provision and security were assured for the whole population. However, as we have shown, over the following decades relationships between the state and citizens have shifted in complex ways that have undermined the basis of this social contract. The drivers of these shifts include growing social and health inequalities, unprecedented transnational migration and 'statelessness', the climate and environmental crises and the continuing dominance of neoliberal policies shrinking the role of the state as a provider of health and welfare services. However, the COVID-19 pandemic has paused this trajectory, as the role of states has expanded (at least temporarily) with countries borrowing and spending money to prevent the destruction of existing social and economic infrastructures.

As we have shown, ideals of citizenship are imbued in various policy frameworks and everyday health practices, creating powerful notions of different forms of citizenship. These ideals and forms have major political ramifications. Indeed, some groups and individual citizens are judged and evaluated differently from others, based on citizenship regimes which demand performances of particular activation, morality, culture and emotion. Many struggle to live up to these expectations, but some citizens – individually and collectively – are especially stigmatized, designated as risky and treated with suspicion (Veltkamp and Brown, 2017) or contempt. This marginalization, stigma and distrust can be experienced over multiple generations. Significant groups of citizens may therefore come to feel as outsiders in relation to the state, whereby the relationship between citizen and state is marked by a reciprocated distrust.

This breakdown in state–citizen relations in high-income countries has important effects on health in many domains, from lower vaccine uptake to lower levels of acccessing services, to greater levels of violence directed towards healthcare professionals. The effects of these undermined relations are apparent in attempts by national governments to limit the spread of the SARS-CoV-2 virus, where cooperation with guidelines/regulations and vaccine uptake are lower in some communities. In many cases these effects of low trust – reflective of and arguably a product of a 'fractured society' that has been ravaged by financial capital in the post-1970s era (Scambler, 2018) – may add to, and compound, existing health inequalities, as explored in Part 1 of this volume.

It is important to note here that much of the published critical sociological literature on citizenship discussed so far emanates from the Global North and high-income countries in particular. These arguments cannot therefore be simply transferred to the context of low- and middle-income countries with a history of colonialism. Nor can they readily illuminate the situation of the millions of displaced people around the globe: refugees, asylum seekers and residents of informal settlements who make up the often-stateless *nomadic proletariat* (Scambler, 2018). These people are driven by a toxic mix of poverty, conflict, discrimination, genocide, environmental degradation and climate change to live in a *state of exception* where the laws applying to citizens are not recognized (Diken and Lausten, 2005).

However, some common elements can be found in an emerging literature exploring changing citizenship regimes associated with the health and welfare policies being implemented by governments in the Global South, including cash transfer schemes and universal healthcare. In the context of growing inequalities and the minimal support involved, these developments are seen by some to offer 'a biopolitics not of care but of "bare life"' (Prince, 2017: 157). Others view them as explicitly framed by arguments about justice and the rightful share of citizens, conceived as active recipients (Ferguson, 2009). Recent research in French Guiana (*Guyane* in French) has illuminated how the power dynamics underpinning these social processes play out in particular local contexts, pointing to the pivotal role of colonialism. The study describes the drivers of a public policy shift from biological and chemical mosquito control by local authorities to awareness-raising campaigns focusing responsibility on domestic spaces, resembling the 'active' citizenship narratives in the Global North. But it also identified a strong demand from the local population for mosquito control by public authorities to continue. As the authors note: 'This reciprocal passing of responsibility is exacerbated by the colonial past and heritage of slavery in these multi-ethnic overseas territories located over 7000 km from the seat of the French government ... politically France but culturally Latin-America and historically colonial' (Mieulet and Claeys, 2014: 581).

Together with the Black Lives Matter movement, the COVID-19 pandemic as a social, and not just health, crisis has shattered Marshall's framing of citizenship. Shortly before these two events, Fraser (2017) appositely called for a new paradigm that brings together progressive forces concerned with *recognition* of identity rights with a continued acknowledgement of class inequalities, which demands a redistribution of material, economic and social *resources*. To this should be added the critical need to incorporate the legacy of colonialism into debates about the meaning of citizenship, as well as to consider the complex web of inequalities which further marginalize the position of undocumented migrants. We have sought to show how a sociological lens can contribute to these debates, within and between national regimes and welfare systems. For example, various authors have described a biological format of citizenship at the intersection of health risk, bio-scientific understandings of healthy populations and a responsibilizing of citizens for their bodies, health and risk reduction

(Setälä and Väliverronen, 2014). Historical neglect of particular groups, glaringly highlighted amid COVID-19, can help us understand lived experiences of disenfranchizement and its effects on health, (dis)trust and other barriers to health and healthcare. An attentiveness to how the culturalization of citizenship and an increased biological lens may be fostering new or deepening processes of sub-citizenship would highlight the adverse consequences of these processes for equity in the experience of health and well-being, in access to care and for democracy. As Prince (2017: 157) argues, equally important questions also need to be asked about how health and welfare reforms in the Global South 'are shaping new collectives of care and citizenship, forms of obligation and solidarity, and a re-evaluation of the role of the state'.

See also: Consumerism; Managerialism; Neoliberalism; Pandemics and Epidemics; Place; Stigma.

REFERENCES

Calnan, M. and Gabe, J. (2001) 'From consumerism to partnership? Britain's National Health Service at the turn of the century', *International Journal of Health Services*, 31 (1): 119–131.

Diken, B. and Lausten, C.B. (2005) *The Culture of Exception: Sociology Facing the Camp.* London: Routledge.

Ferguson, J. (2009) 'The uses of neoliberalism', *Antipode*, 41 (1): 166–184.

Forster, R. and Gabe, J. (2008) 'Voice or choice? Patient and public involvement in the National Health Service in England under New Labour', *International Journal of Health Services*, 38 (2): 333–356.

Fraser, N. (2017) 'From progressive neoliberalism to Trump – and beyond', *American Affairs*, I (4): 46–64.

Lewis, R. and Gillam, S. (2001) 'The National Health Service Plan: further reform of British health care', *International Journal of Health Services*, 31 (1): 111–118.

Marshall, T.H. (1950) *Citizenship and Social Class and other Essays.* Cambridge: Cambridge University Press.

Mieulet, E. and Claeys, C. (2014) 'The implementation and reception of policies for preventing dengue fever epidemics: a comparative study of Martinique and French Guyana', *Health, Risk & Society*, 16 (7–8): 581–599.

Prince, R. (2017) 'Universal health coverage in the Global South: new models of healthcare and their implications for citizenship, solidarity, and the public good', *Michael*, 14: 153–172.

Rogers, A. and Pilgrim, D. (1989) 'Mental health and citizenship', *Critical Social Policy*, 9 (26): 44–55.

Scambler, G. (2018) *Sociology, Health and the Fractured Society: A Critical Realist Account.* London: Routledge.

Setälä, V. and Väliverronen, E. (2014) 'Fighting fat: the role of "field experts" in mediating science and biological citizenship', *Science as Culture*, 23 (4): 517–536.

Simmons, H. (2020) *Surveillance of Modern Motherhood: Experiences of Universal Parenting Courses.* Cham: Palgrave Macmillan.

Tonkens, E. and Duyvendak, J.W. (2016) 'Introduction', in J.W. Duyvendak, P. Geschiere and E. Tonkens (eds), *The Culturalisation of Citizenship*. London: Palgrave.

Veltkamp, G. and Brown, P. (2017) 'The everyday "risk work" of Dutch child-healthcare professionals: inferring "safe" and "good" parenting through trust, as mediated by a lens of gender and class', *Sociology of Health & Illness*, 39 (8): 1297–1313.

Walby, S. (1994) 'Is citizenship gendered?' *Sociology*, 28 (2): 379–395.

SUGGESTED FURTHER READING

- Hamilton, M. (2014) 'The "new social contract" and the individualisation of risk in policy', *Journal of Risk Research*, 17 (4): 453–467.

Focusing especially on the UK and Australia, this article explores the changing relationship between the state and its citizens and how policies framed through risk have shifted additional responsibility onto the shoulders of citizens while making rights conditional upon active attempts to 'improve' the self.

- Sparke, M. (2017) 'Austerity and the embodiment of neoliberalism as ill-health: towards a theory of biological sub-citizenship', *Social Science & Medicine*, 187: 287–295.

This article describes pathways through which austerity and other policy shifts associated with neoliberalism have become embodied globally in ill-health. Research on these processes is combined with the development of a theory of the resulting forms of biological sub-citizenship that have developed and which contribute to ill-health.

- Tonkens, E. (2012) 'Working with Arlie Hochschild: connecting feelings to social change', *Social Politics*, 19 (2): 194–218.

This article discusses how particular configurations of welfare state policies assume and foster specific ways of feeling and caring. This institutionalization of care through 'citizenship regimes' may then lead to tensions when policies shift in ways which are out of keeping with prevailing 'feeling rules' and care norms.

- Scambler, G. (2020) 'Covid-19 as a "breaching experiment": exposing the fractured society', *Health Sociology Review*, 29 (2): 140–148.

This paper argues for a politically engaged sociology. Scambler uses Garfinkel's notion of a 'breaching experiment' to describe how the pandemic is disrupting neoliberal governance and exposing dimensions of what he terms the 'fractured society'. Following a critique of the UK government's pandemic response, he considers possible scenarios for a post-fractured society, drawing on Fraser's concepts of 'reactionary' versus 'progressive populism'.

54

Social Movements and Health

Nick Crossley

Social movements, including health movements, are '(1) Informal networks, based on (2) shared beliefs and solidarity, which mobilise around (3) conflictual issues, through (4) the frequent use of various forms of protest' (Della Porta and Diani, 1999: 16).

The concept 'social movements' is used widely and in varying ways both within and outside of social science, not least by activists within social movements themselves. This variation in use makes it impossible to arrive at criteria which are both sufficiently inclusive and sufficiently exclusive to give a precise definition that is suited to all cases. Like 'games', as defined by Wittgenstein (1953), 'social movements' share 'family resemblances' and are clearly identifiable as such but they are very difficult to pin down (Crossley, 2002). However, the above definition, by Della Porta and Diani (1999), captures many properties of movements deemed important by contemporary analysts.

Examples of movements include the environmental movement, feminist movements, the global justice and anti-war movements, whose mobilizations enjoyed a high profile in the first decade of the 21st century, and a variety of movements mobilized around conflicts concerning health and medicine. I return to these health conflicts and movements shortly. First, however, we must unpick 'social movements' in more detail.

The informal networks to which Della Porta and Diani (1999) refer might be networks of individual activists but they might equally be networks of 'social movement organizations' (SMOs). They are often networks of both. An SMO, in turn, might be anything from a formal organization with paid workers and subscribing members to a loose cluster of activists experimenting with new ways of living and alternative social practices; for example, a feminist commune or alternative therapeutic community, such as those of the anti-psychiatry movement (Crossley, 2006). Likewise, addressing Della Porta and Diani's (1999) second criterion, the extent to which beliefs are shared and solidarity achieved can be highly variable, not only between movements but across time and context. Factional infighting is by no means uncommon. Finally, the forms of protest that Della Porta and Diani refer to are highly variable also, including everything from petitions and marches through various forms of obstruction to the political violence of al-Qaida and related groups. Generally, however, 'social movements' operate outside of institutionalized channels, putting pressure upon government, insofar as that is the target of their actions, by means of symbolic challenges to its legitimacy. This distinguishes them from political parties, that seek to effect political change by becoming elected within government, and from lobby and pressure groups that tend to work through the official channels of the political system.

Contemporary ways of analysing social movements draw from two, once distinct but now merged schools, the European and the American, each of which is itself widely recognized to be the culmination of a history of paradigmatic shifts. Both traditions draw from Marxism to varying degrees. However, the key European writers, such as Habermas (1987) and Touraine (1981), who I will discuss first, before turning to the American tradition, follow Marx more directly. In so doing, European writers seek to identify where the key fault-lines of society lie and which movement will emerge from the conflicts surfacing around that fault-line, constituting itself as the agent of change for its epoch. They reject Marx's own answers to these questions, which identify class relations as the fault-line of (capitalist) society and the working class as the agent of historical change, arguing that capitalism has moved on and that the working class has been incorporated within it. But they remain focused on the questions, suggesting that the contradictions of society have been displaced rather than resolved and that 'new social movements' which took to the political stage in the late 1960s have replaced the working class as society's key agents of change (see also the Suggested Further Reading, notably Edwards, 2014).

This argument is pertinent to health movements because both Touraine (1981) and Habermas (1987) recognize health-related movements amongst the new social movements. Habermas, in particular, theorizes their emergence as resistance to a 'colonization of the lifeworld' by both the state and economy; a colonization whose form includes the birth and growth of the welfare state in the latter half of the 20th century, with its implications in terms of surveillance and regulation of conduct. The aforementioned anti-psychiatry movement of the 1960s, which sought to resist the power of psychiatrists (as agents of the state) to define normality and deny the liberty of those deemed 'mentally ill', might be one example of this (Crossley, 2006). Fat activists, who challenge obesity discourse and related attempts to 'enforce' an ideal of slimness, would be another (Cooper, 2016). And activism focused upon the intersexed would be another still (Crocetti et al., 2020).

However, the distinction between 'new' and 'old' movements posited in the work of Habermas, Touraine and others has been hotly contested (Edwards,

2004) and 'health' was a focus of social movement activism long before the 1960s. Indeed, the establishment of welfare states and related forms of public healthcare provision in the West were in many cases and many ways influenced by the campaigns of working class and women's movements in the late 19th and early 20th centuries, and the campaigns of bourgeois reform movements before them. The latter included, for example, the 'lunacy reformers' who campaigned for reform of the private market in 'madhouses' during the early 19th century (Crossley, 2006). Furthermore, many of the issues apparently associated with the 'old' social movements, including issues relating to health, have resurfaced in 21st-century movements, often alongside the supposedly 'new' issues – which are no longer new, if they ever were (Crossley, 2003). Contemporary protests and movements often focus upon economic inequalities at various levels (global, national and local), highlighting, amongst other things, their deleterious effects upon the health of the poor. In many cases, moreover, these inequalities intersect with political identities both old and new, including racial identities – which have become increasingly prominent in recent years, particularly with the Black Lives Matter movement (for example, see *The Lancet* editorial of 13 June 2020). Issues relating to quality of care, which have occasioned movement mobilization, also fall into this category (Waring and Crompton, 2017).

In contrast to the European focus on 'the' agent of change in any given historical juncture, the American school has tended to recognize a plurality of movements in play at any time and is more concerned to identify the mechanisms that explain, for example, how movements form and recruit members, their effects and efficacy. This 'school' too must be approached through its history. It underwent a paradigm shift in the 1970s when a new generation of scholars launched a fierce attack upon their predecessors, who, they claimed, had characterized protest as an irrational 'crowd' response to 'structural strain' on behalf of previously atomized individuals (Crossley, 2002). In contrast, the new generation has deemed activists rational (often in a 'rational choice' sense), has claimed that they are usually well-embedded in social networks and has focused upon the impact of the availability of resources and 'political opportunities' on mobilization.

This paradigm was itself subject to attack in the 1990s, however, when a successive generation criticized its rational choice assumptions and neglect of such issues as culture and emotion (Crossley, 2002). Protest and campaigning are not mere irrational outbursts, the new generation agreed, but neither are they an outcome of pure economic rationality. It is important to understand the role of different emotions, identities and cultural practices both within movements and within their wider environments. This move has also involved a merging of the European and American schools, with most movement scholars now borrowing insights from both (Edwards, 2014).

New developments within the field have also included a small body of literature addressing movements focused variously upon issues of health, medicine and/or medicalization. There are a small number of case study monographs addressing specific movements (for example, Cooper, 2016; Crossley, 2006) as well as broader reflections upon health and medical movements as a sub-type of movement in general (Brown and Zavestoski, 2005). The area remains ripe for further analysis, however, as there has been a proliferation of health movements of various kinds in recent years. As noted above, mobilization around health issues, whether by bourgeois reform, working-class or women's movements, is by no means new and has played an important role in shaping health provision at various points in its history. However, the enormous expansion of healthcare provision in Western societies over the last 60 years, with the related extension of the remit of health professionals and the sheer growth of what is technically possible, have provoked many further and diverse mobilizations.

In some part conflicts centre upon the allocation of resources. Medical capability outstrips what the medical profession and the wider society which funds it can afford to provide, prompting an inevitable competition over the available resources by both 'disease specific' movements and groups and movements representing wider constituencies (for example, women, children, older people, specific ethnic groups). Where this is simply a matter of lobbying for funds it is not technically social movement activism. As noted above, social movement activism utilizes extra-government means to achieve its ends. Many routine resource-related health campaigns do use such means, however, and some take on an additional aspect when they address such issues as the practices of major pharmaceutical companies. These are social movements.

Beyond resource issues, 'medicalization' of conditions has also proved a major issue of contention, especially in relation to disability and 'mental illness'. In the case of mental illness, for example, a succession of movements involving both medical professionals and 'patients' have sought to challenge medical categories, authority and language, arguing that the difficulties experienced by those labelled 'mentally ill' are not symptoms of an illness and should not be treated as such (Crossley, 2006). In this case, furthermore, where 'survivors' (as radicalized 'patients' have re-labelled themselves) can be incarcerated and 'treated' against their own will with electro-convulsive therapy (controlled electric shocks) and mind-altering drugs, both of which can have deeply debilitating side-effects, issues of personal liberty have been predominant too. As often happens, however, these movements have provoked counter-movements that argue that the more libertarian position called for by the critics of medicalization leads to neglect of both vulnerable individuals and the family members who seek to support them, and thus a great deal of personal misery (Crossley, 2006). Thus, conflicting movements and SMOs compete, generating a 'field of contention' around psychiatric practice.

Where disability activists and psychiatric survivors challenge medicine for, in their view, wrongly identifying their difficulties as illnesses, other movements, like the counter-movements in mental health, attack medicine for failing to recognize illness where, they claim, it exists. Important examples include mobilizations around both chronic fatigue and Gulf War syndromes. What both share in common, however, and share also with a range of other health-related movements, including most famously the movement mobilized around HIV/AIDS (Epstein, 1996), is a championing of lay knowledge and the patient perspective relative to medical knowledge. Activists have argued that the experience of the 'patient' is or rather should be a legitimate source of knowledge with respect to both definitions of illness and measurement of the efficacy and value of treatments. They have challenged the monopoly and authority which the medical profession enjoys in relation to these matters.

In some cases this challenge coincides with the shift towards a consumerist ethos within health provision, introduced by neoliberal policy-makers. And some campaigners recognize – often with ambivalent feelings – that neoliberal health reforms have opened certain doors to them in their quest to break medical monopolies and promote the view of those on the receiving end (Crossley, 2006). Their critique is generally more fundamental than that of the consumer-focused agenda of neoliberalism, however, and the language of consumerism is in many cases alien to them.

As the capacities of medicine expand and perhaps events such as the recent COVID-19 pandemic become more common, we should expect that these and other health-political issues will become more prominent in the public sphere, along with the movements that champion them. Health never has been and never will be a matter of politically/morally neutral knowledge and intervention. It is a central facet of our well-being and thus of our political life. Sociologists have been waking up to this for some time now but lines of communication between medical sociologists and social movement analysts remain relatively thin. It is time for more sustained dialogue between these branches of the discipline and for a more comprehensive review both of what health-related social movements involve and what their analysis might entail.

See also: Consumerism; Disability; Lay Knowledge; Medicalization.

REFERENCES

Brown, P. and Zavestoski, S. (eds) (2005) *Social Movements in Health*. Oxford: Blackwell.

Cooper, C. (2016) *Fat Activism*. London: HammerOn.

Crocetti, D., Arfini, E.A.G., Monro, S. and Yeadon-Lee, T. (2020) '"You're basically calling doctors torturers": stakeholder framing issues around naming intersex rights claims as human rights abuses', *Sociology of Health & Illness*, 42 (4): 943–958.

Crossley, N. (2002) *Making Sense of Social Movements*. Buckinghamshire: Open University Press.

Crossley, N. (2003) 'Even newer social movements?' *Organisation*, 10 (2): 287–305

Crossley, N. (2006) *Contesting Psychiatry*. London: Routledge.

Della Porta, D. and Diani, M. (1999) *Social Movements*. Oxford: Blackwell.

Edwards, G. (2004) 'Habermas and social movements: what's new?' In N. Crossley and J.M. Roberts (eds), *After Habermas*. Oxford: Blackwell.

Epstein, S. (1996) *Impure Science*. Berkeley: University of California Press.
Habermas, J. (1987) *The Theory of Communicative Action, Vol II*. Cambridge: Polity.
Touraine, A. (1981) *The Voice and the Eye*. New York: Cambridge University Press.
Waring, J. and Crompton, A. (2017) 'A movement for improvement?' *Sociology of Health & Illness*, 39 (7): 1083–1099.
Wittgenstein, L. (1953) *Philosophical Investigations*. Oxford: Blackwell.

SUGGESTED FURTHER READING

- Edwards, G. (2014) *Social Movements and Protest*. Cambridge: Cambridge University Press.

An up-to-date introduction to key movements and issues in social movement studies.

- Keefe, R.H., Lane, S.D and Swarts, H.J. (2008) 'From the bottom up', *Journal of Health & Social Policy*, 21 (3): 55–69.

An interesting paper exploring the effectiveness of a number of movements in transforming medical practice.

- Landzelius, K. (2006) 'Editorial. Introduction: patient organisation movements and new metamorphoses in patienthood', *Social Science & Medicine; Special Issue: Patient Organisation Movements*, 62 (3): 529–537.

Landzelius introduces a collection of articles addressing a range of different health movements and the meanings of patienthood.

55

Medicines Regulation

Jonathan Gabe

Medicines regulation refers to the role of the state in regulating the safety and efficacy of medicines.

Over recent decades medical sociology has paid increasing attention to medicines and their production by the pharmaceutical industry and how the state controls which medicines are available for consumption, their safety, efficacy and price. Below we focus on safety and efficacy issues, with particular reference to the UK and the USA (a discussion of the state's role regarding pricing can be found in Suggested Further Reading). Before proceeding, however, we need to mention some of the key concepts which have been employed to understand the relationship between the pharmaceutical industry and the state and provide a brief history of medicine's regulation.

Informed by political sociology and the political economy of medicines, the focus has been on the way in which the interests of the state and pharmaceutical industry may disadvantage consumers in various ways. Particular attention has been given to the possibility of 'regulatory capture', where the government agency responsible for regulating the pharmaceutical industry comes to represent that industry rather than the 'public interest' (Abraham, 1995). The extent to which the relationship between government regulators and drug companies can be characterized in terms of 'corporatism' and 'corporate bias' is also receiving attention. Corporatism refers to whether drug companies have been granted semi-official status, giving them 'internal representation' in executive decision-making structures, thereby enabling them to assist government to implement policies that directly affect them (Wiktorowicz et al., 2012). Corporate bias is demonstrated by the industry having privileged access to and influence over the state, not afforded to any other interest group (Abraham, 2009). Light et al. (2013) have also introduced the related concept of 'institutional corruption', which refers to the distortion of the responsibility of regulators to make sure that new drugs do more good than harm. Examples in support of their claim include the approval of new drugs which are at best a little better than existing medicines, failing to ensure adequate testing for serious risks and inadequately protecting the public from harmful side-effects of new medicines. They argue that such distortions benefit commercial interests at the expense of public health.

In order to explore these issues a brief history of medicines regulation in the UK and the USA will be provided. This account will illustrate differences in the degree of corporatism, corporate bias, institutional corruption and regulatory capture in the two countries and the possible reasons for these. Reference will also be made to the Europeanization of medicine's regulation and the extent to which the agency established to harmonize standards of regulatory evaluation across Europe has adopted the UK approach to regulation with its attendant consequences.

In the UK, before the 1960s, the safety and efficacy of medicines were, for the most part, unregulated by the state. Pharmaceutical companies could sell drugs as remedies, as long as they were unadulterated, at prices that the market could bear. Regulation was thus by the market, with drugs usually only falling out of favour if it became clear that they were toxic or ineffective. The government trusted the pharmaceutical industry to test their products for safety and efficacy before bringing them to market. In the early 1960s this trust was breached when reports started to be published about the disastrous side-effects of the sedative Thalidomide. It was found that drugs could destroy lives as well as save them (Abraham and Lewis, 2002). To restore public confidence in medicines, the UK government introduced regulatory mechanisms to check that new medicines were safe and effective before they were introduced to the market. From the start, however, the government agreed that information submitted by the manufacturers would be treated as confidential, thereby sealing off the regulators from public scrutiny. It was also accepted that the review process should be rapid, so as not to delay the introduction of possibly valuable drugs (Abraham, 2009). Producers' interests thus remained dominant, with citizens' rights of security in healthy medications being circumscribed.

In 1968 the Medicines Act was passed which provided the basis for contemporary UK medicines regulation. This Act, which came into force in 1971, required the Department of Health (now the Department of Health and Social Care), advised by a new Committee on Safety of Medicines (CSM), to become legally responsible for assessing drug safety and efficacy. Members of the CSM were permitted to hold consultancies and shares in pharmaceutical companies, allowing a low level of differentiation between the regulators and these companies (Abraham, 2009). Under the Act, pharmaceutical companies were required for the first time to obtain approval from the government for the marketing of new medicines. As before, however, it was agreed that all information about new drug applications should be treated as confidential. Moreover, information on adverse drug reactions was withheld from citizens, including lawyers and journalists, on the grounds that they lacked the medical expertise to interpret such information. Citizens' rights to health thus remained limited in the face of producer interests and medical power.

Since the 1970s the pharmaceutical industry has attempted to maintain its influence over the regulatory authorities through close consultation about regulations on data requirements for product licenses. It has also complained regularly about the length of time taken to get decisions from regulators. In the 1980s, these concerns were heeded by a Conservative government that was keen to reduce state intervention in the economy, in line with its neoliberal agenda. In 1981 it reduced the amount of toxicological data drug companies were required to submit to the regulators before getting approval to conduct clinical trials; and in 1989 it set up the Medicines Control Agency (MCA) in response to industry claims that regulators were inefficient and reluctant to approve drugs quickly. The MCA was to be funded by the industry through the licence fee charged and run as a business, selling its regulatory services to the industry and promoting itself as the fastest licensing authority in the world (Abraham, 2009). In effect, then, the UK government had decided to reform the regulatory authorities as a new neoliberal, corporatist partnership between industry and regulators. Consumers continued to be excluded despite attempts over the period to extend their rights through legal action against certain pharmaceutical companies, in the face of drug disasters such as Opren (prescribed for arthritis sufferers) and Ativan (for anxiety) (Medawar, 1992).

This corporatist partnership between industry and regulators has also shaped the process of Europeanization of medicines regulation. This process dates back to 1965 when the European Community, now the European Union (EU), made provision for regulating medicines in the Community. It acquired greater urgency in the 1990s when European governments and industrialists realized that an integrated EU-wide pharmaceutical market was needed if European drug companies were to be competitive on the world stage (Abraham, 1997). Common technical standards were agreed and a committee of European experts – the Committee for Proprietary Medicinal Products (CPMP) – was established, with representatives from each of the national regulatory bodies. Under this system pharmaceutical companies were encouraged to seek simultaneous approval for their products in more than one Member State. Once a drug had been approved by one Member State, other Member States were encouraged to accept this decision. This body was incorporated into the European Medicines Agency (EMA) in 1995, as one of its core scientific advisory committees. The EMA is funded by the EU and the pharmaceutical industry. From 1995 its recommendations became binding on Member States, as can be seen when these states accepted the EMA's assessment that AstraZeneca's vaccine to protect people from COVID-19 was safe, despite concerns in March 2021 that it caused blood clots. When the EU established the EMA it also agreed, under pressure from the drug companies, to introduce strict timescales surrounding approval decisions. National regulatory agencies now compete for licensing fees from the industry by presenting themselves as the fastest in approving drugs. Acting primarily on the basis of this economic imperative increases the chances that scientific checks, needed to provide adequate levels of drug safety, are undermined (Abraham and Lewis, 2002) and the likelihood of institutional corruption enhanced. Under this neoliberal model the regulatory science on which decisions are based remains secret, despite challenges from transnational consumer organizations for greater openness. As in the UK, which since Brexit is no longer involved in EMA decision making, the same arguments are used about the need for secrecy in order to protect valuable intellectual property from commercial competitors. Thus it can be argued that corporate bias towards the drugs industry at the national level has been reproduced supra-nationally.

Such corporate bias is also apparent in post-marketing surveillance of adverse drug reactions (ADRs) to long-term use of medicines. Such surveillance is based on pharmacovigilance: 'the science of collecting, monitoring, researching and evaluating information on ADRs to identify and prevent harm' (Wiktorowicz et al., 2012: 165). In the EU and the UK, drug companies have been allowed to negotiate the basis of evidence used in pharmacovigilance. This is because the EMA and the UK MCA, and its successor (since 2003 the Medicines and Health-care-products Regulatory Agency (MHRA)), lack the resources to undertake independent research. European and UK regulators are reliant on drug companies to establish their own pharmacovigilance systems to monitor their products, thereby allowing the industry to influence regulatory decisions (Wiktorowicz et al., 2012). Delays in submitting the results of such post-marketing surveillance by pharmaceutical companies to the EMA (as found in the case of cancer drugs; Salcher-Konrad et al., 2020), with few if any penalties for such failings, means that there is little chance of the regulators subsequently revoking approval.

In general terms medicines regulation is rather different in the USA, mainly as a result of a different political environment. Regulation started much earlier than in the UK and the rest of Europe. Since 1938 drug manufacturers have been required to obtain permission to market a new product from the American drug regulatory authority, the Food and Drug Administration (FDA). In the late 1950s the industry was exposed to embarrassing criticism during congressional hearings conducted by Senator Kefauver. The result was the 1962 Kefauver-Harris Amendment to the 1938 Act. Thereafter, manufacturers had to provide substantial evidence of effectiveness as well as safety and the FDA was required to withdraw approval already granted for a drug if it lacked evidence of efficacy (Light, 2010). The FDA was thus specifically required by Congress to protect the public from ineffective as well as unsafe drugs. In addition, as a result of the passing of the 1967 US Freedom of Information Act, members of the public now had the right to information about the FDA's grounds for approving a new drug and records of its meetings with particular drug companies. Drug regulators in the USA therefore operate in a political climate in which consumers have much greater opportunity to examine the extent to which regulators are protecting their interests instead of operating primarily in the interests of the drug industry. Moreover, the litigious nature of US society means that the relationship between the regulators, the drug industry and consumers is much more adversarial than is the case in the UK (Abraham, 1997).

Opportunities for regulatory capture still exist, however, as was recognized by Congress in the 1970s. It acknowledged that the FDA, during the Nixon administration, had become more 'industry-friendly' and had sought to neutralize medical scientists within the organization who were felt to be adversarial towards the pharmaceutical industry. In response, Congress prohibited FDA scientists from joining the industry for two years after leaving the Administration. In the 1980s, in the face of the neoliberal political agenda of the Reagan and Bush Senior administrations, the FDA was pressurized to limit its regulatory activities in order to avoid harming the drug industry's competitiveness. However, congressional committees reminded the FDA that it could be called to account and required to demonstrate that it was acting in the 'public interest' by subsequently investigating some of its regulatory decisions. These procedural checks, combined with the ability of consumer groups to use the Freedom of Information Act to examine the basis for regulatory decisions, generally made the FDA much more cautious about embracing the values of the drugs industry than has been the case in the UK.

However, pressure from the Reagan and Bush Senior administrations in the late 1980s and 1990s for the FDA to reduce its regulatory burden and adapt a 'lighter touch' regulatory approach, like that of the UK, resulted in the FDA being less cautious. This was illustrated through its adoption of accelerated approval of drugs intended to treat serious or life-threatening conditions in response to industry concerns – a policy which was subsequently followed in the EU. For Light et al. (2013) such accelerated approvals, with shorter review times, has resulted in a substantial increase in serious adverse reactions in patients, and as such is illustrative of institutional corruption. For Davis and Abraham (2011) this policy change reflects a 'tentacled corporate bias', with the industry stretching its influence by seeking a range of strategic partnerships with various elements of the state. However, they also acknowledged the role of patients' groups and the medical profession in successfully demanding accelerated drug approvals. This suggests that a tentacled theory of corporate bias needs to be modified to take account of demands from such interest groups, as they helped to cement a smooth partnership between industry and the state.

While the case of accelerated drug approval suggests a convergence in regulatory–state relations between the USA, UK and EU, the case of pharmacovigilance highlights some continuing differences. As noted above, UK and EU policy in this area demonstrates the role of corporatism. In the USA, however, a more pluralist approach is apparent, with industry as just one research partner. The FDA has the funds to commission independent epidemiological research on adverse drug reactions to specific drugs, which allows it some managerial discretion. It is also subject to congressional oversight.

In sum, it seems that there is some movement in the direction of corporate bias in the USA as well as in the UK, although important differences remain. In the USA regulators still operate in a more adversarial climate and the political checks and balances reduce opportunities for regulatory capture and corporatism. In the UK and EU countries a culture of secrecy continues to prevail and corporatism and industrial capture are more apparent. There is, however, increasing pressure from consumer organizations and patient groups in Europe which may eventually threaten the stability of the relationship between the regulators and the pharmaceutical industry. Time will tell how successful this more active citizenship is in making regulators in Europe more accountable. Future empirical research might also consider the role of such active citizens in the Global South as well as the Global North and explore this theme especially in relation to the availability, safety and efficacy of medicines in general and vaccines intended to protect people against COVID-19 in particular.

See also: Citizenship and Health; Consumerism; Pharmaceuticalization.

REFERENCES

Abraham, J. (1995) *Science, Politics and the Pharmaceutical Industry*. London: UCL Press.

Abraham, J. (1997) 'The science and politics of medicines regulation', in M.A. Elston (ed.), *The Sociology of Medical Science and Technology*. Oxford: Blackwell Publishers.

Abraham, J. (2009) 'The pharmaceutical industry, the state and the NHS', in J. Gabe and M. Calnan (eds), *The New Sociology of the Health Service*. London: Routledge.

Abraham, J. and Lewis, G. (2002) 'Citizenship, medical expertise and the capitalist regulatory state in Europe', *Sociology*, 36 (1): 67–88.

Davis, C. and Abraham, J. (2011) 'Desperately seeking cancer drugs: explaining the emergence and outcomes of accelerated pharmaceutical regulation', *Sociology of Health & Illness*, 33 (5): 731–747.

Light, D.W. (2010) 'The Food and Drug Administration: inadequate protection from serious risks', in D.W. Light (ed.), *The Risks of Prescription Drugs*. New York: Columbia University Press.

Light, D.W., Lexchin, J. and Darrow, J.J. (2013) 'Institutional corruption of pharmaceuticals and the myth of safe and effective drugs', *Journal of Law, Medicine & Ethics*, 41 (3): 590–600.

Medawar, C. (1992) *Power and Dependence: Social Audit on the Safety of Medicines*. London: Social Audit.

Salcher-Konrad, M., Naci, H. and Davis, C. (2020) 'Approval of cancer drugs with uncertain therapeutic value: a comparison of regulatory decisions in Europe and the United States', *The Millbank Quarterly*, 98 (4): 1219–1256.

Wiktorowicz, M., Lexchin, J. and Moscou, K. (2012) 'Pharmacovigilance in Europe and North America: divergent approaches', *Social Science & Medicine*, 75 (1): 165–170.

SUGGESTED FURTHER READING

- Calnan, N. (2020) *Health Policy, Power and Politics. Sociological Insights.* Bingley: Emerald.

The chapter in this book on 'Rationing, Regulation and Big Pharma' provides an excellent account of the relationship between the state and the pharmaceutical industry, focusing on the pricing of medicines. The primary consideration is the English NHS, but there is also a discussion of regulatory policies in the USA, Brazil, Cuba and New Zealand.

- Webster, A. and Wyatt, S. (eds) (2020) *Health, Technology and Society: Critical Inquiries.* Basingstoke: Palgrave Macmillan.

The section of this book on 'Regulation and Governance' includes a summary and update of Davis and Abraham's work on pharmaceutical regulation. These authors examine how the regulation of innovative pharmaceuticals in the USA and EU in the neoliberal era has been misdirected because of corporate bias.

- Lexchin, J., Graham, J., Herder, M. et al. (2021) 'Regulators, pivotal clinical trials, and drug regulation in the age of COVID-19', *International Journal of Health Services*, 51 (1): 5–13.

An interesting discussion of what counts as a pivotal trial when deciding whether to approve a new drug in the USA, Canada and the EU and how differences between regulators in these countries reflect different regulatory cultures. The authors suggest that as new medicines and vaccines for COVID-19 come up for approval, transparency in how pivotal trials are interpreted will be critical in determining how these treatments should be used.

56

Evaluation

Nicholas Mays

> *Evaluation refers to the use of social research methods to assess the extent to which a policy, programme or service is implemented and achieves its goals.*

Evaluation in the health field involves assessing, in a structured and rigorous way, whether public health programmes and healthcare achieve their intended goals, including improving health and quality of life, and at what cost. Evaluation is applied to varying degrees to assess the value of many areas of public policy such as education, welfare benefits, transport and penal systems. However, the high costs and high political profile of modern health and healthcare systems have made evaluation an increasingly important feature of health policy-making. Payers such as businesses funding health insurance for their workers and governments providing publicly financed healthcare have become increasingly interested in assessing the value of their expenditure on both curative and public health measures (for example, restrictions on smoking). Clinicians too have increasingly espoused the concept of 'evidence-based health care' (Gray, 1997), which includes undertaking randomized clinical trials to assess the effectiveness of drugs and procedures (see below).

Evaluation research has evolved in a number of ways, most notably:

1. Increased use of experimental research in which investigators explicitly design an intervention, such as a new treatment, and apply it under pre-specified conditions to a chosen group or groups of patients. Randomized controlled trials (RCTs), described below, are perhaps the best-known type of experiment undertaken in health and medicine.
2. Development of methods for the synthesis of findings from individual evaluations, such as meta-analysis of RCTs of the effectiveness of treatments.

3. Development of methods of economic evaluation that attempt to quantify the costs and benefits of programmes and policies.
4. Increased use of administrative data in evaluation research, such as patient contacts, but also in the last decade 'big data' from other sources such as internet searches, social media and smartphone usage to enable rapid evaluation of innovations, potentially at low cost (UNDP, 2013).
5. Alongside exclusively positivist and experimental approaches to programme evaluation, the gradual adoption of a wider range of more sociologically informed, interpretative approaches, including realist and participatory methods. The latter are designed to stimulate democratic dialogue and empower stakeholders; the former encourage a focus on identifying the common theories of change that underpin seemingly different programmes.

Though evaluation is a form of social research, it is usually commissioned to provide policy-makers and implementers with instrumental knowledge to meet their needs, which typically include understanding the value of policies, programmes and services. Sometimes, value is inferred from the description and quantification of a range of costs and benefits related to the goals of the programme expressed in 'naturally occurring units' (for example, hospital bed days averted by a hospital-at-home scheme). At other times, formal economic methods are used to estimate either the monetary value (as in cost–benefit analysis) or the 'utility' (as in cost–utility analysis) of an intervention (Weimer and Vining, 2017), so that disparate programmes can be compared on the same measurement scale. The most high-profile form of cost–utility analysis is cost per quality-adjusted life year (QALY) analysis. It can be used to calculate both the non-monetary value of the health gains generated by different treatments for the same condition and, more ambitiously, the relative value of treatments for different conditions to guide priority setting and subsequent resource allocation (Drummond et al., 2015).

Contemporary health policy and programme evaluations typically use a range of research methods, both qualitative and quantitative, drawing on insights from psychology, sociology, economics, statistics, epidemiology, anthropology, policy science and basic clinical sciences. The nature, range and combination of methods reflect wider trends in the social sciences towards more interpretative approaches and the increasing use of 'mixed' methods in which qualitative and quantitative data are triangulated as well as contrasted (Bell and Aggleton, 2016).

Evaluation can, in principle, contribute to decisions throughout the policy process. It can be used prospectively at the design stage to help model the likely impacts of different approaches to achieving a policy goal. It can be used during the implementation stage to identify the conditions for successful implementation (known as 'process' or 'formative' evaluation), and later to measure the impact of the programme or policy (known as 'summative' or outcome evaluation). If an intervention is novel, the evaluation process may well start with a formative evaluation looking at the feasibility and acceptability of the programme, followed by an efficacy evaluation looking at its impact under optimal conditions and then a summative (cost) effectiveness evaluation looking at its impact under ordinary conditions.

A classic, still valuable framework for organizing the evaluation of health and social services was developed by Donabedian (1966). He distinguished between the structure, process and outcome of services. An evaluation of structure typically focuses on the adequacy of facilities, equipment, staffing, funding and organization. A simple example would be examining the number of general practitioners per capita. Such evidence might help to assess geographical equity in availability of doctors between different parts of a country. However, it would ultimately not be possible to determine what the optimal number of doctors should be without asking questions about what services general practitioners provide and their results. This leads to Donabedian's second type of evaluation: examination of process. Processes are activities such as history taking, examination, diagnostics, treatment, follow-up and coordination that constitute care, including the quality of the relations between patients and clinicians. The final dimension of Donabedian's framework focuses on outcomes. Outcomes are the effects in terms of health change that result from the structures and processes of health services. Outcomes of healthcare have frequently been assessed in terms of survival rates. However, outcome measures more appropriate to the role performed by contemporary health services include assessment of the impact of services from the user's point of view upon pain, disability, health-related quality of life, reassurance and the ability to cope with health problems – all outcomes that are more complex to measure.

The method that has proved most reliable in evaluating the effectiveness of healthcare is the RCT. With their informed consent, patients are randomly allocated to receive either the novel treatment, or a placebo, or the best available alternative treatment. The purpose of randomization is to minimize the possible influence on outcomes of factors other than the treatments under study, such as severity of illness between patient groups. Randomization makes it very likely that such factors are equally present in the intervention and control groups.

The RCT has proved its value particularly in relation to pharmaceuticals. An especially valuable feature of drug trials is that both patient and clinician are unaware of which treatment the patient is receiving. This so-called 'double-blind' trial substantially reduces risks of biased results. However, many other interventions in health and care services cannot be subject to the double-blind trial. For example, it may be desirable to evaluate the advantages of a nurse prescribing drugs instead of a general practitioner, compare hospital- with home-based rehabilitation after a surgical procedure, or compare self-help groups with health professionals in their ability to provide counselling, support and advice for people with long-term conditions. In these situations, the options being compared are not like drugs. Drugs are now delivered in formats that completely standardize the active ingredient for each dose. By contrast, the 'active ingredients' that make a nurse practitioner, hospital at-home scheme or self-help group effective in improving health outcomes may be multi-faceted and may vary enormously from one setting to another. In addition, it is frequently impossible to 'blind' service users and staff to the intervention.

For these sorts of reasons, for a long time, sociologists rejected the experimental approach to the evaluation of behavioural, social and population-based ways to improving health, despite this being a potentially powerful evaluation design (Oakley, 1998). Although some sceptics still argue that RCTs are simply infeasible for assessing social policies and community-based interventions, there are grounds for claiming that such trials of social and public health policies are not only feasible but an ethical imperative. Evaluation can be deemed essential because such programmes cannot be assumed to be benign, and some have unexpected negative consequences contrary to common-sense. For example, school-based driver education programmes provided before young people reach the age when they are legally permitted to learn to drive have been shown in RCTs to lead to increased crash and injury rates. Participants in these programmes typically pass their driving tests at younger ages than non-participants, and younger age is strongly related to higher accident rates (Roberts and Kwan, 2001). As a result, pragmatic trials of more complicated whole programmes of care or public health interventions that compare real-life alternatives are increasingly being undertaken. Such evaluations typically collect data on a range of effects or outcomes over a considerable period of time, but also include data on the process of implementation (feasibility) and the acceptability of programmes to individuals and communities. They may also include non-health effects at a societal level, including spill-over impacts in other sectors such as the economy (Smith and Petticrew, 2010).

Considerable attention has thus been devoted to developing methods for evaluation of these so-called 'complex' interventions and programmes. The UK Medical Research Council's guidance on the evaluation of complex interventions – recently updated to take into account emerging theoretical, methodological and practical concerns – identifies 'complexity' in terms of the 'properties of the intervention itself, such as the number of components involved; the range of behaviours targeted; expertise and skills required by those delivering and receiving the intervention; the number of groups, settings, or levels targeted; or the permitted level of flexibility of the intervention or its components' (Skivington et al., 2021: 2). As a result, the active elements of complex interventions are subject to more variation than, say, drugs or even surgical procedures. Though more challenging to evaluate, evaluations of such interventions may not require fundamentally different methods from simpler evaluations, as long as the analyst is not too concerned to discover how a programme has its effect (i.e. the intervention is treated as a 'black box' receiving inputs and then generating outputs and outcomes).

Where there is more interest in the precise operation of a programme, with a view to optimizing its delivery, evaluation designs such as RCTs need to be adapted and/or supplemented by other methods such as qualitative research that can explain how and why interventions improve outcomes. Only when 'the active ingredients' (for example, specific skills or ways of organizing services) of a new way of providing care are uncovered by more detailed qualitative study is it possible to reproduce such effects outside the original evaluative study.

With these considerations in mind, there has been considerable interest in the 'realist' approach to evaluation, developed by Pawson and Tilley (1997) as a more sociologically informed response to the challenges inherent in evaluating complex behavioural and social programmes. Realist evaluations aim to answer the question: 'what works for whom in what circumstances, in what respects and how?' The approach is based on three fundamental sociological insights. First, social programmes are 'theories' in the sense that they are based on implicit or explicit causal propositions about how to produce change. Second, similar programmes have variable effects when implemented across different settings. Third, the local context of each setting influences the ability of the mechanisms underlying programmes to produce the outcomes desired (i.e. programmes are socially embedded). Realist evaluations attempt to develop and test empirically the range of 'context–mechanism–outcome' configurations relevant to understanding the impact of a particular programme or policy.

However sophisticated its design, methods and theoretical underpinning, the contribution of evaluation as an applied social science is largely dependent on the institutions and political imperatives faced by decision-makers (Boaz et al., 2019). Health policies are rarely initiated with evaluation at the forefront of either planning or implementation. Programmes are often not articulated with sufficiently clear objectives for straightforward evaluation and are frequently rolled out before their effects can be definitively assessed. As a result, evaluations often have to focus on inputs, outputs, user experience and professional views, rather than being able directly to attribute 'final' outcomes (for example, health improvements) to specific policies.

It is also important to recognize that much of healthcare evaluation practice is premised on the modernist Enlightenment assumption that action can be studied and then adapted on the basis of a single rational, objective evaluation to improve its effectiveness and efficiency (for example, a health economic evaluation of practices of the New Public Management). However, there are postmodern approaches that posit multiple competing rationalities and forms of knowledge, reflecting the interests of particular groups (Greenhalgh and Russell, 2010). From their perspective, not only is knowledge seen as contingent and far from universal (i.e. there is no single, simple 'truth' about a programme waiting to be uncovered), but evaluation practice is seen to require the participation of a far wider range of players in order to ensure that all relevant 'voices' are heard. The role of the evaluator is thus to negotiate between different versions of truth and value rather than produce a summative account.

Policy evaluation has perhaps never been more important or more challenging than during the COVID-19 pandemic. There is an urgent need worldwide to evaluate the pervasive direct and, possibly more significant, indirect, consequences of the COVID-19 pandemic and especially of the early responses implemented by governments around the world. Critics argue that an 'unprecedented public health experiment occurred without sufficient consideration of the social, political, and economic consequences' (Caduff, 2020: 468). Given the huge social and economic costs (including damage to the health of people with conditions other than COVID-19) of the societal lockdowns that were commonplace, it is vital to be able to identify the policies which stand the best chance of minimizing the risks of the virus while generating the least long-term social and economic harm.

See also: Lay Knowledge; Managerialism; Quality of Life.

REFERENCES

Bell, S. and Aggleton, P. (eds) (2016) *Monitoring and Evaluation in Health and Social Development: Interpretive and Ethnographic Approaches.* London: Routledge.

Boaz, A., Davies H., Fraser, A. and Nutley, S. (eds) (2019) *What Works Now? Evidence-Informed Policy and Practice.* Bristol: Policy Press.

Caduff, C. (2020) 'What went wrong? Corona and the world after the full stop', *Medical Anthropology Quarterly*, 34 (4): 467–487.

Donabedian, A. (1966) 'Evaluating the quality of medical care', *Milbank Memorial Fund Quarterly*, 44 (3): 169–179.

Drummond, M.F., Sculpher, M.J., Claxton, K. et al. (2015) *Methods for the Economic Evaluation of Health Care Programmes*, 4th edn. Oxford: Oxford University Press.

Gray, J.A. (1997) *Evidence Based Healthcare.* London: Churchill-Livingstone.

Greenhalgh, T. and Russell, J. (2010) 'Why do evaluations of eHealth programs fail? An alternative set of guiding principles', *PLoS Med* 7 (11): e1000360

Oakley, A. (1998) 'Experimentation and social interventions: a forgotten but important history', *British Medical Journal*, 317: 1239–1242.

Pawson, R. and Tilley, N. (1997) *Realistic Evaluation.* London: SAGE.

Roberts, I.G. and Kwan, I. (2001) 'School-based driver education for the prevention of traffic crashes', *Cochrane Database of Systematic Reviews*, Issue 3. Online: www.cochranelibrary.com/cdsr/doi/10.1002/14651858.CD003201/epdf/full

Skivington, K., Mathews, L., Simpson, S.A. et al. (2021) 'A new framework for developing and evaluating complex interventions: update of Medical Research Council guidance', *British Medical Journal*, 374: n2061.

Smith, R.D. and Petticrew, M. (2010) 'Public health evaluation in the twenty-first century: time to see the wood as well as the trees', *Journal of Public Health*, 32 (1): 2–7.

UNDP (2013) *Innovations in Monitoring & Evaluation.* Discussion Paper. Prepared for the 3rd International Conference on National Evaluation Capacities, 29 September–2 October 2013, São Paulo, Brazil. Online: www.outcomemapping.ca/download/UNDP%20Discussion%20Paper%20Innovations%20in%20Monitoring%20and%20Evaluation.pdf

Weimer, D.L. and Vining, A.R. (2017) *Policy Analysis: Concepts and Practice*, 6th edn. London and New York: Routledge.

SUGGESTED FURTHER READING

•   Raine, R., Fitzpatrick, R., Barratt, H. et al. (2016) 'Challenges, solutions and future directions in the evaluation of service innovations in health care and public health', *Health Services and Delivery Research*, 4 (16).

This is a book-length collection of essays by leading researchers summarizing recent developments in a range of quantitative and qualitative methods of evaluation of policies, programmes and interventions in healthcare and wider public health with particular emphasis on more complex changes. The essays cover the evolution of RCTs and other quantitative approaches, evaluation of the equity consequences of interventions and measurement of outcomes from the service user's perspective. The volume also includes chapters on the evaluation of major system change from an organizational and managerial perspective, and understanding the importance of context in evaluation, including the contribution of qualitative research.

- Moore, G.F., Audrey, S., Barker, M. et al. (2015) 'Process evaluation of complex interventions: Medical Research Council guidance', *British Medical Journal*, 350: h1258.

This is an authoritative summary of how to study change processes with a view to understanding how and why health and healthcare programmes produce their effects. Sociologically trained researchers in evaluation teams often lead this aspect of a wider evaluation, which can include a RCT or some form of quasi-experimental approach to measuring the effectiveness of the programme. It complements the general UK Medical Research Council guidance on the evaluation of complex interventions (Skivington et al., 2021), cited above.

- Davidoff, F., Dixon-Woods, M., Leviton, L. and Michie, S. (2015) 'Demystifying theory and its use in improvement', *BMJ Quality & Safety*, 24 (3): 228–238.

A good discussion of the contribution of theory to the evaluation of the effectiveness of health service improvement programmes that is equally applicable to other types of programmes and interventions. The paper helpfully distinguishes the nature and role of grand theory, mid-range theory and programme theory.

- Bonell, C., Fletcher, A., Morton, M. et al. (2012) 'Realist randomised controlled trials: a new approach to evaluating complex public health interventions', *Social Science & Medicine*, 75 (12): 2299–2306.

This article argues that it is possible to undertake social science-informed RCTs which embody the principles of realist evaluation, thereby bridging two seemingly different and much debated traditions in policy and programme evaluation.

57

Malpractice

Jonathan Gabe

> Malpractice refers to improper treatment or culpable neglect of a patient by a health service professional.

Malpractice is often discussed in the context of regulating doctors' behaviour and, in particular, the ways in which doctors are held accountable for their mistakes or errors. Various types of regulatory control have been introduced in Great Britain. These range from self-regulation through the General Medical Council (which is responsible for adjudicating on allegations of professional misconduct and revalidating doctors' licence to practise) and medical audit (continuous peer review of practice) to regulation as a result of individual patients making complaints or seeking legal redress through the courts. The focus here will be on the last form of regulation – malpractice litigation.

Malpractice litigation is based on common law, particularly torts of negligence. The term 'tort' is derived from Norman French and means a wrong or wrongdoing. Tort law is based on the view that people owe a duty of care to others and should avoid harming or injuring those they come into contact with. In the case of medicine, this means that a doctor has caused harm to a patient as a result of failing to act in accordance with their profession's customary standards (Dingwall and Hobson-West, 2006). In bringing a case of malpractice a plaintiff needs to prove that there was negligence and that this negligence caused or contributed to damage or injury.

Medical negligence claims have grown considerably in Britain in the last 30 years. There was a sharp increase in claims in the 1990s with a 72 per cent increase between 1990 and 1998. The cost of settlement grew from £50 million in 1990 to £294 million in 2000–1. These costs have continued to rise since the millennium, reaching £787 million in 2009–10 (Feinmann, 2011) and £1.28 billion in 2011–12 (Dyer, 2012). In 2016–17 damages cost the National

Health Service (NHS) £1.6 billion and 10,600 new claims were recorded – double the number a decade earlier. It has been estimated that annual spend on claims will reach £3.2 billion by 2020–21, with claims rising faster than NHS funding. This rise is adding to the significant financial pressures already faced by many NHS Trusts (National Audit Office, 2017).

Most negligence claims are for small sums of up to £25,000, with amounts in excess of £250,000 being claimed by a relatively small number of plaintiffs. Hospital specialties most likely to be claimed against are Obstetrics and Gynaecology, Orthopaedics and Accident and Emergency. Doctors working in these specialties tend to be sued for negligence as a result of misdiagnosis, often leading to a delay in treatment or inappropriate treatment. The other main cause of negligence relates to technical or surgical mistakes made before, during or after an operation (National Audit Office, 2001). Doctors working in Obstetrics and Gynaecology are particularly prone to large claims because damage at birth (for example, brain damage) carries with it lifetime costs in terms of health care. A single claim in this area can now run into millions of pounds, with such high-value birth injury claims growing at 9 per cent a year between 2006–7 and 2016–17.

In the past, hospital doctors in Britain subscribed to a medical defence organization (MDO) to cover possible liability for damages. As membership fees escalated in the 1980s Health Authorities found themselves subsidizing their staff. In 1990, the British government responded by requiring Health Authorities and Trusts to meet the full cost of negligence actions. Since 1995 the NHS Litigation Authority (NHSLA) (now known as NHS Resolution) has taken responsibility for claims against Trusts. To start with, Trusts could identify an excess figure and accept responsibility for meeting the cost of claims below this figure. Since 2002, however, the NHSLA has taken full responsibility for dealing with claims against the NHS. Such arrangements, however, only apply to the NHS in England. Since political devolution in 1999 NHS bodies in Scotland and Wales have put in place their own fault-based schemes (Stephen et al., 2012).

It has been suggested that the medical profession has responded to this state of affairs by being more defensive in its medical practice. This defensive medicine has involved hospital doctors ordering treatments, tests and procedures (or on occasion withholding them) primarily to protect themselves from criticism or potential litigation (Carrier et al., 2010). Fears about being sued are also said to have encouraged GPs to make practice changes such as deciding not to treat certain conditions, increasing diagnostic testing, engaging in more detailed note taking and giving patients more detailed explanations (Summerton, 2000). In the USA there is also evidence of physicians attempting to recognize 'suit-prone' patients in the consultation, in order to reduce the likelihood of litigation. Patients who appear to be 'dependent', 'demanding', 'self-styled experts' or 'subservient' are all seen as potentially malpractice-prone. However, there is an inconsistency in such perceptions. Patients who are deferential and those who are consumerist and want to take responsibility for decisions about their health seem to be perceived as equally problematic. This seeming ambivalence among physicians actually reveals a reluctance to accept a reduction in authority, standing and control. Consequently, exhortations for doctors to provide more information and share decisions with patients in order to minimize the threat of litigation may fall on deaf ears.

The rapid increase in medical negligence claims in recent decades has led many commentators to talk about a medical litigation 'crisis'. Reference is regularly made to the USA where the total cost of malpractice claims has risen faster than inflation. Doctors in Britain (and the USA) tend to blame the growth of consumerism for encouraging patients to complain and take legal action if they feel their rights and expectations have not been met. Reference is also made to the greed of lawyers who have benefited financially from the rapid increase in claims. Such lawyers are said to have sought out patients and touted for business. Certainly there is evidence of lawyers in Britain advertising in NHS hospitals on the basis of 'no win, no fee' in the hope of finding clients who might claim for road- or work-related injuries. 'No win, no fee' was introduced in Britain in 1995 to help remove financial barriers to individuals accessing legal services. Subsequent amendments reduced the risks for lawyers, who could claim up to twice their legal fees for cases they won. The resulting growth in claims was, however, curbed by follow-up measures (National Audit Office, 2017). In the USA physicians also criticize lawyers for their ignorance of medicine and the application of a confrontational, argumentative approach to solve what they perceive as medical disputes (Hupert et al., 1996).

In so far as there is a crisis, it is necessary to ask 'crisis for whom'? For doctors the crisis is one of increasing negligence claims, proactive lawyers and assertive patients. For patients, on the other hand, the crisis may be one of loss of confidence in the medical profession and a lack of sufficient resources to take negligent doctors to court. Certainly there is evidence that when patients (and their relatives) do take legal action, intense emotions are aroused that continue to be felt long after the original injury. For these patients the decision to seek legal redress is determined not just by the original injury but also by a desire to hold doctors to account and to get an adequate explanation for their concerns. Patients can be traumatized further when health professionals fail to take complaints seriously and label their patients negatively for taking action (Vincent, 2010).

Some commentators have nonetheless questioned the extent to which increased medical negligence represents a crisis. Dingwall and Hobson-West (2006) have argued that we should not take the claims of doctors that they are facing a crisis at face value. Instead they suggest that the increase in malpractice claims should be seen as part of a wider cultural shift, which is affecting the professions in general, not just medicine. Accountants, architects, engineers and veterinary surgeons have all seen their liability claims increase in frequency and severity in recent times. The medical profession's response is therefore best seen as a moral panic and a symbolic expression of discontent with wider social and cultural changes that are affecting all professions.

Regardless of whether other professions are facing increased litigation, it can nonetheless be argued that the increase in medical negligence claims does represent a challenge to medical authority that has real consequences for the doctor–patient relationship. While malpractice as a regulatory tool may empower some patients and lead some doctors to make more considered decisions, it may also have the unintended consequence of encouraging doctors to undertake unnecessary tests and of undermining the trust necessary for the shared decision-making and patient partnership advocated by policy-makers. Despite this, medical negligence action does have a role as a regulatory tool in that it encourages at least some public discussion of standards. The recent decline in the NHS's performance against key waiting time standards may increase the risk of future claims in England. This likelihood is enhanced further as a consequence of the COVID-19 pandemic, which has had a significant knock-on effect on waiting times. Future research is needed to explore the impact of the pandemic on malpractice in Britain and elsewhere.

See also: Consumerism; Medical Autonomy, Dominance and Decline.

REFERENCES

Carrier, E.R., Reschovsky, J.D., Mello, M. et al. (2010) 'Physicians' fears of malpractice lawsuits are not assuaged by Tort reforms', *Health Affairs*, 29 (9): 1585–1592.

Dingwall, R. and Hobson-West, P. (2006) 'Litigation and the threat to medicine', in D. Kelleher, J. Gabe and G. Williams (eds), *Challenging Medicine*. 2nd edn. London: Routledge.

Dyer, C. (2012) 'NHS bill for compensation exceeds £1bn for the first time', *British Medical Journal*, 345: e4638.

Feinmann, J. (2011) 'Why sorry doesn't need to be the hardest word', *British Medical Journal*, 342: d3258.

Hupert, N., Lawthers, A.G., Brennan, T.A. and Peterson, L.M. (1996) 'Processing the tort deterrent signal: a qualitative study', *Social Science & Medicine*, 43 (1): 1–11.

National Audit Office (2001) *Handling Clinical Negligence Claims in England*. London: The Stationery Office.

National Audit Office (2017) *Managing the Costs of Clinical Negligence in Trusts*. London: The Stationery Office.

Stephen, F., Melville, A. and Krauser, T. (2012) *A Study of Medical Negligence Claims in Scotland*. Edinburgh: Scottish Government.

Summerton, N. (2000) 'Trends in negative defensive medicine within general practice', *British Journal of General Practice*, 50 (456): 565–566.

Vincent, C. (2010) *Patient Safety*, 2nd edn. Chichester: Wiley-Blackwell.

SUGGESTED FURTHER READING

- Annandale, E. (1989) 'The malpractice crisis and the doctor–patient relationship', *Sociology of Health & Illness*, 11 (1): 1–23.

A classic study of the implications of the malpractice crisis for patient care at the micro level of the doctor–patient relationship in the USA. Drawing on commentary in medical journals, it reveals the way in which doctors have been encouraged to give more information to patients and involve them in decision-making in the face of this crisis. While this change may benefit patients, it may also draw attention away from medical practice to the patient as the source of negligent injury and reduce the latter's chances of gaining compensation for real medical errors.

- Ocloo, J.E. (2010) 'Harmed patients gaining a voice: challenging dominant perspectives in the construction of medical harm and patient safety reforms', *Social Science & Medicine*, 71 (3): 510–516.

A useful analysis of how the discussion of medical harm is focused mainly on clinical markers and individual agency reflecting the medical model. It is argued that this approach fails to capture the full experience of harmed patients and their perception of medical power and accountability, and that a broader framework for addressing patient safety is needed. The paper is based on an analysis of data collected from self-help groups set up as a result of medical harm and from individuals affected by medical harm attending a residential workshop.

- Winance, M., Barbot, J. and Parizot, I. (2018) 'From loss to repair. A study of body narratives in patient claims for medical injury', *Sociology of Health & Illness*, 40 (1): 53–66.

An interesting study of the different ways in which patient complainants perceive and describe their body which has been damaged by medical activity and how it might be repaired or compensated. The data are made up of complaints filed with the French out-of-court settlement mechanism.

INDEX

A

Abraham, J., 103, 106, 107–8, 110, 368, 369, 370, 371, 372
action, 5–6, 115
active citizenship, 357–8
activism *see* social movements
activity spaces, 49
actor-network theory (ANT), 238
actors, xx, 46, 49, 99, 100, 106, 109, 111, 236, 255, 288, 324, 335
actual social identity, 123
adult risk factors, 65
adverse childhood experience, 65–6, 67, 68
adverse drug reactions (ADRs), 369, 372
advertising, 101, 108, 284, 384
age, 188; *see also* old age
ageing, 77–83, 196, 205
agency, 26–7, 62–3, 85–6, 195, 209, 231, 335
alcohol consumption, 18, 26, 47, 60, 66, 218, 219
alcoholism, 99, 100, 102, 247
allied health professions *see* professions allied to medicine
allostatic load, 61
alternative medicine *see* complementary and alternative medicine (CAM)
analytical categories, 40–1
Annandale, E.C., 231–2, 272
antibiotics, 4, 171, 202, 225
anti-categorical approach, 41
apps, 130, 189, 236, 241, 242, 243, 244, 256

architectural care assemblage, 335
Armstrong, D., 115, 116, 118, 262, 332
arthritis, 141–2, 154, 157, 370
artificial intelligence (AI), 190, 235, 256
asexuality, 31, 32, 33
asset flows, 62
assisted dying, 194–5, 196, 257
asthma, 123, 143, 219, 238
AstraZeneca, 370
asylum seekers, 359
Atkinson, P., 205, 209
attachment theory, 68
augmentation, 109
austerity, 13, 92, 144, 149, 150, 358
austerity policies, 12, 18, 124, 338
Australia, 25, 28, 163, 171, 303,
autism, 212, 249
autonomy *see* medical autonomy

B

bacteria, 3–4, 5
bacteriology, 202
Bambra, C., 12, 13–14, 86
bare life, 359
Beck, U., 81, 164, 262, 277
behaviour, 114; *see also* deviant behaviour; health behaviour; illness behaviour; risk behaviour
Bell, S., 110, 376
Bendelow, G., xiii, 129, 137
Berg, M., 238, 333
Bernstein, J., 305, 306

healthcare settings, 28
healthcare systems, 14, 28, 60, 194, 235–6, 278, 356
healthcare workers, 28, 282, 297–8; *see also* care workers; migrant healthcare workers
healthicization of sleep, 189
health-related quality of life (HRQL), 181–4
healthy life expectancy (HLE), 11–12
Hedgecoe, A., 248, 250, 255
hegemonic masculinity, 324–5
heroin, 110
heroin recovery, 188
Herzlich, C., 216, 217–18
heterosexuality, 31–2, 33, 34, 35
hierarchists, 161
Higgs, P.F., 80, 81
HIV/AIDS, 3, 4, 6, 19, 34, 42, 101, 123, 154, 177, 262–3, 366
Hobson-West, P., 382, 384
Hochschild, A., 134, 135, 316–17, 318, 319, 320, 326
Homeopathy, 311, 312
homosexuality, 31, 32, 33–4, 101, 247; *see also* gay marriage
horizontal stratification, 273
hospice movement, 194
hospitals, 331–6, 337–8, 338–9
Human Genome Project (HGP), 248
Hunter, D.J., 343, 344, 346
Huntingdon's disease, 250
hypertension, 42, 182

I

idiopathic pain, 136
ill health, 78, 80, 147, 149, 168, 218,
Illich, I., 101
illness
  as deviance, 168
  social construction of, 209–10
illness behaviours, 60, 114–16, 118, 119, 170, 216
illness narratives, 136, 153–9, 231
immigrant populations, 264

impairment, 144, 147, 148, 149, 150, 151
income inequality, 13, 61, 92, 93
Independent Treatment Centres, 338
India, 28, 107, 123, 223, 249, 303, 304, 310, 312
individual interventions, 261, 263
individualism, 13, 47, 60, 86, 161, 202, 218, 311
inequality, 6, 80–1, 150, 242; *see also* gender inequalities in; health inequalities; income inequality; social inequalities; structural inequalities
infectious disease, 3–4, 47, 53, 54, 78, 170, 196
infertility, 231
influenza, 3, 4
informal care, xxi, 323–8
informal networks, 91, 362
information literacy, 352
information technology (IT), 235, 333–4
informed consent, 255
informed trust, 278
Ingleby, D., 261, 263, 264
insomnia, 111
institutional corruption, 369, 371, 372
institutional trust, 91, 278, 280
institutionalization, 79, 100, 116, 194, 279
instrumental emotional labour (EL), 318
interactional dominance, 176
inter-categorical approach, 41, 42
interdependence, 164, 263, 283, 299, 323, 324
intergenerational conflict, 79
International Classification of Functioning, Disability and Health (WHO), 149
International Monetary Fund, 84, 304
internet, 107, 108–9, 116, 241, 278, 352, 376
interpersonal trust, 278, 280, 294
intersectionality, 38–45, 80–1
intra-categorical approach, 41